Health system performance comparison

An agenda for policy, information and research

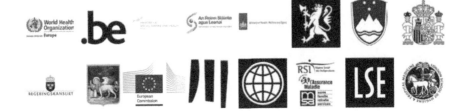

The European Observatory on Health Systems and Policies supports and promotes evidence-based health policy-making through comprehensive and rigorous analysis of health systems in Europe. It brings together a wide range of policy-makers, academics and practitioners to analyse trends in health reform, drawing on experience from across Europe to illuminate policy issues.

The European Observatory on Health Systems and Policies is a partnership between the World Health Organization Regional Office for Europe, the Governments of Belgium, Finland, Ireland, the Netherlands, Norway, Slovenia, Spain, Sweden and the Veneto Region of Italy, the European Commission, the European Investment Bank, the World Bank, UNCAM (French National Union of Health Insurance Funds), the London School of Economics and Political Science, and the London School of Hygiene & Tropical Medicine.

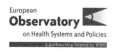

European
Observatory
on Health Systems and Policies
a partnership hosted by WHO

Health system performance comparison

An agenda for policy, information and research

Edited by

Irene Papanicolas and Peter C. Smith

Mc
Graw
Hill
Education

Open University Press

Open University Press
McGraw-Hill Education
McGraw-Hill House
Shoppenhangers Road
Maidenhead
Berkshire
England
SL6 2QL

email: enquiries@openup.co.uk
world wide web: www.openup.co.uk

and Two Penn Plaza, New York, NY 10121-2289, USA

First published 2013

A catalogue record of this book is available from the British Library

ISBN-13: 978-0-33-524726-4 (pb)
ISBN-10: 0-33-524726-1
eISBN: 978-0-33-524727-1

Library of Congress Cataloging-in-Publication Data
CIP data applied for

Typesetting and e-book compilations
by RefineCatch Limited, Bungay, Suffolk

Printed and bound by CPI Group (UK) Ltd, Croydon, CR0 4YY

European Observatory on Health Systems and Policies Series

The European Observatory on Health Systems and Policies is a unique project that builds on the commitment of all its partners to improving health systems:

- World Health Organization Regional Office for Europe
- Government of Belgium
- Government of Finland
- Government of Ireland
- Government of the Netherlands
- Government of Norway
- Government of Slovenia
- Government of Spain
- Government of Sweden
- Veneto Region of Italy
- European Commission
- European Investment Bank
- World Bank
- UNCAM
- London School of Economics and Political Science
- London School of Hygiene & Tropical Medicine

The series

The volumes in this series focus on key issues for health policy-making in Europe. Each study explores the conceptual background, outcomes and lessons learned about the development of more equitable, more efficient and more effective health systems in Europe. With this focus, the series seeks to contribute to the evolution of a more evidence-based approach to policy formulation in the health sector.

These studies will be important to all those involved in formulating or evaluating national health policies and, in particular, will be of use to health policy-makers and advisers, who are under increasing pressure to rationalize the structure and funding of their health system. Academics and students in the field of health policy will also find this series valuable in seeking to understand better the complex choices that confront the health systems of Europe.

The Observatory supports and promotes evidence-based health policy-making through comprehensive and rigorous analysis of the dynamics of health care systems in Europe.

Series Editors

Josep Figueras is the Director of the European Observatory on Health Systems and Policies, and Head of the European Centre for Health Policy, World Health Organization Regional Office for Europe.

Martin McKee is Director of Research Policy and Head of the London Hub of the European Observatory on Health Systems and Policies. He is Professor of European Public Health at the London School of Hygiene & Tropical Medicine as well as a co-director of the School's European Centre on Health of Societies in Transition.

Elias Mossialos is the Co-director of the European Observatory on Health Systems and Policies. He is Brian Abel-Smith Professor in Health Policy, Department of Social Policy, London School of Economics and Political Science and Director of LSE Health.

Richard B. Saltman is Associate Head of Research Policy and Head of the Atlanta Hub of the European Observatory on Health Systems and Policies. He is Professor of Health Policy and Management at the Rollins School of Public Health, Emory University in Atlanta, Georgia.

Reinhard Busse is Associate Head of Research Policy and Head of the Berlin Hub of the European Observatory on Health Systems and Policies. He is Professor of Health Care Management at the Berlin University of Technology.

European Observatory on Health Systems and Policies Series

Series Editors: Josep Figueras, Martin McKee, Elias Mossialos, Richard B. Saltman and Reinhard Busse

Published titles

Regulating entrepreneurial behaviour in European health care systems
Richard B. Saltman, Reinhard Busse and Elias Mossialos (eds)

Hospitals in a changing Europe
Martin McKee and Judith Healy (eds)

Health care in central Asia
Martin McKee, Judith Healy and Jane Falkingham (eds)

Funding health care: options for Europe
Elias Mossialos, Anna Dixon, Josep Figueras and Joe Kutzin (eds)

Health policy and European Union enlargement
Martin McKee, Laura MacLehose and Ellen Nolte (eds)

Regulating pharmaceuticals in Europe: striving for efficiency, equity and quality
Elias Mossialos, Monique Mrazek and Tom Walley (eds)

Social health insurance systems in western Europe
Richard B. Saltman, Reinhard Busse and Josep Figueras (eds)

Purchasing to improve health systems performance
Josep Figueras, Ray Robinson and Elke Jakubowski (eds)

Human resources for health in Europe
Carl-Ardy Dubois, Martin McKee and Ellen Nolte (eds)

Primary care in the driver's seat
Richard B. Saltman, Ana Rico and Wienke Boerma (eds)

Mental health policy and practice across Europe: the future direction of mental health care
Martin Knapp, David McDaid, Elias Mossialos and Graham Thornicroft (eds)

Decentralization in health care
Richard B. Saltman, Vaida Bankauskaite and Karsten Vrangbæk (eds)

Health systems and the challenge of communicable diseases: experiences from Europe and Latin America
Richard Coker, Rifat Atun and Martin McKee (eds)

Caring for people with chronic conditions: a health system perspective
Ellen Nolte and Martin McKee (eds)

Nordic health care systems: recent reforms and current policy challenges
Jon Magnussen, Karsten Vrangbæk and Richard B. Saltman (eds)

Diagnosis-related groups in Europe: moving towards transparency, efficiency and quality in hospitals
Reinhard Busse, Alexander Geissler, Wilm Quentin and Miriam Wiley (eds)

Migration and health in the European Union
Bernd Rechel, Philipa Mladovsky, Walter Devillé, Barbara Rijks, Roumyana Petrova-Benedict and Martin McKee (eds)

Successes and failures of health policies in Europe: four decades of divergent trends and cenverging challenges.
Johan P. Mackenbach and Martin Mckee (eds)

Contents

Foreword by Zsuzsanna Jakab   ix
Foreword by Paola Testori Coggi   xi
Foreword by Mark Pearson   xiii
List of contributors   xv
List of tables, figures and boxes   xvii
Abbreviations   xxiii

one   *Introduction*   **1**
         Irene Papanicolas and Peter C. Smith

two   *International frameworks for health system
         comparison*   **31**
         Irene Papanicolas

three   *International comparisons of health systems*   **75**
         Irene Papanicolas and Peter C. Smith

four   *Benchmarking: lessons and implications for
         health systems*   **113**
         Andy Neely

five   *Comparing population health*   **127**
         *Marina Karanikolos, Bernadette Khoshaba, Ellen Nolte and
         Martin McKee*

six	***Comparing health services outcomes***	*157*
	Niek Klazinga and Lilian Li	
seven	***Conceptualizing and comparing equity across nations***	*183*
	Cristina Hernández-Quevedo and Irene Papanicolas	
eight	***Measuring and comparing financial protection***	*223*
	Rodrigo Moreno-Serra, Sarah Thomson and Ke Xu	
nine	***Understanding satisfaction, responsiveness and experience with the health system***	*255*
	Reinhard Busse	
ten	***Comparative measures of health system efficiency***	*281*
	Jonathan Cylus and Peter C. Smith	
eleven	***Commentary on international health system performance information***	*313*
	Nick Fahy	
twelve	***Conclusions***	*335*
	Irene Papanicolas and Peter C. Smith	
	Index	373

Foreword from WHO

The 2008 Tallinn Charter underlined the importance attached to strengthening health systems by WHO European Region Member States. It included a commitment to promoting 'transparency and accountability for health system performance, to produce measurable results' and to 'foster cross-country learning and cooperation'. International comparison of health system performance is indeed becoming increasingly prevalent, driven by growing availability of comparable datasets and increasing demand for transparency and accountability.

International comparison can be one of the most powerful drivers of health systems improvement by influencing policy-makers. However, if the comparison is partial or relies on inadequate analysis, it can give rise to seriously misleading signals, resulting in inappropriate policy responses. It is therefore essential that – if the full potential of international comparison is to be realized – policy-makers and analysts need to be made aware of the associated opportunities and pitfalls. This timely and authoritative book offers an important summary of the current 'state of the art' on international comparison of health systems. It forms part of a programme of work initiated by the European Observatory on Health Systems and Policies that will assess current data sources and methodology, and seek to promote greater understanding of the potential offered by international comparison of health systems. It offers a rich source of material for policy-makers, their analytic advisors, international agencies, academics and students of health systems.

Zsuzsanna Jakab
Regional Director, WHO Regional Office for Europe

Foreword from the European Commission

Health is clearly among the most precious treasures we can have.

What do we mean by health? The capacity to live a full, active and breathing life.

Where does our health come from? It is the result of a complex interaction between our genetic, the environment we live in, the society we are part of and our lifestyles. Thus, health systems are not at the origin of our health. But they play a fundamental role: they help people maintain and improve their own health.

That's why it is so important to make sure that health systems perform at their best. And, in order to lead them to their best performance, we have to understand how they work: this is the goal of health systems performance assessment.

Knowing how our systems work is always a necessity. But it is even more imperative in these times of economic turmoil and fiscal constraints. Healthcare expenditure has grown steadily in most European countries, and governments are becoming increasingly concerned in achieving higher levels of efficiency, matching financial sustainability with high quality delivery of healthcare.

However, as the authors of this volume properly highlight, performance is not only about efficiency; other dimensions are also crucial. This book gives great attention in analysing and understanding how health systems can be effective in improving the health status of the populations, how they can be attentive to equity, how they are responsive to patients' expectations, and how they ensure their financial protection.

All these dimensions fit perfectly in the overarching values of universality, access to good quality care, equity, and solidarity that have been widely accepted in the work of the European Union.

For all these reasons, I am particularly glad to welcome this book, which shows, in a comprehensive and clear manner, the progresses that have been made in assessing the performance of health systems and indicates the road for further improving our knowledge in this field.

Paola Testori Coggi
Director General, DG Health and Consumers, European Commission

Foreword from the OECD

International agencies have an important role to play in promoting the comparison of health system performance across countries. The OECD has for many decades been the prime source of international comparative data on health system characteristics, and in 2002 we initiated a system of Health Care Quality Indicators. The intention has been to complement and coordinate efforts of national and other international bodies, and to offer policy makers and other stakeholders a toolkit to stimulate cross-national learning. We are pleased that the European Observatory on Health Systems and Policies has produced this book to examine the 'state of the art' on international comparison. We are seeking annually to expand the scope of the HCQI project, and to improve the quality of the data, and our member states are finding the material we provide increasingly helpful.

This book offers a great deal of valuable material to help identify priorities for future developments in the work of the OECD and our partner international agencies.

Mark Pearson, Head of the Health Division,
Directorate of Employment, Labour and Social Affairs,
Organisation for Economic Co-operation and Development

List of contributors

Reinhard Busse
Professor Dr. med. MPH, Dept. Health Care Management, University of Technology Berlin/European Observatory on Health Systems and Policies

Jonathan Cylus
Research Fellow, European Observatory on Health Systems and Policies, LSE Health

Nick Fahy
Independent consultant and researcher

Dr Cristina Hernández-Quevedo
Technical Officer, European Observatory on Health Systems and Policies, LSE Health

Marina Karanikolos
Research Fellow at the European Observatory on Health Systems and Policies and the London School of Hygiene and Tropical Medicine

Bernadette Khoshaba
Research Fellow at the London School of Hygiene and Tropical Medicine

Niek Klazinga
(MD PhD) is coordinator of the Health Care Quality Indicator work at the OECD in Paris. He is also professor of Social Medicine at the Academic Medical Centre at the University of Amsterdam.

Lilian Li
Is a health economist who at the time the chapter was written was working at the Health Division of the OECD in Paris and is presently working for the National Clinical Guideline Centre at the Royal College of Physicians in London.

Martin McKee
Professor of European Public Health at the London School of Hygiene and Tropical Medicine and Research Director at the European Observatory on Health Systems and Policies

Dr Rodrigo Moreno-Serra
MRC Research Fellow, Business School and Centre for Health Policy, Imperial College London

Professor Andy Neely
Director, Cambridge Service Alliance, University of Cambridge

Ellen Nolte
Director of the Health and Healthcare Research Programme at RAND, Europe and Honorary Senior Lecturer at the London School of Hygiene and Tropical Medicine

Irene Papanicolas
Lecturer in Health Economics, Department of Social Policy, London School of Economics and Political Science

Peter C. Smith
Is Professor of Health Policy, Imperial College Business School

Dr Sarah Thomson
Senior Research Fellow, European Observatory on Health Systems and Policies; Senior Research Fellow and Deputy Director, LSE Health

Dr Ke Xu
Team Leader, Health Care Financing, WHO Regional Office for the Western Pacific

List of tables, figures and boxes

Tables

1.1	Performance measurement implications of setting health system boundaries	14
1.2	Selected examples of international comparisons in the area of equity	18
1.3	Main indicators for fairness in financing	21
2.1	Health system boundaries in international HSPA frameworks	34
2.2	Health system objectives	36
2.3	Conceptualizations of key terms	38
2.4	Conceptualizations of health system architecture	42
2.5	Classification of frameworks	47
A1	Dimensions in the Behavioural Healthcare framework	53
A2	WHO 2000 Index of Health System achievement	59
A3	OECD and WHO performance framework objectives and measurement dimensions	59
A4	Key indicators of performance	61
A5	Dimensions in HCQI health care system framework	65
A6	Four goals of a high performance health care system	67
A7	The six building blocks of a health system	69
3.1	Main data collection efforts of WHO	79
3.2	Existing OECD health care quality indicators	82
3.3	Main categories for the ECHI indicator set	83
3.4	Examples of EU funded projects in comparative health system performance research	86

3.5   Evaluation areas and indicators of the Euro Health
      Consumer Index (2009)   89
3.6   Evaluation areas of HCP specialized indices   91
3.7   Criticisms of the *World Health Report 2000*   98
4.1   Implications of benchmarking purpose for benchmarking activity 118
5.1   Common measures of population health   133
6.1   Health status measures used in the PROMs questionnaires (UK) 175
7.1   Selected ethical paradigms applied to equity   185
7.2   Some evidence on social determinants of health in Europe   187
7.3   Long-term concentration indices and mobility indices, 2005–2007 200
7.4   Main areas of equity measurement   212
7.5   Areas of equity research with limited data for international
      comparisons   214
8.1   Main indicators of financial protection in health systems   249
9.1   Satisfaction with country's health care system or availability of
      quality health care in city/area in EU15 countries plus Switzerland
      and Norway (in %), various surveys 1996–2011; countries sorted
      according to results of 2008 survey   258
9.2   Definition, grouping and weights of responsiveness dimensions
      in *WHR2000* and number of questions used to measure it in two
      subsequent population surveys   260
9.3   WHO dimensions of responsiveness and questions used to
      measure it in two population surveys   261
9.4   Questions used in Picker responsiveness survey, sorted according
      to WHO responsiveness domains and whether they address
      expectations or patient experience   264
9.5   Expectations for and rating of choice of different types of
      providers in eight European countries, 2002; countries
      sorted from left to right by responsiveness rating   265
9.6   Patients reporting problems with hospital, 1998–2000 (%);
      available countries sorted by overall evaluation from left to right,
      dimension sorted by average percentage from low to high   267
9.7   Evaluations of general practice care in four different surveys;
      countries sorted from top to bottom by rating in 2009   268
9.8   Evaluation of general practice care in six European countries with
      data for 1998 and 2009 (% with positive rating); countries sorted
      from left to right by overall evaluation in
      2009, items from top to bottom by average across countries
      in 2009   270
9.9   Example questions and results from Commonwealth Fund's
      International Health Policy Surveys, 2010 (adults with health
      care encounter) and 2011 ('sicker adults')   273
9.10 Important questionnaires/studies/surveys/rankings with questions
      on patients' and citizens' experience; sorted by date of first use 274
10.1 An example of an incremental cost per QALY league table   285
10.2 Sample of efficiency indicators   290
10.3 Categorization and examples of total and partial indicators   291

10.4 Contributions of main explanatory variables to cross-country differences. Differences in life expectancy at birth between countries and the OECD average for each variable, expressed in years, 2003   298

12.1 Types of frameworks   337
12.2 Main indicators for health service outcomes   345
12.3 Main indicators for equity   350
12.4 Measurement of financing function   353
12.5 Key resources and challenges   359

Figures

1.1 Five-year period survival rates 1991–2002 for colorectal and breast cancer from *Eurocare 4* data   3
1.2 Orthopaedic bed days per 100 000 aged over 65 in the NHS and Kaiser   6
2.1 Performance measurement implications of setting health system boundaries   35
A1 Framework for Assessing Behavioral Healthcare   52
A2 WHO (2000) framework   56
A3 Control Knobs framework, 2004   62
A4 OECD HCQI, 2006   64
A5 Commonwealth Fund framework, 2006   66
A6 WHO (2007) framework   68
A7 Atun framework, 2008   70
A8 IHP framework, 2008   71
3.1 Summary of variations in costs of appendectomy   95
4.1 The benchmarking cycle   124
5.1 Major factors leading to ischaemic heart disease   130
5.2 Breast cancer survival, incidence and mortality in Australia, Canada, Denmark, Norway, Sweden and the UK   138
5.3 Amenable mortality in OECD countries, 2007   147
6.1 Admission-based and patient-based in-hospital case-fatality rates within 30 days after admission for AMI, 2009 (or nearest year)   163
6.2 Reduction in in-hospital case-fatality rates within 30 days after admission for AMI, 2000–09 (or nearest year)   165
6.3 Avoidable hospital admission rates, 2007   169
6.4 Schizophrenia readmissions to the same hospital, 2009 (or nearest year)   171
6.5 Bipolar disorder readmissions to the same hospital, 2009 (or nearest year)   172
6.6 Mammography screening, percentage of women aged 50–69 screened, 2000–09 (or nearest year)   174
7.1 Lorenz curve for health status   194

7.2   Concentration curve for an indicator of health limitations   195
7.3   Concentration curves to measure inequity in utilization   207
7.4   Kakwani index: pre-tax income and taxes   209
8.1   Per capita gross national income and out-of-pocket payments
       as a share of total health expenditures, 164 countries (2007–08)   228
8.2   Catastrophic spending incidence and DTP3 immunization
       coverage among 1-year-olds, 87 countries (various years)   239
8.3   Catastrophic spending incidence and percentage of births
       attended by skilled personnel, 79 countries (various years)   240
10.1 The production process in hospital care   282
10.2 Went to the ER for a condition that could have been treated
       by a regular doctor, among sick adults, 2005   292
10.3 Five-year relative survival rate and availability of mammography
       machines in a recent year   293
10.4 Appendectomy: comparison of costs by country   293
10.5 Comparing DEA and panel data regression results   300
10.6 A more realistic model of efficiency?   308
12.1 Country rankings for DALE and amenable mortality   344
12.2 An example of events within an episode of care   348

Boxes

1.1   The power of international comparisons to influence policy: cancer
       services in England   3
1.2   Efforts at mutual learning: Kaiser Permanente and the English
       National Health Service   5
1.3   The role of international organizations in HSPA   8
1.4   Policy and methodological debates arising from *WHR2000*   10
1.5   Lessons of benchmarking for health systems   13
1.6   Avoidable Mortality in European Health Systems (AMIEHS)   17
1.7   Health Care Quality Indicators (HCQI)   18
1.8   Conflicting notions of efficiency   23
3.1   Dimensions of quality of care   81
3.2   Overview of the ten vignettes   94
3.3   Examples of vignette questions used in the WHS   96
5.1   Sudden infant death syndrome prevention in the UK   131
5.2   Explaining differences in mortality trends from IHD   136
7.1   Measures of health outcomes   188
7.2   Example of a vignette   190
7.3   Potential sources of socioeconomic gradient   191
7.4   Construction and application of the mobility index   198
7.5   Examples of unmet need questions in multi-country health surveys   205
11.1 Communicable diseases: a model for data on health systems?   315
12.1 Health system design – an important variable in international
       comparisons of health system performance   338

12.2 Effective coverage   341
12.3 PERFECT, EuroHOPE and ECHO projects   348
12.4 Financing arrangements in health systems   353
12.5 Interpreting performance information across settings   355
12.6 Using diagnostic-related groups (DRGs) for efficiency comparisons   357
12.7 Different perspectives on performance   363
12.8 Possible sources of variations in cross-country performance
      indicators   364

Abbreviations

ADL	activities of daily living
AIDS	acquired immunodeficiency syndrome
AMI	acute myocardial infarction
AMIEHS	Avoidable Mortality in European Health Systems
APQC	American Productivity and Quality Centre
ARD	ageing-related disease
BFB	Bang-For-Buck adjusted score
BMI	body mass index
CABG	coronary artery bypass graft
CC	concentration curve
CHF	congestive heart failure
CI	concentration index
CISID	Centralized Information System for Infectious Diseases
COPD	chronic obstructive pulmonary disease
CT	computed tomography
DALE	disability-adjusted life expectancy
DALY	disability-adjusted life year
DEA	data envelopment analysis
DEPLESET	demographic, economic, political, legal and regulatory, epidemiological, sociodemographic and technological
DFLE	disability-free life expectancy
DMDB	Detailed Mortality Database
DRG	diagnosis-related group
DTP3	diphtheria–tetanus–pertussis

ECDC	European Centre for Disease Prevention and Control
ECHI	European Community Health Indicators
ECHIM	European Community Health Indicators Monitoring
ECHIS	European Core Health Interview Survey
ECHP	European Community Household Panel
EFQM	European Foundation for Quality Management
EGIPSS	Évaluation globale et intégrée de la performance des systèmes de santé
EHR	electronic health record
EHSS	European Health Survey System
ESS	European Social Survey
EU	European Union
EU15	EU Member States prior to 2004
EU-SILC	European Union Statistics on Income and Living Conditions
EUNetPaS	European Network for Patient Safety
FNORS	National Federation of Regional Health Observatories, France
GDP	gross domestic product
GHO	Global Health Observatory
GNP	gross national product
GP	general practitioner
HAART	highly active antiretroviral therapy
HALE	health-adjusted life expectancy
HBS	Household Budget Survey
HCP	Health Consumer Powerhouse
HCQI	Health Care Quality Indicators
HFA-DB	European Health for All database
HiT	Health Systems in Transition
HIV	human immunodeficiency virus
HMDB	Hospital Morbidity database
HOPIT	hierarchical ordered probit
HS	health system
HSMR	hospital standardized mortality rate
HSPA	health systems performance assessment
HSR	health services research
HTA	health technology assessment
ICD	International Classification of Disease
ICHI	International Compendium of Health Indicators
ICT	information and communication technology
IHD	ischaemic heart disease
IHP+	International Health Partnership and Related Initiatives
IHPS	International Health Policy Survey
IHSN	International Household Survey Network
ISARE	Indicateurs Santé Régionaux d'Europe
ISCO	International Standard Classification of Occupations
LSMS	Living Standard Measurement Study
MCS	multi-country survey
M&E	monitoring and evaluation
MI	mobility index

MRI	magnetic resonance imaging
NDPHS	Northern Dimension Partnership in Public Health and Social Wellbeing
NHA	national health accounts
NHCSG	Nordic hospital comparison study group
NHS	National Health Service
NICE	National Institute of Clinical Excellence
NOMESKO	Nordic Medico-Statistical Committee
OECD	Organisation for Economic Co-operation and Development
OMC	Open Method of Coordination
PAsQ	European Network on Patient Safety and Quality of Care
PATH	Performance Assessment Tool for Hospitals
PDQ-39	Parkinson's Disease Questionnaire
PPP	purchasing power parity
PPS	Prospective Payment System
PROM	patient-reported outcome measure
PSI	patient safety indicator
QALY	quality-adjusted life year
RAI	resident assessment instrument
RAPIA	Rapid Assessment Protocol for Insulin Access
RII	relative index of inequality
RIVM	National Institute for Public Health and the Environment (The Netherlands)
SAH	self-assessed health
SDR	standardized death rate
SEER	Surveillance Epidemiology and End Results
SF36	Short Form 36
SFA	stochastic frontier analysis
SHA	System of Health Accounts
SHARE	Survey of Health, Ageing and Retirement in Europe
SIDS	sudden infant death syndrome
SII	slope index of inequality
SMR	standardized mortality ratio
SPRG	Scientific Peer Review Group
SYSRA	systemic rapid assessment
TB	tuberculosis
TECH	Technological Change in Health Care
THL	National Institute for Health And Welfare (Finland)
UPI	unique patient identifier
WHO	World Health Organization
WHO-MCS	WHO Multi-Country Survey Study on Health and Responsiveness
WHOSIS	WHO Statistical Information System
WHR	World Health Report
WHR2000	World Health Report 2000
WHS	World Health Survey
YLL	years of life lost

chapter one

Introduction

Irene Papanicolas and Peter C. Smith

1.1 Introduction

Individual nations are increasingly seeking to introduce more systematic ways of assessing the performance of their health systems and of benchmarking performance against other countries. They recognize that without measurement it is difficult to identify good and bad service delivery practice, or good and bad practitioners; to design health system reforms; to protect patients or payers; or to make the case for investing in health care. Measurement is central to securing accountability to citizens, patients and payers for health system actions and outcomes. This focus on assessment coincides with the enormous increase in the capacity for measurement and analysis seen in the last decade, driven in no small part by massive changes in information technology and associated advances in measurement methodology.

However, notwithstanding major progress by organizations such as the European Commission, the Organisation for Economic Co-operation and Development (OECD), the Commonwealth Fund and the World Health Organization (WHO), as well as by individual countries, performance comparison efforts are still in their early stages and there are many challenges involved in the design and implementation of comparison schemes.

The state of current developments in performance measurement was comprehensively surveyed in the book *Performance measurement for health system improvement* that followed the 2008 WHO European Ministerial Conference on Health Systems in Tallinn (Smith et al., 2009). The book identifies the important sources of international comparison noted above but also highlights the limitations of many performance assessment initiatives in terms of both scope and policy usefulness. The difficulties of interpreting performance information from a health system policy perspective are highlighted and attention is also drawn to the danger that comparison can lead to serious policy errors if not accompanied by careful commentary on the implications of variations for health system improvement and reform.

Properly conducted country comparisons of performance may provide a rich source of evidence and exert powerful influence on policy. However, the growing appetite for cross-country performance comparisons and benchmarking amongst countries, citizens and the media gives rise to new risks. Caution is required as initiatives that rely on poorly validated measures and biased policy interpretations may lead to seriously adverse policy and political impacts.

Hence, there is an increasing need to harness the potential of comparative health systems performance assessment (HSPA), building on credible initiatives and strengthening both the methodologies and policy analysis. This should include highlighting not only the 'policy uses' but also the 'policy abuses' of comparisons. In other words, as well as drawing out the information content and potential of performance measures, researchers should indicate what *cannot* be inferred from the analysis, showing the limitations of current measures and suggesting fruitful future improvements.

This volume seeks to summarize the current 'state of the art' of health system comparison, identifying data and methodological issues, and exploring the current interface between evidence and practice. It also draw's out the priorities for future work on performance comparison, in the development of data sources and measurement instruments; analytic methodology; and assessment of evidence on performance. It conclude's by presenting the key lessons and future priorities that policy-makers should be taking into account.

1.2 Why perform international comparisons?

There are numerous challenges in carrying out international comparisons of health system performance, first and foremost among which is the limited availability of comparable data. However, international comparisons also provide vast potential for both within and cross-country learning. Through comparative assessments of performance, policy-makers are provided with a benchmark that allows them to identify in which areas they are performing above or below expectations. Even more importantly, it provides them with an impetus to understand what is driving reported performance, as well as guidance on where to look for potential solutions.

Sceptics may argue that there is little merit in the comparison of health systems that have diverse organization and funding arrangements, and which serve different populations. However, most health systems have similar goals and face similar challenges, such as demographic change, limited resources and rising costs. Countries have applied diverse strategies to address these challenges and may even find that existing structures and organizations find them better or worse placed to cope with them. Thus, the major benefit of international comparisons is their potential to provide a snapshot comparison of different experiences or even act as an "experimental laboratory for others" (Nolte, Wait & McKee, 2006). These comparisons offer the possibility of exploring new and different options; the potential for mutual learning and even policy transfer; and the opportunity to reconsider and reformulate national policy in the light of comparative evidence (Box 1.1).

Box 1.1 The power of international comparisons to influence policy: cancer services in England

According to Ham (2009), cancer is a major issue in English health policy, not only because of the large burden of the illness but also resulting from evidence that the quality of cancer care in the UK has fallen behind that of other countries. In a review of English health policy specifically concerned with cancer services, Richards (2010) outlines key steps in the development and implementation of a comprehensive national cancer programme. Instrumental to the policy focus on cancer was comparative evidence emerging in the 1990s from the *Eurocare* studies, which identified poor survival rates in the UK relative to the rest of Europe.

According to Richards (2010), one of the first actions taken in 1997 by the new Labour Government was to raise the profile of waiting times for cancer treatment, an issue already highlighted in their election manifesto. In line with this, a retrospective baseline audit of waiting times for patients diagnosed with cancer in England was commissioned by the Department of Health and this confirmed the size of the problem. As a result, monitoring programmes and referral guidelines were set up to support the implementation of a 'two week wait' target for patients with suspected cancer to see a specialist (DOH, 2000; Spurgeon, Barwell & Kerr, 2000). Moreover, dedicated funds to improve the quality of cancer care were directed towards the health system.

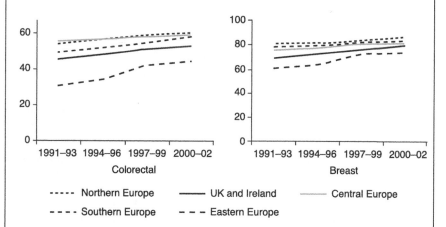

Figure 1.1 Five-year period survival rates 1991–2002 for colorectal and breast cancer from *Eurocare 4* data

Source: Richards, 2010.

Despite these actions, by early 1999, there was agreement that the pace of change for cancer was not fast enough and more negative evidence was emerging from the *Eurocare* programme. In response, the then Prime Minister, Tony Blair, convened a summit meeting on cancer and openly acknowledged that England and Wales lagged behind Europe on cancer survival rates and that cancer was to be declared a top priority (Richards, 2010). Following the summit, a number of actions to improve cancer care were taken, which led in 2000 to the development of the NHS Cancer Plan, an ambitious, long-term, comprehensive plan that aimed to raise the level of cancer services to among the best in Europe.

While interest in international health system comparisons as a way to inform national health policy is not new (Goldmann, 1946; Mountin & Perrott, 1947; Nolte, Wait & McKee, 2006), recent years have seen a growth in the publication and dissemination of this type of information (Smith et al., 2009). The increased interest in international health system comparison can be attributed to several factors. On the demand side, global social developments such as films, television and the Internet, as well as travel and migration, have given the citizens and patients of many countries an image of life in other nations. This exposure has put health systems around the world under pressure to deliver what is available elsewhere, as citizens increasingly recognize that their own health systems could be improved (Roberts et al., 2008). Schoen et al. (2005) note from evidence of international surveys that negative user experiences of health systems put increased pressure on governments to seek out alternative policy options from other countries. Rising expectations are also combined with reduced levels of trust in public institutions, and specifically the health profession, from whom increasing audit and proof of accountability are demanded (Power, 1999; Smith, 2005).

At the European level, another major driver behind the increased use of comparison is the development of health care legislation aimed at making cross-border health care for European Union (EU) citizens possible. This directive makes it easier for EU citizens to get medical treatment in another EU Member State and ensure that at least some of the costs are reimbursed in their own country. However, the directive emphasizes that Member States retain responsibility for providing safe, high-quality care on their territory, and that care should be provided according to their own standards of quality and safety. Indeed, there are various comparative assessment initiatives taking place at the European level, such as the European Community Health Indicators Monitoring (ECHIM) project at national level, and the Indicateurs Santé Régionaux d'Europe (ISARE) projects at regional level. These projects seek to develop and improve health indicators as well as implement health monitoring in the EU and all its Member States.

On the supply side, advances in information technology have made it much cheaper and easier to collect and process data. As a result, many countries have developed national repositories of health information or national performance assessment programmes. Indeed, several systems often coexist in many countries. In the United States, there are several performance measurement initiatives, constructed by different institutional bodies and targeted at different areas of the health system. For example, the Dartmouth Atlas project documents variations in medical resources using Medicare data, the Commonwealth

Fund documents state variations on different benchmarks collected through its State Scorecard, and there are also other projects, such as the Healthy People 2020 initiative, which measures performance in preventative services and determinants of health.

International benchmarks can help national strategies in formulating national policy programmes and priorities. For example, the Commonwealth Fund has developed the National Scorecard on U.S. Health System Performance to measure the performance of the United States health system (Schoen & How, 2006; McCarthy et al., 2009). The Scorecard assesses how well the United States health system performs relative to what is achievable through the assessment of key dimensions of performance in relationship to benchmarks and over time, set according to the levels achieved internationally (from a set of six other industrialized countries). In 2008, the Dutch National Institute for Public Health and the Environment (RIVM) conducted a similar exercise that assessed Dutch performance using the European Community Health Indicator (ECHI) shortlist, benchmarked against EU Member States (Harbers et al., 2008).

In a similar vein, success stories from other systems, especially when based on effective restructuring through the use of performance data (such as the United States Veterans Health Administration) encourage other nations to emulate these efforts and contribute to the spirit of mutual learning (Kerr & Flemming, 2007; Veillard et al., 2009). As more and better data are collected, analysis of the factors contributing to differential performance becomes more feasible and the analysis of variation more meaningful. Comparisons are usually made amongst peer groups that share similar organizations, goals and challenges, as well as employing similar data collection mechanisms. In these circumstances the learning opportunities are more obvious and the comparisons more robust (Box 1.2).

Box 1.2 Efforts at mutual learning: Kaiser Permanente and the English National Health Service

In 2002, Richard Feachem and colleagues published a performance assessment comparing the English National Health Service (NHS) with the California-based non-profit-making health maintenance organization Kaiser Permanente (Feachem, Sekhri & White, 2002). The aim of the study was to challenge notions about efficiency in the NHS as stated in the NHS Plan 2000, namely that: "The NHS gets more and fairer health care for every pound invested than most other health care systems." They concluded that Kaiser achieved better outcomes for similar inputs and sparked a sharp national debate (Shapiro & Smith, 2003). Critics argued that the basis on which the costs between the two organizations had been compared, and the different populations served, might explain the conclusions reached (Himmelstein & Woolhandler, 2002; Talbot-Smith et al., 2004). The authors argued that these debates confirmed rather than undermined the findings, as follow-up work indicated that

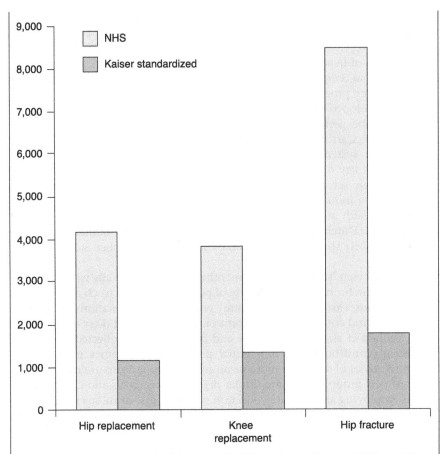

Figure 1.2 Orthopaedic bed days per 100 000 aged over 65 in the NHS and Kaiser
Source: Ham, 2005.

differences observed were indeed adjusted for currency and purchasing differences between the two countries (Feacham & Sekhri, 2004).

Moreover, follow-up work by Ham et al. (2003), conducted in order to better understand the reasons for the findings in the original work, found that bed day use in the NHS was three times that of Kaiser. According to the article, Kaiser Permanente was able to achieve this lower utilization of acute bed days through better integration of care, more active management of patients, use of intermediate care, self-care, and medical leadership specialists per 100 000 population than in the NHS (Ham et al., 2003).

Subsequent studies (Light & Dixon, 2004; Ham, 2005) used data to analyse and explain differences and possible areas of improvement for the NHS. In order to take the learning process further, the NHS Modernisation Agency arranged for senior NHS managers and clinical leaders to visit Kaiser in order to understand better how they delivered care. The following areas where the NHS could learn from Kaiser's experience were identified (Ham, 2010):

- integration of care
- focus on chronic care
- population management
- self-management support
- leadership development.

The knowledge from these areas has been piloted in three areas (Birmingham and Solihull, Northumbria and Torbay), which are known as Beacon sites and have been identified as making a concerted effort to adapt the learning from Kaiser in relation to the populations they serve (Ham, 2006, 2010). These sites have made progress in improving their services. Moreover, comparisons amongst the three sites have also provided important lessons to guide future policy-makers as to what factors promote better policy learning.

1.3 International comparisons of what?

The starting point of most international comparisons is the creation of a conceptual framework on which to base the collection of information and which can be used as a heuristic in the understanding of the health system. A theoretical framework is necessary to assist organizations in defining a set of measures that reflect key objectives and then, in turn, making an appropriate assessment of performance. In the last decade, numerous conceptual frameworks have been created for health system performance assessment at the international level (Jee & Or, 1999; Murray & Frenk, 2000; Hurst & Jee-Hughes, 2001; Aday et al., 2004; Arah et al., 2006; Commonwealth Fund, 2006; Kelley and Hurst, 2006; Atun & Menabde, 2008; IHP, 2008; Roberts et al., 2008). While these frameworks have varied purposes, they all aim to provide a better understanding of what a health system is, its goals, and the underlying structure and factors that drive its performance.

At any level – regional, national or international – a good performance assessment framework will assist in the collection and interpretation of performance data for health system improvement. In order for a framework to serve this purpose, it is important that it: takes into account the perspectives of all relevant stakeholders; clearly defines objectives of the health system; embraces all the salient components of the health system; and is sustainable enough to encourage a dynamic assessment process.

There are distinct differences between international and national frameworks. International frameworks must inevitably reflect a global 'consensus' on the major goals and constituents of the health system, and will be aimed at a broad range of stakeholders. International organizations can play only a limited role in changing policy, thus their performance measurement efforts are targeted at the areas in which they can exert influence, such as holding nations to account and influencing system reform (Box 1.3). National governments, on the other hand, play a fundamental role in the stewardship of their health systems. Their function varies considerably in practice, ranging from seeking to manage the entire system to merely playing a role in its regulation. Nevertheless, their ability to influence policy and the performance of the system is profound. National frameworks may therefore need to reflect the stewardship arrangements and organizational idiosyncrasies of the country. Yet, notwithstanding the differences in their ultimate objectives, international and national frameworks are usually constructed similarly in terms of the performance goals they identify and the dimensions of the health system they measure.

When determining the objectives that should underpin an international framework, there must first be agreement over what activities the health system encompasses and the boundaries of the health system. Narrow boundaries can

Box 1.3 The role of international organizations in HSPA

The role of international organizations in HSPA is explicitly addressed in the WHO report, *Everybody's Business: Strengthening health systems to improve health outcomes*, where the organization recognizes itself as a producer of global norms, standards and guidance. This responsibility includes: "[the production of] health systems concepts, methods and metrics; synthesizing and disseminating information on 'what works and why', and building scenarios for the future" (WHO, 2007).

In an attempt to further clarify why there is demand for such a function from policy-makers, regulators, governments, citizens and other stakeholders, Veillard et al. (2009) identify three main roles of international health system performance comparisons:

- enforcing accountability
- developing strategy
- assisting countries in mutual learning.

International organizations play a key role in holding policy-makers to account, by using international data to draw comparisons between similar countries and offering the public and the media the ability to scrutinize them. International comparisons can also prompt countries to develop a national strategy, or framework, to improve performance in a systematic way.

Finally, the provision of comparative data at an international level allows countries to learn from the experiences of their peers. While HSPA exercises have become increasingly popular since the publication of the *World Health Report 2000* (*WHR2000*), they have not always been met with approval. Historically, professional, practical and political barriers hindered early efforts at performance measurement (Speigelhalter, 1999). Even today, debate arises about the role international organizations should play in addressing the strategic health policy issues that nations face when deciding how to structure or reform their health systems (Williams, 2001a).

be better aligned with identifiable accountability relationships and can target performance improvement initiatives at relevant actors. However, they can also introduce severe problems of attribution, because many of the determinants of health lie outside those narrow boundaries. Broader boundaries therefore present a more comprehensive understanding of all the factors that determine health but may embrace factors that are beyond the control of health ministers and other accountable individuals.

Ultimately, the boundaries should be drawn, taking these factors into account, to be aligned with the main objective of the performance assessment exercise itself. Irrespective of how narrow or broad the boundaries are, it should be made clear what activities are included. One criticism of past frameworks has been the way in which they have treated the areas of public health and health promotion (Arah et al., 2003). Some frameworks have excluded them entirely, while others have failed to specify whether or not they are included. Yet, many of the most commonly used performance indicators of population health specifically reflect system performance in these areas.

Despite differences in the boundaries set by different international frameworks, the key objectives outlined are almost universally acknowledged as being:

- the health conferred on citizens by the health system
- the health system's responsiveness to citizen preferences
- the financial protection offered by the health system
- the health system's productivity (Smith, Mossialos & Papanicolas, 2008).

'Health' includes broad notions of the level of health of the population, as well as the health outcomes secured after a course of treatment. 'Responsiveness' captures dimensions of the health system concerned with patients' interactions with the health-care system, such as the health system's respect for patient dignity, autonomy and prompt service, as well as ensuring good communication, access to social support during care, quality of basic services and choice of provider. 'Financial protection' indicates the extent to which the system protects people from financial hardship in times of ill health. 'Productivity' refers to the extent to which the resources used by the health system are used efficiently in the pursuit of effectiveness.

Furthermore, in addition to the measurement of the overall attainment a health system achieves in each of these areas, most existing frameworks also highlight the importance of equity or fairness, expressed in terms of the *distribution* of health outcomes, responsiveness and payment within the population.

There is general acceptance that a framework should incorporate functions – such as (but not limited to): service delivery; health workforce; information; medical products; vaccines and technologies; financing; stewardship – as key building blocks of any health system. However, it is less clear what role such functions should play in any framework, and how they can be systematically compared across countries, as they are likely to take different forms in different health systems. Chapter 2 considers in more detail the differences in boundaries, objectives and functions identified by various international frameworks, and seeks to identify the areas of debate, the challenges underlying such debates and the prospects for resolution.

1.4 Lessons from international comparisons to date

Lessons from international comparisons in health

International health system comparisons provided by multilateral institutions, such as WHO or the OECD, have generated much interest since the publication of the *World Health Report 2000* (*WHR2000*; WHO, 2000). While desultory performance measurement efforts had occurred long before *WHR2000*, dating back over a century, this publication highlighted the potential for cross-country learning from the scrutiny of comparable data. Careful examination of experiences associated with such initiatives offers considerable scope for international learning.

By way of example, Box 1.4 suggests some of the policy and methodological debates that arose from *WHR2000*. Some of the key issues were:

1. the lack of data available to conduct this type of analysis;
2. the methodological limitations surrounding the use of a 'single number' measure of whole health system performance;
3. the ranking of countries.

Notwithstanding the many legitimate concerns about the principles and methods underlying the report, *WHR2000* without question played an important role in drawing the attention of policy-makers and academics to the issues surrounding health performance assessment and comparison.

Amongst the numerous subsequent efforts to draw international comparisons of health systems, some have again focused on overall health system performance, such as the Commonwealth Fund's International Scorecard (Davis, Schoen & Schoenbaum, 2007) and the *Euro Health Consumer Index* (HCP, 2007, 2008, 2009), while others have focused on specific areas of performance, such as

Box 1.4   Policy and methodological debates arising from *WHR2000*

The publication of *WHR2000* had an enormous and far-reaching impact. Immediately following its publication it was picked up by much of the mainstream media.

Policy abuses

While the report was instrumental in highlighting the potential for international comparisons to bring the discussion of health system performance to the forefront of national policy, there were examples of instances where comparative information was misinterpreted or misused.

- The report generated a discussion about the merits of ranking countries, especially given limitations in the availability and comparability of the underlying data used to construct the performance indicators.
- Regarding the measurement of responsiveness and efficiency, there were concerns about the publication of results based on patchy data and new, untested methodological techniques.

- The report generated a discussion about the merits of offering 'single number' measures of whole health system performance, and generated awareness of potential methodological limitations and the limited scope for policy action.
- The report might also distract policy-makers from seeking out and remedying the parts of their system requiring attention. An example that was used to illustrate the misuse of the report for national policy was in Spain. The Spanish health care system was ranked third best in Europe and yet on the day the report was released there were demonstrations against the Spanish health care authorities over long waiting lists and short consultation times. The Health Minister showed the WHO report to the protesters as proof of their unjustified complaints and demands (Navarro, 2000).

Policy uses

In academic circles, the report created debate around the methodological and ideological issues underlying the performance assessment framework adopted by WHO (Navarro 2000; Almeida et al., 2001; Murray & Frenk, 2001; Murray et al., 2001; Navarro 2001a, 2001b; Williams, 2001a, 2001b). This debate led to important advances in the area of performance measurement and an improved ability to conduct international comparisons of health systems. Some of the most notable advances directly linked to these discussions were:

- The report explicitly recognized that there are multiple goals for health systems, which is useful to realize for policy purposes and also in thinking about the trade-offs between goals (Anand et al., 2003).
- The report allowed for the development of the concept of 'responsiveness', a term which encompasses the whole patient experience, covering not only the interpersonal process between practitioner and patient but also the interaction of the health system with the population it serves (Valentine & Salomon, 2003).
- The report highlighted the lack of any comparable data on responsiveness and led to the construction and implementation of the *World Health Survey*, which now provides cross-national information on responsiveness for 70 countries.
- The report recognized the importance of measuring health system efficiency, highlighting the need to consider health system outputs relative to what can be attained for given inputs.
- The report attracted unprecedented media coverage, generating public interest in health policy and health system performance. The news was still reaching various popular media outlets even years after publication. In 2009, a YouTube video entitled 'We're number 37' was released; it contained a song referring to the rank 37 that the United States had received in the report.

the OECD Health Care Quality Indicators project on quality (OECD, 2010) and the EU funded *HealthBasket* project on comparative efficiency (Busse, Schreyögg & Smith, 2008). Chapter 3 summarizes and assesses the main health system comparative performance efforts implemented to date and considers the key issues for international comparison that can be drawn from these experiences.

Lessons from other sectors

When considering how international comparisons can be most beneficial for health systems, it is important to look beyond what has been done in the health sector and to learn from the experience of benchmarking efforts in other areas of the public and private sectors. Globally, there is widespread interest in and take up of benchmarking. Yet, there are various forms of benchmarking that have different aims in mind and offer different lessons. A key distinction can be made between performance benchmarking and practice benchmarking. Performance benchmarking concentrates on establishing performance standards, while practice benchmarking is concerned with identifying the reasons why organizations achieve the level of performance they do. Evidence suggests that performance benchmarking is more prevalent than practice benchmarking, although it can be argued that practice benchmarking is more beneficial in the long run. Chapter 4 discusses these issues in more depth.

As well as the political challenges of benchmarking, there are also practical challenges. Deciding what and how to benchmark, which organizations to compare with and how to ensure comparability with them, what data to use and whether these data are robust, all affect the value of benchmarking. It is noteworthy that, particularly in practice benchmarking, one does not always seek out perfect organizational comparability. Indeed, when focusing on how to improve processes within organizations and to encourage innovation, it is often helpful to compare organizations from very different sectors. One of the original proponents of benchmarking, Xerox, compared itself with L.L.Bean, a mail order company, because Xerox wanted to improve its warehousing and distribution processes and L.L.Bean was recognized as being excellent in these areas.

Clearly, there are challenges associated with benchmarking as well as benefits to be obtained. Some organizations consider that they have achieved no benefit from their benchmarking activities, while others claim the reverse. An important distinction between these two groups appears to be the extent to which the benchmarking focuses on strategic priorities, involves clear and careful planning, and adopts new practice selectively in line with organizational needs. Box 1.5 summarizes some of the major lessons for health systems from the general benchmarking experience.

1.5 How to compare key domains of performance

Performance measurement evaluates the extent to which a health system meets its key objectives. Most HSPA efforts focus on the common dimensions

Box 1.5 Lessons of benchmarking for health systems

From what is known of benchmarking in other sectors, five implications can be extended to benchmarking efforts in the health system:

1. Health benchmarks should focus on practice as well as performance.
2. Health benchmarks should not be used simply to evaluate and compare performance.
3. Benchmarks need to be grounded in a broader change process.
4. The benchmarking process itself needs to be well structured and planned, and designed to engage people in making change in their organizations.
5. The designers of health benchmarking systems need to consider very carefully the link between resource allocation and benchmark performance if they are to avoid dysfunctional behaviour.

Adapted from: Chapter 4.

of measurement discussed above, such as health improvement, health status, responsiveness, financial protection, equity and efficiency. Table 1.1 lists the key dimensions of HSPA efforts, why it is important for these dimensions to be measured and also the key comparison areas of interest to policy-makers.

The range and content of available performance data vary considerably between countries. This has inevitably led to variations in the measurement of key goals and functions, even within similar frameworks. Also, countries direct different degrees of effort towards collecting new information to fill in the gaps in their frameworks as opposed to using information that is readily available. In practice, many countries and organizations have been investing money and effort in generating good quality information that adequately measures the dimensions in which they are interested. Canada, for example, has committed extensive resources to creating new surveys that will collect the data specifically required by their framework. Moreover, health indicators are designed and developed in a way that is closely tied to the development of information systems. This means that the entire performance measurement system is mutually reinforcing, in a way that theory would recommend (Wolfson & Alvarez, 2002). A key issue for any system is the effort and resources put into data collection, leading to tensions between the scope, quality, timeliness, relevance and cost of the available performance information.

At the international level, WHO also carefully selected the indicators it chose to operationalize its framework in *WHR2000*, in most cases trying to construct a new measure that would best reflect the identified objective. While some of these indicators were heavily criticized – and undeniably inadequate – the efforts to reduce the reliance on readily available information were laudable. The OECD has also pursued a careful selection process in choosing the indicators for its Health Care Quality Indicators (HCQI) framework, with very strict requirements to ensure comparability across countries, which has led to delays in the collection and pubication of indicators in the past (Armesto, Medeiros & Wei, 2008). Similarly, the Nordic Collaboration, working together

Table 1.1 Performance measurement implications of setting health system boundaries

Dimension	Motivation for international comparison	Areas of interest for comparison
Population health	● To provide a comparison of health within and across countries considered from a broad, aggregated perspective, which includes the contribution of many risk factors for disease as well as the delivery of health care. ● To provide a comparative assessment of how health systems contribute to the population's health.	● Life expectancy ● Mortality by age group and condition ● Morbidity ● Avoidable mortality ● Population risk factors
Health service outcomes	● To provide a comparative assessment of how health services assist individuals in realizing their potential health.	● Performance of different areas of the health services (e.g. preventative care, primary care, secondary care, long-term care, mental health) ● Health service outcomes ● Health service processes
Equity	● Provides an assessment of inequalities in health amongst different population/ demographic/social groups within and between countries. ● Provides an assessment of inequalities in access and/ or utilization of services amongst different population/ demographic/social groups within and between countries. ● Provides an assessment of inequalities in the financing of health services amongst different population/demographic/social groups within and between countries. ● Provides an assessment of inequalities in responsiveness of health services amongst different population/demographic/social groups within and between countries.	● Distribution of health status by population/demographic/ social groups ● Distribution of access/ utilization of health services by population/demographic/ social groups ● Progressivity of financing system ● Distribution responsiveness of health services by population/demographic/ social groups

Dimension	Motivation for international comparison	Areas of interest for comparison
Fairness in financing	• To provide a comparative assessment of the extent to which citizens are protected from the financial consequences of illness.	• Fairness of financing • Out-of-pocket spending • Catastrophic expenditures on health care • Impoverishing expenditures on health care
Responsiveness	• To provide a comparative assessment of how satisfied health systems leave the patients they come into contact with.	• Patient satisfaction • Patient choice • Respect for patients' dignity • Prompt attention to medical needs

with the National Institute for Health And Welfare in Finland (THL), formerly STAKES, is investing in developing better indicators for measuring efficiency. For a discussion about the progress and challenges involved in developing international health system performance information, see Chapter 11.

One of the difficulties in conducting a well-rounded performance comparison across the many dimensions of the health system is that progress in the development of data collection techniques in the different dimensions of health performance varies. Some areas, such as population health, can be quite reliably captured through established indicators, while other areas, such as efficiency, are in earlier stages of development. Moreover, some dimensions of health systems are harder to capture due to their complex and intangible nature, in particular multifaceted concepts like responsiveness. In undertaking international comparisons, it is important to have a broad idea of the strengths and limitations of the existing metrics and how useful they are for the purposes of assessing system performance and helping design system reforms. Some of the key measurement issues for each dimension listed in Table 1.1 are summarized below. These various dimensions are considered in more detail in Chapters 5 to 10, with each chapter covering one of the dimensions.

Population health

Without question, the main aim of any health system is to improve the health of the population it serves. Thus, population health is often the first area considered when evaluating the performance of a health system, requiring aggregated data on the health status and health improvement of the population (Chapter 5). Principal indicators in this area include measures such as life expectancy at particular ages, age-standardized mortality, premature or infant mortality, years of life lost and disability-adjusted life years (DALYs), all of which capture generic information on population health. These types of measures take a broad perspective, measuring the effect on the health of the population of many risk factors for disease as well as the delivery of health care. This perspective can be attractive from a political point of view because it demonstrates the role that broader determinants of health play in determining health status. However, it also creates major methodological challenges in seeking to attribute changes in health to any particular policy or factor.

Consequently, without discarding the broader approaches, more recent research has focused on measuring the contribution of health services to improved health. This has led to the development of concepts such as avoidable mortality and the use of tracer conditions. Tracer conditions are an evaluative technique where carefully selected health problems are used to infer the quality of elements within the overall health system (Nolte, Bain & McKee, 2009). In order to be used as a tracer, a health problem should have adequate prevalence, a known epidemiology, be relatively easy to diagnose, require treatment to the extent that lack of treatment or inappropriate treatment would result in functional impairment and have a natural history that varies with utilization and quality of health services used (Kessner, Kalk & Singer, 1973). Some conditions used as tracers have been diabetes (Nolte, Wait & McKee, 2006), cervical cancer and hypertension (Neuhauser, 2004).

A similar concept is that of avoidable mortality, which refers to deaths that are considered avoidable with appropriate and timely medical care, or preventable by population-based interventions. Avoidable mortality can be further broken down into subsets of *amenable mortality*, which refers to conditions where "it is reasonable to expect death to be averted even after the condition develops" and *preventable mortality*, which includes deaths from conditions that can be prevented by population-based interventions but where the contribution of health care may be limited once the condition has developed (Nolte & McKee, 2004). Recent work in this area has considered how avoidable mortality can be measured in different countries and how metrics can be used in comparative analyses (Box 1.6).

Health service outcomes

Health systems can also be compared through the health outcomes achieved specifically through health care. Even though the achievement of good outcomes is the fundamental purpose of health care (Porter, 2010), there are still distinct challenges in being able to measure the contribution of health services to health outcomes (Chapter 6). Outcomes are inherently condition-specific and multidimensional. This poses a measurement challenge even without the extra difficulties associated with ensuring comparability across organizations and even nations, such as adjustment for differences in service provision or population characteristics. Moreover, health services include numerous and diverse organizational structures and settings, ranging from family care doctors providing single services, to specialized hospitals and long-term care facilities. To date, most measures of health service outcomes capture only a limited range of the activities and services that make up the health care system.

The most commonly used indicators of the contribution of health services to health outcomes refer to a limited set of areas, such as mortality (through indicators such as standardized hospital mortality rates or disease-specific health

Box 1.6 Avoidable Mortality in European Health Systems (AMIEHS)

Funded under the European Union Public Health Programme, the AMIEHS project, led by Erasmus Medical University and coordinated jointly with the London School of Hygiene & Tropical Medicine, brings together partners in seven EU countries with the aim of creating better comparable indicators with which to measure the contribution health care makes to the population and how this varies among countries. The project aims to develop a set of avoidable mortality-based indicators that can be used in future surveillance of the performance of health systems in Europe.

The project aims to undertake the following initiatives which will assist policy-makers and researchers with the understanding, measurement and use of avoidable mortality indicators in Europe:

- to conduct a systematic review of the literature to assess to what extent causes of death can be considered avoidable;
- to gather in-depth information on the introduction of medical innovations in seven countries;
- to develop a set of avoidable mortality-based indicators that is agreed upon; and
- to prepare an electronic atlas of avoidable mortality in 25–30 countries in Europe (http://survey.erasmusmc.nl/amiehs/maps/J45_J46/atlas.html).

Source: AMIEHS, 2012.

---

outcome measures), patient safety (adverse events, never events or sentinel events), and complications (through readmissions and avoidable admissions). More recently, patient-reported outcome measures (PROMs) have also been routinely used to attempt to address some existing measurement gaps. Much less prevalent are outcome measures in areas such as disability or discomfort, especially at the international level, although the OECD Quality Indicators project is an important resource in this area (Box 1.7).

In some performance assessment initiatives, health care process measures may be used instead of, or in conjunction with, outcome measures. There are various benefits to using process measures; they are faster and easier to collect, and are based on actions or structures known to be associated with good practice. However, unless used together with outcome measures, they are less meaningful to most stakeholders and may not be appropriate for more complex patient settings where standards or guidelines for single diseases can be misleading.

Equity

The concept of equity in health is the principle of equal (or equitable) health outcomes (for example, quality-adjusted life expectancy). Various factors outside the health care system have an impact on equity in health status, including

Box 1.7 Health Care Quality Indicators (HCQI)

The HCQI project, led by the OECD, was initiated in 2001 with the aim of measuring and comparing the quality of health service provision in the different OECD countries. Over the years, the HCQI project has grown into a robust source of internationally comparable data on the quality of care, as well as a forum for policy-makers and researchers to assist in the improvement of quality measurement. The project has focused on producing comparable indicators in key areas of health care, such as primary care, acute care, mental health care, cancer care, patient safety and patient experience.

Most data are collected from administrative databases, registries and population surveys. Following the compilation of the data, considerable efforts are undertaken to refine the methodology of data assessment and collection procedures, such as assessment of data quality, refinement of technical specifications, enhanced data collection guidelines and questionnaires, and the harmonization of approaches to age/gender standardization. Currently, there are nearly 40 indicators that are routinely collected and reported for at least some Member States every two years.

Source: OECD, 2010.

socioeconomic factors, demographic factors and genetics (Chapter 7). In the literature, the analysis of equity is often conducted separately for *substantive equity* (the wider study of disparities in health across groups) and *procedural equity* (the study of equity within the health system) (Aday et al., 2004). International comparisons in these areas have shown that, while inequities in health status related to socioeconomic factors exist in most countries, these have variable magnitude. With regard to procedural equity, different financing and structural arrangements of health systems have been found to lead to differences in equity (Table 1.2). These findings are useful to countries in their policy-making as they seek to establish which factors and policies are associated with improved equity.

One of the main challenges associated with the comparison of substantive and procedural inequalities is the availability of comparable data across countries.

Table 1.2 Selected examples of international comparisons in the area of equity

Countries compared	Evidence	Reference
Substantive equity		
United Kingdom and United States	Based on self-reported illnesses and biological markers of disease, US residents are much less healthy than their English counterparts and these differences exist at all points of the socioeconomic distribution.	Banks et al. (2006)

Countries compared	Evidence	Reference

Substantive equity

Countries compared	Evidence	Reference
Belgium, Czech Republic, Denmark, England and Wales, Estonia, Finland, France, Hungary, Italy, Lithuania, Norway, Poland, Slovenia, Spain, Sweden, Switzerland	Inequalities in health associated with socioeconomic status are present in all countries, but their magnitude is highly variable.	Mackenbach et al. (2008)
Denmark, Finland, Norway, Sweden	Health inequalities are present in all Nordic countries for both men and women.	Lahelma et al. (2002)
Austria, Belgium, Denmark, Finland, France, Germany, Greece, Ireland, Italy, Luxembourg, Netherlands, Portugal, Spain, UK	Income-related inequalities in health exist in all countries, both in the short and long term.	Hernández-Quevedo et al. (2006)

Procedural equity

Countries compared	Evidence	Reference
Denmark, Ireland, Italy, Netherlands, Spain, Switzerland, UK, US	Based on Household Survey data, horizontal equity in the delivery of health care is assessed for eight countries using two different methods.	van Doorslaer & Wagstaff (1992)
Denmark, France, Ireland, Italy, Netherlands, Portugal, Spain, Switzerland, UK, US	Concludes that different types of health care financing systems have different levels of progressivity. Tax-financed systems tend to be proportional or mildly progressive; social insurance systems are regressive; and private systems are even more regressive.	Wagstaff & van Doorslaer (1992)
Australia, Austria, Belgium, Canada, Denmark, Finland, France, Germany, Greece, Hungary, Ireland, Italy, Mexico, Netherlands, Norway, Portugal, Spain, Sweden, Switzerland, UK	Inequities exist in physician utilization favouring the rich in about half the countries studied. In most countries there is no inequity in the distribution of general practitioner visits across income groups, but there is evidence of pro-rich inequity in specialist visits in all countries.	van Doorslaer et al. (2006)
Bangladesh, China (Taiwan), Indonesia, Japan, Republic of Korea, Kyrgyzstan, Nepal, Philippines, India (Punjab), Sri Lanka, Thailand	In all territories, higher-income households contribute more to the financing of health care. The better-off contribute more as a proportion of ability to pay in most low- and lower-middle-income territories.	O'Donnell et al. (2008)

These types of analyses require, at the very minimum, comparable data on health status and socioeconomic factors. Extending the study to procedural equity also requires comparable data on the interaction of individuals with the health care system (such as utilization, access, financing and need). Most comparable data of this sort are available in the form of surveys collected across a group of countries, but the subjective nature of many data collection mechanisms may give rise to concerns of comparability.

Financial protection

The area of financial protection is often studied separately from equity, and looks specifically at the extent to which people are protected from the financial consequences of ill health and the use of medical care (Chapter 8). The last decade has witnessed a growing interest in the ability of health systems to protect citizens in this way, culminating in the publication of the World Health Report 2010 (WHO, 2010), which firmly emphasizes the need for health systems to move towards universal 'coverage' of their populations. Yet, determining the most appropriate set of policies for the improvement of financial protection in a nation will depend on its particular context; that is, the extent and determinants of financial risk in a particular health system. Useful measurement tools have been developed to assist policy-makers with these goals (Table 1.3).

The emphasis of most cross-country studies in the area of financial protection has been on the extent of out-of-pocket payments present in a health system or on the incidence of 'catastrophic' health payments, relative to some threshold of household income, and 'impoverishing' health payments, relative to some pre-defined poverty line. However, such metrics ignore the likelihood that some households are unable even to secure access to needed services because of financial constraints (Moreno-Serra, Millett & Smith, 2011). The limited scope of existing studies has meant that conclusions about system-wide determinants of differences in financial protection levels across countries have often been based on descriptive or anecdotal evidence. A major challenge is to move beyond the immediate expenditure on health care, to trace the longer-term implications for households' wealth and savings.

Patient experience

WHO developed and proposed the concept of responsiveness, which it defined as aspects of the way individuals are treated, and the environment in which they are treated, during health system interactions (Valentine & Salomon, 2003). This notion emphasizes the importance of goals other than health improvement, such as the communication between patients and their providers, and the satisfaction of patients with the treatment they receive. Eight associated dimensions, or domains, are collectively described as responsiveness goals for health care processes and systems. The domains are: dignity, autonomy, confidentiality, communication, prompt attention, quality (of) basic amenities,

Table 1.3 Main indicators for fairness in financing

Main indicators	Policy uses	Limitations
Catastrophic and impoverishing health payments	Catastrophic spending indicators can offer a useful picture of the extent to which citizens in a health system suffer hardship due to the costs of health care services. Impoverishing health payment indicators allow system comparisons in terms of the number of people being pushed into poverty, relative to a minimum living standard, due to illness.	• Provide only limited insights into what the major determinants of inadequate financial protection are in a given context. • Do not inform as to whether factors related to health care play a relevant role for the measured extent of financial protection and, if so, which individuals are more affected by such barriers. • A lack of work investigating the various aspects related to access to health services as determinants of financial protection levels means that the comparison of incidence of catastrophic or impoverishing spending across countries can only result in speculative conclusions about system-wide determinants of differences in financial protection levels across countries.
Out-of-pocket payments	A simple strategy to gain some insight into how far citizens in a health system are protected against the financial consequences of illness is to look at the contribution of private health spending to the financing of the system.	• Cross-country examinations of the relative importance of out-of-pocket expenses for funding the health system can convey helpful insights for performance comparisons of financial risk. • Measuring and comparing the actual extent of financial protection across health systems would require the analyst to examine micro-data relating households' out-of-pocket health expenses to some metric in terms of their living standards.
Index of fairness of financial contribution (WHO, 2000)	The notion of fairness of financial contribution developed in *WHR2000* is based on the premise that a fair health system ensures that households make health care payments according to their ability to pay rather than risk of illness, hence being protected against the risk of falling into poverty – or being deterred from seeking care – due to health care costs.	• The indicator is unable to discriminate: between countries where health payments are progressive or regressive; the extent to which inequalities are due to horizontal inequity or vertical inequity; or between the different proportions of national income going to health care systems.

Adapted from: Chapter 8.

access to social support networks during treatment (labelled 'social support'), and choice (of health care providers).

Both responsiveness and satisfaction are terms that aim to capture the degree to which health systems are successful in responding to the expectations of their patients or the population they serve. Increasingly, health service reforms in many countries have been placing explicit emphasis on improving responsiveness to patients and increasing both population and patient satisfaction. However, lack of a clear definition, or even terminology, in this area makes it difficult to agree on what to measure. National indicators related to the area of patient experience usually refer to the patient/carer experience or the coordination of care, but may include a variety of different dimensions, probably reflecting national policy preoccupations, making it difficult to use this information for cross-country comparisons.

However, there are patient surveys focusing on the collection of information relating to patient experiences available at the international level (Chapter 9), such as the population satisfaction questions in *Eurobarometer* surveys (European Commission, 1996, 1998, 1999, 2000, 2002); the Picker Institute's development of patient experience surveys (Coulter & Cleary, 2001; Jenkinson, Coulter & Bruster, 2002); the EUROPEP instrument to assess general practice (Grol et al., 2000); the World Health Report 2000 (WHO, 2000), as well as work by the Commonwealth Fund (Schoen et al., 2007). While these data are collected in many countries, given their subjective nature and lack of clarity on the concept, there is some concern about the validity of drawing comparisons across countries and across surveys.

Self-reported data may be prone to measurement error, where bias results from groups of respondents, for example defined by socioeconomic characteristics, systematically varying in their reporting of a fixed level of the measurement construct. The degree of comparability of self-reported survey data across individuals, socioeconomic groups or populations has been debated extensively, usually with regard to health status measures (for example, Lindeboom & van Doorslaer, 2004; Bago d'Uva et al., 2008). Similar concerns apply to self-reported data on health systems responsiveness where the characteristics of the systems and cultural norms regarding the use and experiences of public services are likely to predominate (Rice, Robone & Smith, 2012).

Efficiency

Systems level efficiency is concerned with understanding how well countries are using the resources at their disposal to achieve valued objectives of their health systems. The need to develop reliable measures of efficiency is important, given the policy problem of trying to decide where limited health system finance is best spent, as well as identifying inefficient providers. In the light of apparently inexorable rises in health care expenditure, concern with the cost–effectiveness of the health system has become a dominant policy concern of many policy-makers. International comparisons in this area are useful for policy-makers; they not only allow the policy-makers to compare what they are achieving relative to other nations that spend similar amounts, but also to identify in which areas of their health system they can achieve the same outcomes with fewer resources (Chapter 10).

The measurement of efficiency can take many forms, from the cost–effectiveness of individual treatments or practitioners, to system level efficiency. Whatever level of analysis is used, a fundamental challenge is the need to attribute both the consumption of resources (costs) and the outcomes achieved (benefits) to the organizations or individuals under scrutiny. The diverse methods used to compare efficiency include direct measurement of the costs and benefits of treatment; complex econometric models that yield measures of comparative efficiency; and attempts to introduce health system outcomes into the national accounts. The experience of *WHR2000* illustrates how difficult this task is at the macro level. Moreover, the accounting challenges of identifying resources consumed become progressively more acute as one moves to finer levels of detail, such as the meso-level (e.g. provider organizations), the clinical department, the practitioner, or – most challenging of all – the individual patient or citizen.

One of the main challenges encountered in this area is the lack of consensus on the conceptualization of efficiency (Box 1.8). While the notion of relating inputs to valued outputs is present in all definitions, valuations can vary across stakeholders because of variations in individual preferences, the decision-making perspective being used, or even because of the level of analysis being applied. This difficulty in conceptualization leads in turn to difficulty in selecting which measures to use for valued outputs. There is an urgent need

Box 1.8 Conflicting notions of efficiency

A number of sometimes conflicting definitions for 'efficiency' exist in the economics and policy literature, and even within health economics itself. Drawing from Chung et al. (2008) and various sources, the following examples of different definitions have been found in the health care literature:

Efficiency of care: "a measure of the cost of care associated with a specified level of quality of care"

(AQA Alliance, 2006)

Efficiency of care: "a measure of the relationship of the cost of care associated with a specific level of performance measured with respect to the other five IOM aims of quality"

(IOM, 2001)

Efficiency of care: "a measurement construct of cost of care or resource utilization associated with a specified level of quality of care"

(National Quality Forum, 2007)

Efficiency: "the relative quantity, mix and cost of clinical resources used to achieve a measured level of quality"

(PBGH & CalPERS, 2006)

Efficiency: "an attribution of performance that is measured by examining the relationship between a specific production of the healthcare system (also called output) and the resources used to create that product (also called inputs)"

(RAND, 2008)

Efficiency: "a measure of the cost at which any given improvement in health is achieved. If two strategies of care are equally efficacious or effective, the less costly one is more efficient."

(Donabedian, 1990)

And specifically referring to efficiency at the health systems level:

Efficiency: "microeconomic efficiency, measured health system productivity as compared to its maximum attainable, macroeconomic efficiency, what effect a change in the level of resources would have on the desired level of health outcomes and responsiveness compared to other goods and services"

(Hurst & Jee-Hughes, 2001)

Efficiency: "technical efficiency (or production efficiency), getting the maximum output for money, and allocative efficiency, producing the right collection of outputs to achieve goals, or being on the production possibility frontier"

(Roberts et al., 2008)

Health systems efficiency: "actual goal attainment achieved related to what could be achieved given the resources available"

(WHO, 2000, 2007)

Efficiency: "production efficiency, the combination of inputs required to produce care and related services at the lowest costs, and allocative efficiency, the combination of inputs that produce the greatest health improvements given the available resources"

(Aday et al., 2004)

Efficient (not wasteful) care: "delivery and insurance administration, delivered at the right time and right setting and where new innovations can be evaluated for both effectiveness and value"

(Commonwealth Fund, 2006)

for clarification on how metrics in this area can be aligned with the needs of policy-makers.

1.6 Conclusions

If undertaken carefully, health system performance comparison offers a powerful resource for identifying weaknesses and suggesting relevant reforms.

The progress that has been achieved is impressive, both in the scope of areas for which comparable international data on health are now available and in the degree to which comparability has been improved. However, the science of international comparison is at a developmental stage. Policy-makers therefore need to be made aware of both the strengths and limitations of health system comparison.

There are various ongoing initiatives and developments that have the potential to yield further and more reliable international comparisons (Chapter 11). One very large area of development is that of information and communication technologies (ICT), often described within the EU context in particular as "e-health". This has the potential to greatly improve the quality, timeliness and scope of data collected at the system level. Moreover, as increasing numbers of people seek health care outside their own country, there is a growing incentive for better comparability at the international level (Busse et al., 2011).

Performance measures by their nature are contestable and all exhibit shortcomings of some sort. However, this does not imply that the search for more and better metrics is futile. Rather, it suggests a need for careful commentaries on the data and better understanding of the reasons for variations. From an international comparative perspective, the crucial requirement is that such metrics should enjoy widespread acceptance and be defined in unambiguous terms that are consistent with most countries' data collection systems. This volume aims at highlighting the state of the art in conceptualization, data collection and interpretation for the key performance dimensions outlined above.

References

Aday, L.A. et al. (2004) *Evaluating the Healthcare System: Effectiveness, efficiency, and equity*, 3rd edn. Chicago: Health Administration Press.

Almeida, C. et al. (2001) Methodological concerns and recommendations on policy consequences of the World Health Report 2000, *The Lancet*, 357: 1692–7.

AMIEHS (2012) *Avoidable Mortality in the European Union: Towards better indicators for the effectiveness of health systems*. Rotterdam: Avoidable Mortality in European Health Systems (http://amiehs.lshtm.ac.uk/, accessed 25 September 2012).

Anand, S. et al. (2003) Report of the Scientific Peer Review Group on health systems performance assessment, in C.J.L. Murray and D.B. Evans (eds) *Health Systems Performance Assessment: Debates, methods and empiricism*. Geneva: World Health Organization.

AQA Alliance (2006) *Principles of "efficiency" measures* (http://www.aqaalliance.org/files/PrinciplesofEfficiencyMeasurement.pdf, accessed 25 September 2012).

Arah, O.A. et al. (2003) Conceptual frameworks for health systems performance: a quest for effectiveness, quality, and improvement, *International Journal for Quality in Health Care*, 15(5): 377–98.

Arah, O.A. et al. (2006) A conceptual framework for the OECD Health Care Quality Indicators project, *International Journal for Quality in Health Care*, 18(Suppl): 5–13.

Armesto, S.G., Medeiros, H. and Wei, L. (2008) *Information availability for measuring and comparing quality of mental health care across OECD countries*. Paris: Organisation for Economic Co-operation and Development (OECD Health Technical Papers, no. 20) (www.oecd.org/dataoecd/53/47/41243838.pdf, accessed 21 September 2012).

Atun, R. and Menabde, N. (2008) Health systems and systems thinking, in R. Coker, R. Atun and M. McKee (eds) *Health systems and the challenge of communicable diseases: Experiences from Europe and Latin America.* Buckingham: Open University Press (European Observatory on Health Systems and Policies Series).

Bago d'Uva, T. et al. (2008) Does reporting heterogeneity bias the measurement of health disparities? *Health Economics*, 17(3): 351–75.

Banks, J. et al. (2006) Disease and disadvantage in the United States and England, *JAMA*, 295(17): 2037–45.

Busse, R., Schreyögg, J. and Smith, P. (2008) Variability in health care treatment costs amongst nine EU countries – results from the HealthBASKET project, *Health Economics*, 17(Suppl 1): S1–8.

Busse, R. et al. (2011) Being responsive to citizens' expectations: the role of health services in responsiveness and satisfaction, in J. Figueras and M. McKee (eds) *Health systems: Health, wealth, society and well-being.* Oxford: Oxford University Press.

Chung, J., Kaleba, E. and Wozinak, G. (2008) *A framework for measuring healthcare efficiency and value.* Working Paper prepared for the Physician Consortium for Performance Improvement (Work Group on Efficiency and Cost of Care) (http://www.ama-assn.org/ama1/pub/upload/mm/370/framewk_meas_efficiency.pdf, accessed 25 September 2012).

Commonwealth Fund (2006) *Framework for a high performance health system for the United States.* New York: The Commonwealth Fund.

Coulter, A. and Cleary, P.D. (2001) Patients' experiences with hospital care in five countries, *Health Affairs (Millwood)*, 20(3): 244–52.

Davis, K., Schoen, C. and Schoenbaum, S.C. (2007) *Mirror, Mirror on the Wall: An international update on the comparative performance of American health care.* New York: The Commonwealth Fund (http://www.commonwealthfund.org/Publications/Fund-Reports/2007/May/Mirror--Mirror-on-the-Wall--An-International-Update-on-the-Comparative-Performance-of-American-Healt.aspx, accessed 3 June 2012).

DOH (2000) *Referral Guidelines for Suspected Cancer.* London: Department of Health.

Donabedian, A. (1990) The seven pillars of quality, *Archives of Pathology and Laboratory Medicine*, 114(11): 1115–18.

European Commission (1996) *Eurobarometer*, 44.3. Brussels: European Commission.

European Commission (1998) *Eurobarometer*, 49. Brussels: European Commission.

European Commission (1999) *Eurobarometer*, 50.1. Brussels: European Commission.

European Commission (2000) *Eurobarometer*, 52.1. Brussels: European Commission.

European Commission (2002) *Eurobarometer*, 57.2. Brussels: European Commission.

Feachem, R. and Sekhri, N. (2004) Reply to 'Questioning the claims from Kaiser', *British Journal of General Practice*, 54: 422.

Feachem, R.G., Sekhri, N.K. and White, K.L. (2002) Getting more for their dollar: a comparison of the NHS with California's Kaiser Permanente, *BMJ*, 324: 135–41.

Goldmann, F. (1946) Foreign programs of medical care and their lessons, *New England Journal of Medicine*, 234: 155–60.

Grol, R. et al. (2000) Patients in Europe evaluate general practice care: an international comparison, *British Journal of General Practice*, 50(460): 882–7.

Ham, C. (2005) Lost in translation? Health systems in the US and the UK, *Social Policy and Administration*, 39: 192–209.

Ham, C. (2006) *Developing integrated care in the NHS: Adapting lessons from Kaiser.* Birmingham: Health Services Management Centre.

Ham, C. (2009) *Health policy in Britain*, 6th edn. Chippenham: Palgrave Macmillan.

Ham, C. (2010) *Working together for health: Achievements and challenges in the Kaiser NHS Beacon Sites programme.* Birmingham: Health Services Management Centre.

Ham, C. et al. (2003) Hospital bed utilization in the NHS, Kaiser Permanente and the US Medicare Programme: analysis of routine data, *BMJ*, 327(7426): 1257–60.

Harbers, M.M. et al. (2008) *Dare to compare! Benchmarking Dutch health with the European Community Health Indicators (ECHI)*. Bilthoven: National Institute for Public Health and the Environment.

HCP (2007) *Euro Health Consumer Index 2007*. Brussels: Health Consumer Powerhouse (http://www.healthpowerhouse.com/media/Rapport_EHCI_2007.pdf, accessed 8 June 2012).

HCP (2008) *Euro Health Consumer Index 2008*. Brussels: Health Consumer Powerhouse (http://www.healthpowerhouse.com/files/2008-EHCI/EHCI-2008-report.pdf, accessed 8 June 2012).

HCP (2009) *Euro Health Consumer Index 2009*. Brussels: Health Consumer Powerhouse (http://www.healthpowerhouse.com/files/Report%20EHCI%202009%20091005%20 final%20with%20cover.pdf, accessed 8 June 2012).

Hernández-Quevedo, C. et al. (2006) Socioeconomic inequalities in health: a comparative longitudinal analysis using the European Community Household Panel, *Social Science and Medicine*, 63(5): 1246–61.

Himmelstein, D.U. and Woolhandler, S. (2002) Getting more for their dollar: Kaiser v the NHS: Price adjustments falsify comparison, *BMJ*, 324(7349): 1332.

Hurst, J. and Jee-Hughes, M. (2001) *Performance measurement and performance management in OECD health systems*. Paris: Organisation for Economic Co-operation and Development Publishing (OECD Labour Market and Social Policy Occasional Paper, no. 47).

IHP (2008) *Monitoring performance and evaluating progress in the scale-up for better health: A proposed common framework.* Document prepared by the monitoring and evaluating working group of the International Health Partnership and Related Initiatives (IHP+), led by the WHO and the World Bank.

IOM (2001) *Crossing the Quality Chasm: A new health system for the 21st century*. Washington, DC: The National Academies Press (Institute of Medicine).

Jee, M. and Or, Z. (1999) *Health outcomes in OECD countries: A framework of health indicators for outcome-oriented policymaking*. Paris: Organisation for Economic Co-operation and Development Publishing (OECD Labour Market and Social Policy Occasional Paper, no. 36).

Jenkinson, C., Coulter, A. and Bruster, S. (2002) The Picker Patient Experience Questionnaire: development and validation using data from in-patient surveys in five countries, *International Journal for Quality in Health Care*, 14(5): 353–8.

Kelley, E. and Hurst, J. (2006) *Health Care Quality Indicators project: Conceptual framework paper*. Paris: Organisation for Economic Co-operation and Development Publishing (OECD Health Working Paper, no. 23).

Kerr, E. and Flemming, B. (2007) Making performance indicators work: experiences of the US Veterans Health Administration, *BMJ*, 335(7627): 971–3.

Kessner, D.M., Kalk, C.E. and Singer, J. (1973) Assessing health quality – the case for tracers, *New England Journal of Medicine*, 288(4): 189–94.

Lahelma, E. et al. (2002) Analysing changes of health inequalities in Nordic welfare states, *Social Science and Medicine*, 55(4): 609–25.

Light, D. and Dixon, M. (2004) Making the NHS more like Kaiser Permanente, *BMJ*, 328(7442): 763–5.

Lindeboom, M. and van Doorslaer, E. (2004) Cut-point shift and index shift in self-reported health, *Journal of Health Economics*, 23(6): 1083–99.

Mackenbach, J.P. et al. (2008) Socioeonomic inequalities in health in 22 European countries, *New England Journal of Medicine*, 358(23): 2468–81.

McCarthy, D. et al. (2009) *Aiming higher: Results from a State Scorecard on Health System Performance 2009*. New York: The Commonwealth Fund.

Moreno-Serra, R., Millett, C. and Smith, P.C. (2011) Towards improved measurement of financial protection in health, *PLoS Medicine*, 8(9): e1001087.

Mountin, J.W. and Perrott, G.S. (1947) Health insurance programs and plans of western Europe: summary of observations, *Public Health Reports*, 62(11): 369–99.

Murray, C.J.L. and Frenk, J. (2000) A framework for assessing the performance of health systems, *Bulletin of the World Health Organization*, 78(6): 717–30.

Murray, C.J.L. and Frenk, J. (2001) World Health Report 2000: A step towards evidence-based health policy, *The Lancet*, 357(9629): 1698–700.

Murray, C.J.L. et al. (2001) Science or marketing at WHO? A response to Williams, *Health Economics*, 10: 277–82.

National Quality Forum (2007) *Measurement framework: evaluating efficiency across episodes of care*. Washington, DC: National Quality Forum.

Navarro, V. (2000) Assessment of the World Health Report 2000, *The Lancet*, 356(9241): 1598–601.

Navarro, V. (2001a) World Health Report 2000: Responses to Murray and Frenk, *The Lancet*, 357(9269): 1701–2.

Navarro, V. (2001b) Science or ideology? A response to Murray and Frenk, *International Journal of Health Services*, 31(4): 875–80.

Neuhauser, D. (2004) Assessing health quality: the case for tracers, *Journal of Health Services Research and Policy*, 9(4): 246–7.

Nolte, E. and McKee, M. (2004) *Does healthcare save lives? Avoidable mortality revisited*. London: The Nuffield Trust.

Nolte, E., Bain, C. and McKee, M. (2009) Population health, in P.C. Smith et al. (eds) *Performance measurement for health system improvement: experiences, challenges and prospects*. Cambridge: Cambridge University Press.

Nolte, E., Wait, S. and McKee, M. (2006) *Investing in health: Benchmarking health systems*. London: The Nuffield Trust.

O'Donnell, O. et al. (2008) Who pays for health care in Asia? *Journal of Health Economics*, 27(2): 460–75.

OECD (2010) *Improving value in health care: measuring quality*. Paris: Organisation for Economic Co-operation and Development (http://www.oecd.org/health/hcqi, accessed on 23 April 2012).

PBGH & CalPERS (2006) *Hospital cost efficiency measurement: methodological approaches*. San Francisco, CA: Pacific Business Group on Health, and Sacramento, CA: California Public Employees Retirement Scheme.

Porter, M.E. (2010) What is value in health care? *New England Journal of Medicine*, 363(26): 2477–81.

Power, M. (1999) *The Audit Society*. Oxford: Oxford University Press.

RAND (2008) *Identifying, categorizing and evaluating health care efficiency measures*. Rockville, MD: Agency for Health Research and Quality (Publication No. 08-0030).

Rice, N., Robone, S. and Smith, P. (2012) Vignettes and health systems responsiveness in cross-country comparative analyses, *Journal of the Royal Statistical Society, Series A*, 175(2): 337–69.

Richards, M. (2010) Improving cancer services: the approach taken in England, in J.M. Elwood and S.B. Sutcliffe (eds) *Cancer Control*. Oxford: Oxford University Press.

Roberts, M.J. et al. (2008) *Getting health reform right: A guide to improving performance and equity*. Oxford: Oxford University Press.

Schoen, C. and How, S.K.H. (2006) *Why not the best? National scorecard on U.S. health system performance*. New York: Commonwealth Fund.

Schoen, C. et al. (2005) Taking the pulse of health care systems: experiences of patients with health problems in six countries, *Health Affairs (Millwood)*, 16(Suppl): 509–25.

Schoen, C. et al. (2007) Toward higher-performance health systems: adults' health care experiences in seven countries, 2007, *Health Affairs (Millwood)*, 26(6): w717–34.

Shapiro, J. and Smith, S. (2003) Lessons for the NHS from Kaiser Permanente, *BMJ*, 327(7426): 1241–2.

Smith, P.C. (2005) Performance measurement in health care: history, challenges and prospects, *Public Money & Management*, 25(4): 213–20.

Smith, P.C., Mossialos, E. and Papanicolas, I. (2008) *Performance measurement for health system improvement: Experiences, challenges and prospects.* Background document for the WHO European Ministerial Conference on Health Systems. Tallinn, Estonia, 25–27 June 2008.

Smith, P.C. et al. (eds) (2009) *Performance measurement for health system improvement: Experiences, challenges and prospects.* Cambridge: Cambridge University Press.

Spiegelhalter, D.J. (1999) Surgical audit: statistical lessons from Nightingale and Codman, *Journal of the Royal Statistical Society*, 162(1): 45–58.

Spurgeon, P., Barwell, F. and Kerr, D. (2000) Waiting times for cancer patients in England after general practitioners' referral: retrospective national survey, *BMJ*, 320(7328): 838–9.

Talbot-Smith, A. et al. (2004) Questioning the claims from Kaiser, *British Journal of General Practice*, 54(503): 415–21.

Valentine, N.B. and Salomon, J.A. (2003) Weights for responsiveness domains: analysis of country variation in 65 national sample surveys, in C.J.L. Murray and D.B. Evans (eds) *Health Systems Performance Assessment: Debates, methods and empiricism.* Geneva: World Health Organization.

van Doorslaer, E. and Wagstaff, A. (1992) Equity in the delivery of health care: some international comparisons, *Journal of Health Economics*, 11(4): 389–411.

van Doorslaer, E. et al. (2006) Inequalities in access to medical care by income in developed countries, *Canadian Medical Association Journal*, 174(2): 177–83.

Veillard, J. et al. (2009) International health system comparisons: from measurement challenge to management tool, in P.C. Smith, et al. (eds) *Performance measurement for health system improvement.* Cambridge: Cambridge University Press.

Wagstaff, A. and van Doorslaer, E. (1992) Equity in the finance of health care: some international comparisons, *Journal of Health Economics*, 11(4): 361–87.

WHO (2000) *World Health Report 2000. Health systems: improving performance.* Geneva: World Health Organization.

WHO (2007) *Everybody's business: Strengthening health systems to improve health outcomes. WHO's framework for action.* Geneva: World Health Organization Document Production Services.

WHO (2010) *World Health Report 2010. Health systems financing: the path to universal coverage.* Geneva: World Health Organization.

Williams, A. (2001a) Science or marketing at WHO? A commentary on World Health 2000, *Health Economics*, 10: 93–100.

Williams, A. (2001b) Science or marketing at WHO? Rejoinder from Allan Williams, *Health Economics*, 10: 283–5.

Wolfson, M. and Alvarez, R. (2002) Towards integrated and coherent health information systems for performance monitoring: the Canadian experience, in P.C. Smith (ed) *Measuring up: Improving health system performance in OECD countries.* Paris: Organisation for Economic Co-operation and Development.

chapter two

International Frameworks for Health System Comparison[1]

Irene Papanicolas

2.1 Introduction

Performance information is essential in assuring a health system's ability to provide improved health to its population. It serves many different purposes, including the promotion of transparency and accountability, determining appropriate treatment for patients, facilitating patient choice and for managerial control and allowing stakeholders to make international comparisons. Whatever the ultimate aim of collecting performance information, in order to reach the desired end-point, users of this information need to be able to understand what data are being collected and how these data relate to the health system architecture and its performance. Yet, as health system performance measurement develops, there is still considerable variation, and often confusion, as to what is being measured. A clear conceptual framework can help to clarify the way in which stakeholders understand health systems; however, the multiple efforts that have been made to meet this need have resulted in considerable debate as to what they propose to measure and how.

Over the last decade, several different conceptual health system frameworks have been proposed (Sicotte et al., 1998; Jee & Or, 1999; Murray & Frenk, 2000; Hurst & Jee-Hughes, 2001; Aday et al., 2004; Commonwealth Fund, 2006; Kelley & Hurst, 2006; Atun & Menabde, 2008; IHP, 2008; Roberts et al., 2008; Klassen et al., 2009). While the ultimate goal of the different frameworks may vary, each attempts to provide a common starting point – a clear and simple conceptualization of the health system – from which its users can make further progress. Yet, what the diverse frameworks betray is a lack of common understanding of what a health system entails. Indeed, the ongoing use of different frameworks by different stakeholders for similar purposes often results in miscommunication, when each party conceptualizes important terms in different ways. Perhaps the most striking of these is the very different understanding different stakeholders have as to what the 'health system' is.

This chapter attempts to review some of the most well-documented of these endeavours, revealing the diversity of approaches taken as well as notable differences in matters of understanding, focus and principle. It is our belief that these matters should be taken into account and carefully considered in any attempt to use a framework as a starting point for performance assessment. This chapter will examine some of the most widely used existing international frameworks, while taking a closer look at the common areas of debate, the challenges behind these and the prospects that need to be considered.

Before concluding the chapter will review how international frameworks can also provide a useful starting point for countries seeking to conduct national health system performance assessments.

2.2 Issues in developing a health system performance assessment framework

This section reviews the *World Health Report 2000* and other large-scale international frameworks that have been developed since, and draws some conclusions from the lessons that this practical experience can offer. The frame for more detailed information on each of the frameworks discussed in this section see Appendix 1.

The WHO 2000 Framework was designed as a conceptual tool that could also be used as an evaluative instrument. While the results of the *WHR2000* performance measurement exercise were subject to large debate, the conceptual framework was successful in providing a clear platform from which this evaluation could be conducted. Indeed, most of the contentious issues surrounding *WHR2000* related to the methods used in analysing and comparing cross-country data, while the conceptual framework behind it largely met with approval (Anand et al., 2003). The WHO 2000 Framework provides a clear conceptual understanding from which to conduct HSPA evaluation by addressing five fundamental questions, laid out in Frenk (2010):

- What are the boundaries of the health system?
- What are health systems for?
- What is the architecture of a health system in terms of its functions?
- How good is a health system in terms of its performance?
- How can we relate health system architecture to performance?

In terms of providing a clear pathway to understanding and evaluating the performance of health systems, we agree that these five questions, or criteria, are essential for all international frameworks. The first three questions touch upon the difficult conceptual questions that the framework is meant to clarify, while the last two consider how helpful the framework can be when used as an assessment tool. We believe a strong framework, and especially a framework that can be used as a basis for international comparison, should provide clear answers to all five of these questions. In order to assess the frameworks listed in Appendix 1, and to disentangle the main challenges associated with constructing and interpreting international frameworks in general, we use these questions as a guide to our assessment.

1. What are the boundaries of the health system?

A key debate when considering international frameworks is how to conceptualize the health system. Should international frameworks reflect national objectives or some form of overarching normative objectives that reflect a kind of international consensus? Central to this debate is the question of where to set the boundaries of the health system. In practice, the frameworks referred to (see Appendix 1) use different expressions to refer to the phenomena they are interested in measuring, as summarized in Table 2.1. These different terms reflect different understandings of where the health system boundaries lie, and what responsibilities lie within the jurisdiction of the health system.

The central point of discussion arises from the recognition that health outcomes are the result of numerous determinants, many of which lie outside the realm that policy-makers can affect. Different frameworks make reference to a wider or narrower set of these determinants. There is relative consensus among authors that herein lies the distinction between the 'health system' and the 'health care system'; the health system encompasses wider determinants of health and the health care system is limited to personal health care services. While most frameworks focus on the health care system, they often refer to, or even include, elements of the wider set of determinants and processes within the boundaries of what they are considering. In particular, there is uncertainty as to where public health and health promotion activities lie.

For example, the OECD (2001) definition unequivocally excludes public health, while the Commonwealth Fund's conceptualization leaves this uncertain. In the OECD HCQI framework, Arah et al. (2006) place public health within the domain of health care services. While Hsiao (2003) does not explicitly mention public health or health promotion, these are included in a definition of the 'health sector' in a later publication of the Control Knobs framework (Roberts et al., 2008). Similarly, Aday et al. (1998) do not explicitly identify these areas but imply that they are included in their definition of behavioural health care, which includes "respectful intervention in human behaviour, behavioural antecedents, and behavioural consequences". The other three definitions (Sicotte, 1998; WHO, 2000, 2007; Atun & Menabde, 2008) are all quite broad, implying an inclusion of not only public health and health promotion but other activities influencing health outcomes as well. WHO's definition of 'health actions' is perhaps the most narrow of these, encompassing only all activities whose primary objective is to improve health, including public health activities, while all others include wider determinants of health.

Depending on how narrowly or broadly the boundaries are set, the causal responsibility in improving health is assigned to different factors (Naylor, Iron & Handa, 2002; Duran et al., 2012), thus influencing the framework's function as an HSPA tool. A wider boundary will not allow the HSPA framework to identify the influence key health system players have on performance,

Table 2.1 Health system boundaries in international HSPA frameworks

Health system boundary

Behavioral Healthcare (1998)
(Behavioural health care)
A continuum of services aimed at promoting physical, mental and social well-being through thoughtful and respectful intervention in human behaviour, behavioural antecedents and behavioural consequences (Aday et al., 1998).

EGIPSS (1998)
(Parsonian organization functions)
Organized systems of action with four functional dimensions: goal attainment; environmental adaptation; production; culture and value maintenance, plus the interchanges taking place between each of these functions and the others (Sicotte et al., 1998).

OMC (2000)
N/A

WHO (2000) & WHO (2007)
(Health actions)
The resources, actors and institutions related to the financing, regulation and provision of health actions, where health actions are any set of activities whose primary intention is to improve or maintain health (Murray & Frenk, 2000; WHO, 2000).

OECD (2001)
(Health care system)
The health care system, not including public health activities or other wider issues (Hurst & Jee-Hughes, 2001).

Control Knobs (2003)
(Health system)
A set of relationships where the structural components (means) and their interactions are associated and connected to the goals the system desires to achieve (ends) (Hsaio, 2003).

Commonwealth Fund (2006)
(Health care services)
The way in which health care services are financed, organized and delivered to meet societal goals for health. It includes the people, institutions and organizations that interact to meet the goals, as well as the processes and structures, that guide these interactions (Commonwealth Fund, 2006).

OECD HCQI (2006)
(Health system, health care)
A health system includes all activities and structures whose primary purpose is to influence health in its broadest sense (in keeping with WHO's definition). Health care refers to the combined functioning of public health and personal health care services (Arah et al., 2006).

IHP (2008)
N/A

Systems Thinking Framework (2008)
(Health system)
A health system is made up of elements that interact together to form a complex system, the sum of which is greater than its parts. The interactions of these elements affect the achievement of health system goals. Although these goals may vary in different countries, essentially many are similar (Atun & Menabde, 2008).

Advantages:
- Easier to hold relative stakeholders to account.
- Identifies areas in which relative stakeholders have the capacity to make changes.

Advantages:
- Provides a more realistic view of all factors that influence health.
- Identifies interactions between sectors, institutions and people that can influence health.

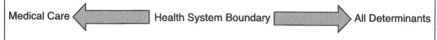

Medical Care ⟵ Health System Boundary ⟶ All Determinants

Disadvantages:
- Most factors influencing health are not included in the framework.
- It may be difficult to disentangle the effect health care has on outcomes from other determinants.

Disadvantages:
- Many determinants indentified are difficult, if not impossible, to change in the short run.
- Does not provide clarity on managerial roles.
- More difficult to assign responsibility and hold stakeholders to account.

Figure 2.1 Performance measurement implications of setting health system boundaries

potentially limiting the framework's ability to hold them to account. Health is the product of a number of determinants, some that can be influenced in the short term (e.g. safety), some that can be influenced directly by actors in the health care system (e.g. improving medical care), and others that require long-term action of actors not directly associated with health (e.g. environmental policy). By reducing the health system to health care alone, actions that have a great impact on health are excluded (such as education or employment). However, including all possible actions is also problematic as it obscures who is responsible for taking action that can drive change (Figure 2.1).

In practice, it seems important to align the definition of the health system as closely as possible to the persons and institutions responsible for improving health, especially if the framework is meant to be a platform for performance assessment. However, acknowledging the wider setting in which it lies will improve the understanding of how the system interacts with the wider economic, political and social surroundings.

2. What are health systems for?

While boundaries are intrinsic to the conceptualization debate, the normative content of international frameworks in defining what health system objectives *should* be trying to achieve is also subject to discussion. The 11 frameworks have defined the health system objectives in terms of several overarching goals. There is some consensus on the broad objectives of the health system, as summarized below (Table 2.2). However, detailed scrutiny indicates greater differences than might at first be evident. For example, WHO considers only the distribution

Table 2.2 Health system objectives

Framework name	Intermediate goals	Final goals
Framework for Assessing Behavioral Healthcare (1998)	• Effectiveness • Efficiency • Equity	• Health and well-being
EGIPSS model (1998)	• Productivity • Volume of care and services • Quality of care and services	• Health improvement • Effectiveness • Efficiency • Equity
OMC (2000)		• Ensuring access to care based on the principles of universal access, fairness and solidarity • Promoting high-quality care • Guaranteeing the financial sustainability of health care
WHO Performance framework (2000)	• Access • Coverage • Quality • Safety	• Level and distribution of health • Level and distribution of responsiveness • Fairness in financing • Efficiency
OECD Performance framework (2001)		• Level and distribution of health • Level and distribution of responsiveness and access • Equity • Macroeconomic and microeconomic efficiency
Control Knobs framework (2003)	• Efficiency • Quality • Access	• Health status • Consumer satisfaction • Risk protection
Commonwealth Fund framework (2006)	• High-quality care • Efficient care • Access • System and workforce innovation and improvement	• Long, healthy and productive lives
OECD HCQI framework (2006)		• Improving health • Macroeconomic efficiency/ sustainability and microeconomic efficiency/ value for money • Equity
WHO Building Blocks Framework (2007)	• Access • Coverage • Quality • Safety	• Level and distribution of health • Level and distribution of responsiveness • Fairness in financing • Efficiency

Framework name	Intermediate goals	Final goals
Systems Thinking Framework (2008)	• Equity • Choice • Efficiency • Effectiveness	• Health • Financial risk protection • Consumer satisfaction
IHP Common Evaluation Framework (2008)	N/A	N/A

of financial contributions, while the OECD also makes a normative statement concerning the absolute level of health expenditure.

The most obvious distinction made between frameworks is their separation of final and intermediate goals. Intermediate goals contribute to the realization of final goals, and often provide valuable information on system performance to that end. Murray and Frenk (2000) note that a goal is *intrinsic* if the level of attainment of that goal is desirable in and of itself, and *instrumental* if it contributes to the attainment of the intrinsic goals. Similarly, Roberts et al. (2008) refer to data about system characteristics as intermediate performance measures; they note that "the features of the system are not in themselves either the root cases of performance difficulties or the manifestations of those difficulties at the level of ultimate outcomes", but are "critical links in the chains that connect root causes to ultimate performance goals".

The only area for which there is apparent consensus is that health is an ultimate goal of the system; yet, here too, there are differences in the conceptualization of health. For example, the Commonwealth Fund refers to a notion of long, healthy and productive lives, while the OECD defines health outcomes as changes in health status brought about by health care, or health system, activities (Table 2.3).

The concept of health used in the frameworks recognizes a holistic view of health status as endorsed by the WHO constitution in 1946. While semantics differ across authors, this idea is treated more consistently than the conceptualization of other terms, particularly quality, equity and responsiveness. In the efficiency domain, all frameworks refer to conventional economic principles of productivity, defined in terms of using available resources to reach their full potential. The Commonwealth Fund, while not explicitly defining efficiency in this way, suggests a similar concept by emphasizing the importance of delivering effective care, with effective technology, in the right setting and avoiding waste. The OECD goes a step further by also including the notion of 'macroeconomic efficiency', which takes into account the relative amount spent on health care as opposed to other sectors. It is not surprising that the notion of efficiency causes difficulty in the conceptual frameworks, as it should reflect the attainment of all other goals relative to what is achievable, given the resources spent and other exogenous influences on goal attainment.

The domains where there is most divergence in concepts relate to quality, responsiveness, access and equity, reflecting their contested nature and the considerable international variation in their interpretation. In particular,

Table 2.3 Conceptualizations of key terms

Health	
Behavioral Healthcare (1998)	Uses WHO (1986) definition: "health is a positive concept emphasizing social and personal resources, as well as physical capacities".
OMC (2000)	Not explicitly defined.
WHO (2000, 2007)	Health of the population at different parts of the life-cycle, including the effects of morbidity and premature mortality.
OECD (2001)	Health outcomes are changes in health status brought about by health care, or health system, activities.
Control Knobs (2003)	Not explicitly defined, but referred to as 'health status'.
Commonwealth Fund (2006)	Health outcomes are defined as the capacity of the health care system to contribute to long, healthy and productive lives.
OECD HCQI (2006)	Not explicitly defined.
Systems Thinking (2008)	Not explicitly defined.

Quality	
Behavioral Healthcare (1998)	Not explicitly defined.
OMC (2000)	Not explicitly defined.
WHO (2000, 2007)	Captured by the average level of health and responsiveness.
OECD (2001)	Captured by levels of attainment of health outcomes and responsiveness.
Control Knobs (2003)	Quality is commonly used in three ways, depending on who is using the term: 1. To denote the *quantity of care* provided to a patient. 2. *Clinical quality*, which involves human inputs (e.g. skill, decision-making); non-human inputs (e.g. equipment and supplies); and production systems (combining human inputs with non-human inputs). 3. *Service quality*, which encompasses hotel services (e.g. food, cleanliness, etc.); convenience (e.g. travel time, waiting time, opening hours, etc.); and interpersonal relations (e.g. whether providers are polite, emotionally supportive and whether patients receive appropriate information and respect).
Commonwealth Fund (2006)	Captured by the provision of the right (effective), coordinated, safe, responsive/patient-centred and timely care.
OECD HCQI (2006)	Captured through the dimensions of accessibility, equity, effectiveness, safety and responsiveness/patient-centredness.
Systems Thinking (2008)	Not explicitly defined.

Efficiency

Behavioral Healthcare (1998)	Defined in terms of *production efficiency* (the combination of inputs required to produce care and related services at the lowest costs) and *allocative efficiency* (the combination of inputs that produce the greatest health improvements given the available resources).
OMC (2000)	Not explicitly defined.
WHO (2000, 2007)	Actual goal attainment achieved related to what could be achieved given the resources available.
OECD (2001)	Defined as *microeconomic efficiency* (measured health system productivity as compared to its maximum attainable) and *macroeconomic efficiency* (what effect a change in the level of resources would have on the desired level of health outcomes and responsiveness compared to other goods and services).
Control Knobs (2003)	Defined as *technical efficiency* (or *production efficiency*; getting the maximum output for money) and *allocative efficiency* (producing the right collection of outputs to achieve goals, or being on the production possibility frontier).
Commonwealth Fund (2006)	Defined as efficient (not wasteful) care delivery and insurance administration, delivered at the right time and right setting and where new innovations can be evaluated for both effectiveness and value.
OECD HCQI (2006)	Defined in terms of microeconomic efficiency, maximizing value for money (or the ratio of quality to costs) and macroeconomic efficiency, finding the right level of health expenditure.
Systems Thinking (2008)	Separated into technical and allocative efficiency (but not explicitly defined).

Responsiveness

Behavioral Healthcare (1998)	Not explicitly defined but notions of consumer satisfaction are encompassed in its definition of equity.
OMC (2000)	Not explicitly defined.
WHO (2000, 2007)	Respect for persons (health system and health provider's respect for dignity, autonomy, confidentiality) and client orientation (right to prompt attention to health needs, basic amenities of health services, access to patient social support networks, choice of institutions providing care).
OECD (2001)	Not explicitly defined but encompasses notions of patient satisfaction, patient acceptability and patient experience, including access.
Control Knobs (2003)	Called *citizen satisfaction* and describes the degree to which citizens are satisfied with the services provided by the health sector.
Commonwealth Fund (2006)	Not explicitly defined but included in definitions of quality and access.
OECD HCQI (2006)	Responsiveness/patient-centredness considers how a health care system treats people to meet their legitimate non–health expectations. This is a component of health care quality.
Systems Thinking (2008)	Not explicitly defined.

(Continued)

Table 2.3 Conceptualizations of key terms *(Continued)*

Equity

Behavioral Healthcare (1998)	Equity assesses the fairness of care delivery, and substantive equity is judged ultimately by the extent to which those health benefits are shared equally across groups in the community.
OMC (2000)	Not explicitly defined.
WHO (2000, 2007)	Captured by the distribution of health and responsiveness across the population as well as fairness of financial contributions.
OECD (2001)	Captured by the distribution of health outcomes, access and financing.
Control Knobs (2003)	Captured by the distribution of performance goals (health status, citizen satisfaction and financial risk protection).
Commonwealth Fund (2006)	Captured by the distribution of health quality, access, and efficiency.
OECD HCQI (2006)	Equity is concerned with the fairness of the distribution of health care across populations and also with the fairness of payment for health care.
Systems Thinking (2008)	Not explicitly defined.

Access

Behavioral Healthcare (1998)	Access is conceptualized as a component of equity, including the availability, organization and financing of services in the health system.
OMC (2000)	Not explicitly defined.
WHO (2000, 2007)	Captured as a determinant of responsiveness.
OECD (2001)	Captured as a component of responsiveness.
Control Knobs (2003)	Captured by two separate notions: *physical availability* (which can be measured by the distribution of available inputs – beds, doctors, nurses) compared to the population; and *effective availability* (which is how easy it is for citizens to get care).
Commonwealth Fund (2006)	Captured by the degree of universal participation and affordability of care.
OECD HCQI (2006)	Accessibility refers to the ease with which health services are reached.
Systems Thinking (2008)	Not explicitly defined.

Note: The EGIPSS model (1998) and IHP Framework (2008) are not included as they are organizational frameworks and thus do not provide detailed definitions on any of the above concepts.

there is a lack of consensus as to where the boundaries of these concepts lie. Responsiveness, equity and access, in particular, seem to overlap. For example, access is considered a component of equity in the Behavioral Healthcare framework; a determinant of responsiveness in the WHO frameworks; and a component of responsiveness in the OECD (2001) framework. Similarly, while equity is concerned with the distribution of performance across the population, the areas of performance being considered vary across frameworks, with the OECD (2001) framework considering the distribution of health outcomes, access and financing; the Commonwealth Fund framework considering the distribution of health quality, access and efficiency; the WHO framework considering the distribution of health and responsiveness across the population, as well as fairness of financial contributions; and the OECD HCQI framework considering the distribution of health care and the fairness of financial contributions. Quality as defined in all frameworks reviewed has to do with the system's attainment of a particular set of goals, however, again there is variation as to which of these goals are considered (Table 2.2).

3. What is the architecture of a health system?

As a performance assessment tool, a framework is useful in clearly outlining the objectives of an organization or system. While it is important to be aware of the ultimate aims of the system, it is essential that the framework also outlines the organizational structure within which these aims are to be achieved. Through a common conceptualization of the structure and workings of a system, stakeholders can work together to understand how the system architecture influences the attainment of goals. This is useful both for comparing different systems to each other (to determine how a different system architecture influences performance), as well as for assessing systems over time (to determine how changes in the system architecture influence performance).

While the different frameworks vary in semantics when describing their conceptualization of the architecture of their health system – whether the health system is constructed in terms of functions, levers, tiers, building blocks, control knobs, etc. – in practice, there is substantial overlap between them (Table 2.4). There are five broad elements considered within the architectures of the frameworks reviewed. Some of these elements always appear, while others are in some cases either not clearly articulated or not included at all:

1. *Service provision*: the organizational setting in which inputs and production processes are structured in order to deliver personal and non-personal health services;
2. *Financing*: the organization, implementation and management of collective revenues to allocate for provider activities;
3. *Resource generation*: the organization, implementation and management of collective revenues to allocate for provider activities;
4. *Leadership/governance*: ensures strategic policy frameworks exist and are combined with effective oversight, coalition building, the provision of appropriate regulation and incentives, attention to system design, and accountability.

5. *Risk factors*: the social, economic, environmental and behavioural transactions influencing health risks.

The health system boundaries set by a particular framework are closely related to the choice of elements considered in that framework. A wider conceptualization of the health system boundaries usually includes broader factors that can influence performance goals, while a narrower conceptualization may leave some of these elements out, or not clearly identify how and where they are considered. For example, while the Commonwealth Fund's ultimate goal is long, healthy and productive lives, it does not consider risk factors as an

Table 2.4 Conceptualizations of health system architecture

Framework	Conceptualization of health system architecture
Behavioral Healthcare (1998)	Constructed in terms of structure, process and outcome, where: • *Structure*: refers to the availability, organization and financing of behavioural health care programmes; the characteristics of the populations to be served by them; and the physical, social and economic environment to which they are exposed; • *Process*: refers to the transactions between patients and providers in the course of actual care delivery, as well as the environmental and behavioural transactions exacerbating behavioural health risks; and • *Outcomes*: consist of the *ultimate outcome* of health care services, which is to enhance the health of individuals and communities; however, this goal is conceptualized as an ongoing process that can be evaluated through the *intermediate outcomes* of effectiveness, efficiency and equity.
OMC (2000)	No conceptualization of health system architecture.

EGIPSS (1998)	Constructed in terms of Parsons' Social Action Theory, in which health systems are conceptualized as organized systems of action with four functional dimensions of action:
	 • Two internal functions:
	   • *Maintaining values*: maintaining values and producing meaning;
	   • *Production*: integrating and stabilizing processes for production;
	 • Two external functions:
	   • *Adapting*: interacting with the environment to acquire the necessary resources and adapting; and
	   • *Achieving goals*: attaining the valued goals of the system.

WHO (2000)	Constructed in terms of health system functions: • *Service provision*: the organizational setting in which inputs and production processes are structured in order to deliver personal and non-personal health services; • *Financing*: the organization, implementation and management of collective revenues to allocate for provider activities; • *Resource generation*: the generation of inputs, such as human resources, physical resources and knowledge, needed to provide services; and • *Stewardship*: the umbrella under which the direction of the health system is defined.

Framework	Conceptualization of health system architecture
OECD (2001)	No conceptualization of health system architecture.
Control Knobs (2003)	Constructed in terms of control knobs: <ul><li>*Financing*: refers to all mechanisms for raising the money that pays for activities in the health sector, including the design of institutions that collect the money and the allocation of resources to different priorities;</li><li>*Payment*: refers to the methods for transferring money to health care providers, and any cases where money is paid directly to patients;</li><li>*Organization*: refers to the mechanisms reformers use to affect the mix of providers in health care markets, their roles and functions, and how the providers operate internally;</li><li>*Regulation*: refers to the use of coercion by the state to alter the behaviour of actors in the health system; and</li><li>*Behaviour*: refers to efforts to influence how individuals act in relation to health and health care, including both patients and providers.</li></ul>
Commonwealth Fund (2006)	Constructed in terms of health system goals: <ul><li>*High-quality safe care*: care is provided in an appropriate, safe, coordinated, responsive and timely manner;</li><li>*Efficient care*: care is delivered at the right time and setting, through an efficient delivery and insurance system, with technologies, devices, products and laboratory testing that have been evaluated for effectiveness and values, and processes put in place for their introduction, surveillance, retesting and re-evaluation over time.</li><li>*Access and equity for all*: care is affordable for the patient and nation, provided equitably according to medical need, and everybody has a minimum level of financial benefit; and</li><li>*System and workforce innovation and improvement*: the system is prepared to deal with shocks, and significantly invests in innovation, research and education with an infrastructure that supports transparency of information and accountability but also balances autonomy and a culture of improvement amongst health care professionals.</li></ul>
OECD HCQI (2006)	Constructed in tiers that illustrate potential causal pathways: <ul><li>*Tier 1: Health*: denotes society's broader health as influenced by health care and non-health care factors;</li><li>*Tier 2: Non-health care determinants of health*: this tier denotes the mostly society-wide, non-health care factors that also influence health;</li><li>*Tier 3: Health care system performance*: this tier denotes the processes, inputs and outcomes of the health care system, as well as its efficiency and equity, recognizing that these may sometimes influence health care determinants. Note that the link between the third and second tiers is captured by primary care/prevention and health promotion; and</li><li>*Tier 4: Health system design and context*: this denotes pertinent country and health system policy and delivery characteristics, which will influence the health system in terms of its costs, expenditure and utilization patterns that must be considered in order to contextualize the findings of the health performance tier.</li></ul>

(Continued)

Table 2.4 Conceptualizations of health system architecture *(Continued)*

Framework	Conceptualization of health system architecture
WHO (2007)	Constructed in terms of health system building blocks: • *Service delivery*: ensures the delivery of effective, safe, quality personal and non-personal health interventions to those who need them, when and where needed, with minimum waste of resources; • *Health workforce*: works in a responsive, fair and efficient way to achieve the best health outcomes possible, given available resources and circumstances; • *Information*: ensures the production, analysis, dissemination and use of reliable and timely information on health determinants, health systems performance and health status; • *Medical products, vaccines and technologies*: ensures equitable access to essential medical products, vaccines and technologies of assured quality, safety, efficacy and cost–effectiveness, and their scientifically sound and cost–effective use; • *Financing*: raises adequate funds for health in ways that ensure people can use needed services and are protected from financial catastrophe or impoverishment associated with having to pay for them; and • *Leadership/governance*: ensures strategic policy frameworks exist and are combined with effective oversight, coalition building, the provision of appropriate regulation and incentives, attention to system design, and accountability.
IHP (2008)	Constructed in terms of a sequence of health system components: • *Inputs and processes*: domestic and international inputs, including funding, improved planning and harmonization practices; • *Outputs*: expected outputs of health reforms or interventions; • *Outcomes*: increased outputs are expected to lead to better outcomes, such as coverage and responsiveness; and • *Impact*: better outcomes are ultimately expected to lead to a better impact, such as improved health. The impact will be influenced by the efficacy of the interventions.
Systems Thinking (2008)	Constructed in terms of levers available to policy-makers when managing the health system: • *Stewardship and organizational arrangements*: refers to the policy environment and the regulatory environment, stewardships function and structural arrangements for purchasers, providers and market regulators; • *Financing*: refers to the collection and pooling of funds; • *Resource allocation and provider payment systems*: refers to the allocation of pooled funds and other available resources (such as human resources, capital investment and equipment) and the mechanism and methods used for paying health service providers; and • *Service provision*: refers to the services provided by the health sector.

element because they do not fall within its narrow health system boundaries. However, we believe that, even when considering narrow boundaries, if an international framework is being used to compare performance across systems, some acknowledgement of the different social, economic, environmental and cultural differences needs to be acknowledged.

As a conceptual framework is fundamental in providing a strategy for health system performance improvement, its construction will help to identify where performance efforts need to be focused. In order to provide a rounded view of performance, it is important that all five structural elements be included within the framework so that stakeholders have a clear vision of what activities can be used, and in what way, in order to strengthen and improve the system goals. If, for example, health promotion or public health activities can improve health system goals, they should be accounted for within the framework, even if they fall outside the boundaries of the health system. Regardless of how narrowly the boundaries of a health care system are set, risk factors will influence the ultimate goals of the system and should therefore be recognized.

4. How good is a health system in terms of its performance?

Most of the frameworks reviewed in this chapter below were constructed with different aims. For example, the Behavioral Healthcare and EGIPSS (*Évaluation globale et intégrée de la performance des systèmes de santé*) frameworks were constructed to provide conceptually sound performance models based on theory; the WHO (2000) and OECD (2001 and 2006) frameworks were created in order to facilitate performance measurement and evaluation efforts; and the Control Knobs (2003), Systems Thinking (2008) and IHP (2008) frameworks were constructed to evaluate specific health system reforms. While the purposes of these frameworks may differ, all frameworks go about achieving their ends by attempting to provide conceptual clarity in analytical, technical and operational thinking for the different stakeholders involved.

However, the ultimate aim of the framework is often fundamental in determining how well it serves as a conceptual or evaluative tool. To better understand this, a distinction needs to be made between a *conceptual health system framework* (HS framework) and a *health system performance assessment framework* (HSPA framework). An HS framework is defined as a generic conceptual tool used to describe a health system. "It defines, describes and explains the health system, its objectives, structural and organizational elements, function and processes" (Shakarishvili, 2009). An HSPA is an actionable performance assessment tool that can be used to map performance information back to the health system's objectives, functions and processes, and thus be used to assess and evaluate the performance of the system. A good conceptual framework could thus provide the basis of a health system performance assessment framework. It follows then that HS frameworks can often lend themselves to becoming suitable HSPA frameworks, regardless of whether this was their initial purpose or not, while frameworks that are created for HSPA purposes may not always make good HS frameworks. For example, the Behavioral Healthcare framework (Aday et al., 1998), which was constructed as a conceptual HS framework, has never been used for performance measurement. However, the conceptual clarity provided by the framework allows the authors to indicate where and how data can be mapped on to the framework, going as far as to highlight what data sets, indicators and levels of detail are most suitable for each area.

Other frameworks created specifically for HSPA purposes, such as the OCM (2000) and IHP (2008) frameworks, are constructed in terms of the data that are available and/or appropriate to collect in order to reflect progress on predefined objectives. However, these frameworks do not provide a clear conceptualization of how these objectives fit back into the health system architecture. This type of framework is often classified as a 'monitoring and evaluation' (M&E) framework. As the name suggests, this type of framework outlines areas in which systematic monitoring and evaluation of progress is undertaken. This provides a snapshot of information at any one point in time and, if conducted over time as an ongoing management activity, can provide information on a regular basis. Evaluation of this information can then provide an in-depth understanding of the activity being monitored (WHO, 2008). Interestingly, M&E frameworks are almost never discussed alongside HS and HSPA frameworks, although, in principle, they have very similar purposes. The key difference is that M&E frameworks are not used to provide a deep understanding of the health system, but rather as a framework outlining what information should be monitored and evaluated in order to assess the achievement of a predefined goal set. Thus, a framework that is an HSPA framework, but not an HS framework, would be classified as an M&E framework.

Hsiao & Sidat (2008) go on to further classify HS frameworks into three categories: descriptive; analytical; deterministic and predictive.[2] A *descriptive* framework provides a basic description of the health system and the components from which it is made, but does not explain why any particular health system would perform better than another. None of the frameworks reviewed in this chapter falls into this category, however, an example is the European Observatory on Health Systems and Policies' Health Systems in Transition (HiT) country profiles, which provide detailed descriptions of European health care systems, including reform and policy incentives. *Analytical* functional frameworks go beyond merely describing what exists in a health system to also analyse the functional components of that system. This type of framework offers a more holistic and deeper analysis of the health system than a purely descriptive framework, but does not reveal the effectiveness of particular policies, reforms or interventions or the interaction between the health system's various functions. *Deterministic and predictive* frameworks differ from analytical functional frameworks in that they try to determine which factors influence the performance of health systems in order to identify which reforms, interventions or policies are most successful. Table 2.5 indicates how we have classified the international frameworks reviewed in this chapter relative to the categories discussed above.

When considering how good a health system is in terms of its performance, the distinction between an HS and an HSPA framework becomes important. An HSPA framework, by definition, is constructed to evaluate performance, and thus will have a more developed method by which to measure how well the health system is performing. While an HS framework can be applied to

Table 2.5 Classification of frameworks

Framework name	Type of framework	HS framework	HSPA framework	M&E framework
Framework for Assessing Behavioral Healthcare (1998)	Analytical	X	X	
EGIPSS model (1998)	Analytical		X	
OMC (2000)	Deterministic		X	X
WHO Performance framework (2000)	Analytical	X	X	
OECD Performance framework (2001)	Analytical	X	X	
Control Knobs framework (2003)	Deterministic	X	X	
Commonwealth Fund framework (2006)	Analytical	X	X	
OECD HCQI framework (2006)	Analytical	X	X	
WHO Building Blocks framework (2007)	Analytical	X	X	
Systems Thinking Framework (2008)	Deterministic	X	X	
IHP Common Evaluation framework (2008)	Deterministic		X	X

performance assessment, it may not have a clear strategy of how this should be done. In both HS and HSPA frameworks, the evaluative capability of the framework will also depend on how explicitly the framework defines what is meant by 'good' performance and even by 'performance'. Performance in this context is commonly understood to reflect the attainment of health system goals. However, of the frameworks reviewed, there are differences in the consideration of exogenous factors. For example, the Commonwealth Fund considers performance to be a measure of the absolute attainment of their four health system goals, while the WHO 2000 framework considers the absolute attainment of goals *relative to the resources available,* as well as their distribution across the population.

This raises two important questions: (1) Should international frameworks measure performance according to national concepts and objectives, or impose some normative principles that the organization itself holds? (2) Should 'good performance' consider only absolute achievement of defined goals, or also encompass some notion of efficiency? With regard to the first question, all frameworks reviewed, apart from the Control Knobs framework (2003), use some guiding normative principles to assess performance, but the chosen concepts differ among the frameworks, reflecting in part the differences in the political, economic and managerial perspectives of the key stakeholders, as well as a lack of clear conceptual development. The second question is related to the first, as it considers the placement and evaluation of efficiency in the attainment of health system goals, and is particularly important when attempting to assess performance comparatively across systems. In order to truly compare how well systems are performing, is it meaningful to look at absolute attainment of goals without considering the resources devoted to this endeavour?

5. How can we relate health system architecture to performance?

In order to relate health system architecture to performance, it is important to understand and analyse the way in which the five health system elements (service provision, financing, resource generation, leadership/governance, risk factors) previously identified are actually carried out. Analysing this information will allow variations in performance to be traced back to one or more of these elements and will ultimately serve as a driver of health system improvements. The first step towards achieving this result is to include all elements in the architecture of the system. The second step involves deciding upon how to measure these elements and which indicators to map onto the framework. Finally, the third – and most difficult – step is to relate the indicators back to the evaluation of performance and establish empirical links, which in turn provide evidence on how changes in these elements can affect performance.

Of the frameworks reviewed, most identify several or all of the five elements that we identify as important to health system architecture. Indeed, most of the recent frameworks now reproduce the same elements, indicating that there is now relative consensus over this. Some of the frameworks are very explicit about relating health system architecture to performance, such as the WHO 2000 and 2007 frameworks, the Control Knobs framework and the OECD HCQI frameworks. While only a few of the frameworks presented have been used for performance assessment, most of them do not map indicators onto the architecture elements. This makes it very difficult for a performance exercise to relate health system architecture to performance. Indeed, while considerable work on how to measure health system goals has taken place, less has been done on measuring the separate elements that make up health system architecture, especially in a standardized way that would facilitate cross-country comparisons.

2.3 Using international frameworks to assess national performance

While the focus of this chapter is on international frameworks rather than national frameworks, it is important to consider the linkages between the two. International frameworks can provide a useful starting point for countries interested in conducting HSPA, and indeed national frameworks are a useful starting point for the development of international frameworks. Many of the frameworks reviewed in this chapter have drawn from national frameworks or HSPA programmes and, in turn, the international frameworks have provided a basis for the creation of national frameworks. This section will review some examples of knowledge exchange that has occurred between selected international frameworks and national frameworks.

As Arah et al. (2003) note, the OECD HCQI framework has borrowed heavily from the Institute of Medicine's national health care quality indicator framework, developed for the United States (IOM, 2001), and the Canadian Health Indicator Framework (CIHI, 1999). The latter has also been adapted in Australia for the European Community Health Indicators (ECHI) Project, and in the WHO and OECD proposal for identifying key economic and social goals for health policy (Murray & Frenk, 2000). Indeed, as shown in Appendix 1, there is considerable borrowing across international frameworks, indicating a convergence in many areas, such as key objectives. Yet, this cross-learning can also extend the other way as national HSPA frameworks also borrow and adapt from established and validated international frameworks. The Kyrgyzstani, Armenian, Portuguese, Estonian, Georgian and Turkish HSPA frameworks all draw heavily from the WHO (2000) framework but are adapted to suit the structure of their own national health systems and key national health system goals (WHO Regional Office for Europe, 2012). The OECD HCQI framework forms the basis of the national framework used to assess health system performance in the Netherlands by the National Institute for Public Health and the Environment (RIVM). Moreover, RIVM assessed their own performance relative to all other EU Member States using ECHIM indicators in the report *Dare to Compare* (Harbers et al., 2008). Similarly, a recent performance assessment of the New Zealand health system, conducted by Gauld et al. (2011) used the Commonwealth Scorecard as a framework.

There is clearly overlap, or even convergence, across national and international health system frameworks and, while these frameworks often provide similar conceptualizations, there are frequently small but important differences.

There are two ways in which to interpret this overlap for future development in this area: the first is that we should move towards the adoption of a common performance framework; the other is that each organization or country conducting an HSPA should construct their own framework that best reflects the key priorities of their own country/organization. There are advantages to each of these approaches. A common framework would facilitate cross-country comparisons and allow assessments to be made on common goals. However, the development of a new framework is an important function in any assessment process, helping to clarify and understand the health system and also to outline key priorities, accountability design and structural differences (such as level of development). These areas are crucial in determining where attention should be focused, what reforms are proposed and, ultimately, the basis upon which the system is judged. In many circumstances, these decisions should be made by the individuals and organizations involved in the health system in order to ensure a transparent and dynamic assessment that responds to current issues and needs.

2.4 Conclusions

Over the last decade much energy has been expended on the creation of international frameworks. While these frameworks have varied purposes, they all aim to provide a better understanding of what a health system is, its goals, and the underlying structure and factors that drive its performance. Indeed, careful examination of the available international frameworks suggests that, over time, a degree of convergence has developed in not only the framework architecture and goals but in the problem areas encountered as well. This suggests that the gains to be had from creating a new framework have progressively decreased in proportion to the effort required to undertake such a task; in other words, there are diminishing returns to creating new international frameworks. Instead, there is a need to clarify those areas where there are longstanding differences in matters of understanding, focus and principle.

One of the main areas of debate that needs to be addressed is that of determining where the boundaries of the health system lie. There can be no right answer to this question, as there are solid arguments to promote the use of both wider and narrower boundaries. However, lack of consensus on this issue makes comparisons across frameworks and national performance assessments difficult. A possible solution to this problem may be to explicitly identify different levels of the health system and attempt to measure the contribution of each of these levels towards the achievement of the performance goals. This is done in the OECD HCQI framework in which the representation of the health system through four tiers allows health care to be placed within a broader conceptualization of the health system in addition to the economic, social and political context of countries. While acknowledging that health care is only one of the wider determinants of health, this structure allows health care performance to be measured without being subsumed within the wider health system model.

There seems to be relative consensus on the goals of health systems; however, there are still differences in interpretation as to what these goals encompass. Some concepts, such as responsiveness, quality and efficiency, tend to mean a combination of different notions, depending on which framework is being used. There is also a lack of consensus as to how the different goals relate to one another; for example; is access part of equity or responsiveness? Or is responsiveness part of equity? Is efficiency included in what we mean by quality, or is quality part of efficiency? This confusion leads to a lack of clarity, which makes the operationalization of frameworks difficult and controversial.

Understanding the architecture of a health system is one of the main purposes of creating a health system framework. Increasingly, more of the same elements are being identified as belonging to the structural foundations of a health system; however, the lack of complete consensus indicates the need to revisit this topic and to ensure agreement across stakeholders. We identify five key elements, namely: service provision, financing, resource generation, leadership/governance and risk factors, which we believe should be included in any framework in order for it to provide a rounded picture of the organizational structure within which a health system operates. Another difficulty to consider when using a framework to inform international comparisons is how to incorporate into the architecture the wider national setting, such as the political system in place or the level of development of a country, which will influence health system decisions.

Finally, in order to use a health system framework for performance assessment, there must be a clear way in which to determine how 'good' a health system is as regards its performance. One question that arises when considering the criteria for determining good performance is whether this implies the absolute attainment of all goals or the attainment relative to resources available; in many of the frameworks reviewed, quality is defined as the absolute attainment of all goals, and efficiency as the output relative to the resources put in. Does this imply that performance is synonymous with quality? Or does it also capture some notion of efficiency? If so, should it also consider notions of allocative efficiency, such as how much a country should spend on health as opposed to other sectors? Finally, in order to use frameworks as heuristic tools they should ultimately be able to relate health system architecture to performance. This means that, apart from clearly identifying the key elements of the health system, these elements should be measured and analysed in order to better understand how much they contribute to health system performance. This requires more effort to be put into clearly defining and measuring the health system elements.

Appendix I: Existing Frameworks

Framework for Assessing Behavioral Healthcare 1998

In 1993, Aday et al. published a framework to assess the effectiveness, efficiency and equity of health care that could be used to guide the current state of the art of health-oriented health services research. This framework was updated in 1998 to recognize the influences of social and individual determinants of health (Aday et al., 1998, 1999, 2004), and named the *Framework for Assessing Behavioral Healthcare*. Figure A1 shows the revised framework, where the shaded boxes indicate the revisions or additions introduced in 1998. The term 'behavioral healthcare' was chosen to emphasize the move away from interpreting health as an understanding of purely physical health to a more holistic concept, such as that endorsed by WHO in its constitution (WHO, 1946). Embracing this idea, Aday et al. (1999) defined behavioural health care as "a continuum of services aimed at promoting physical, mental and social well-being through thoughtful and respectful intervention in human behavior, behavioral antecedents, and behavioral consequences".

The Behavioral Healthcare Framework is organized in terms of the structure, process and outcomes of the health care system, where:

1. *Structure* refers to the availability, organization and financing of behavioural health care programmes; the characteristics of the populations to be served by them; and the physical, social and economic environment to which they are exposed.
2. *Process* refers to the transactions between patients and providers in the course of actual care delivery, as well as the environmental and behavioural transactions exacerbating behavioural health risks.
3. *Outcomes* constitute the *ultimate outcome* of health care services, which is to enhance the health of individuals and communities. However, this goal is conceptualized as an ongoing process that can be evaluated through the *intermediate outcomes* of effectiveness, efficiency and equity, defined in Table A1.

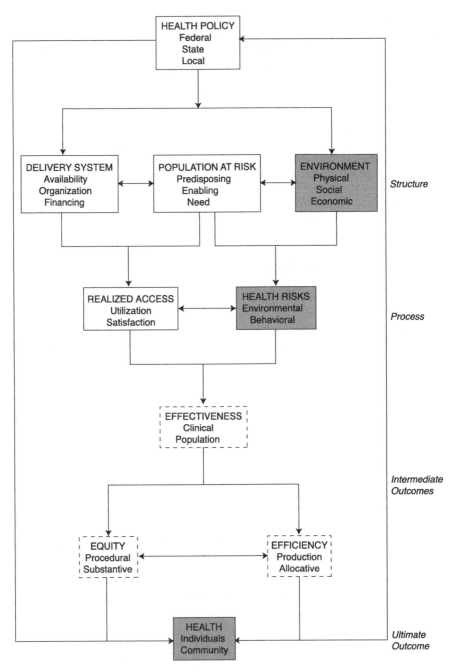

Figure A1 Framework for Assessing Behavioral Healthcare

Source: Aday et al., 1998.

Table A1 Dimensions in the Behavioral Healthcare framework

Effectiveness: the production of behavioural health benefits

Definitions	Methods of assessment
Clinical effectiveness: the impact of care on improvements for individual patients	*System level and institutional level:* • Outcome measures: relapse rates, functioning rates, mental health status, average self-report • Risk adjustment: demographic characteristics, comorbidity rates, risk adjustment systems • Study design: observational/inter-organizational • Data sources: medical records, discharge data, claims data, surveys *Patient level:* • Outcome measures: relapse rates, functioning rates, mental health status, self-reported health • Risk adjustment: patient profiles, comorbidity, diagnoses • Study design: observational/case reports • Data sources: medical records, surveys
Population effectiveness: the role of clinical and non-clinical factors in influencing the health of the population as a whole	*Population/community level:* • Outcome measures: population relapse rates, population functioning rates, mental health status • Risk adjustment: demographic characteristics • Study design: observational/epidemiological • Data sources: population health information system records, surveillance, surveys

---

Efficiency: the cost–effectiveness of producing behavioural health benefits

Definitions	Methods of assessment
Production efficiency: the combination of inputs required to produce health and related services at the lowest costs	*Micro level:* • Estimating production functions • Cost–effectiveness, cost–benefit, and cost–utility analyses
Allocative efficiency: the combination of inputs required to produce the greatest health improvements given the available resources	*Macro level:* • International comparisons of the performance of health care systems in different countries

---

Equity: the distribution of health benefits and costs across groups

Definitions	Methods of assessment
Procedural equity: the fairness of care delivery	*Indicators identified for the following criteria:* participation, freedom of choice, cost–effectiveness, similar treatment, common good, need
Substantive equity: the extent to which health benefits are shared equally across groups in the community	*Indicators identified for the following criteria:* need

---

Adapted from: Aday et al., 1998.

Aday et al. (1999) note that the structure, process and outcomes of behavioural health care can be conceptualized at a macro or a micro level, where the macro level represents a population perspective of the determinants and considers the behavioural health of communities as a whole, while the micro level addresses a clinical perspective on the factors that contribute to the health of individuals at a system, institution or patient level (Aday et al., 1998). In their paper, the authors indicate how these dimensions of behavioural health care should be interpreted and analysed at different levels and in different settings, and go on to consider what types of data and indicators are suitable for measurement and evaluation purposes (Table A1).

Integrated Performance Model for the Health Care System (EGIPSS) (1998)

Researchers at the University of Montreal have worked on creating a global integrated performance model based on Parsons' Social Action theory (Parsons, 1951, 1977). It allows many of the dominant models in organizational performance to be incorporated into the assessment, while taking into account the different operational environment. Parsons' model postulates that for an organization to survive it needs to focus on four functions and the interchange between them. These functions are: the attainment of goals; the production of services; culture and value maintenance; and the adaptation of the organization to its external environment. The push and pull between these dimensions, resulting from the varying preferences of the stakeholders, will result in one of six equilibria (Sicotte et al., 1998; Contandriopoulos et al., 2008).

Their model, called the EGIPSS model (*Évaluation globale et intégrée de la performance des systèmes de santé*), or the *Integrated Performance Model for the Health Care System* takes into account the goals and functions of the health system in addition to other external and internal factors, such as socioeconomic determinants and the culture of the health system itself (Sicotte et al.,1998; Contandriopoulos, Trottier & Champagne, 2008). This framework conceptualizes health systems as organized systems of action with four functional dimensions of action:

- **Two internal functions:**
  - o *Maintaining values:* maintaining values and producing meaning; and
  - o *Production:* integrating and stabilizing processes for production.
- **Two external functions:**
  - o *Adapting:* interacting with the environment to acquire the necessary resources and adapting; and
  - o *Achieving goals*: attaining the valued goals of the system.

The goal attainment function refers to the ultimate goals the system aims to achieve. In the WHO health system framework discussed previously these are: health status; responsiveness; financial fairness; and efficiency. The production function represents the processes that are undertaken in order to achieve the system goals; these are often represented through the dimensions of accessibility, quality and technical efficiency. These two functions are present in most existing frameworks. The adaptation function considers external influences on the system, and how the health system adapts to these influences in order to best serve the system's needs. For example, this could refer to the system's adaptation to the population's health needs, or its capacity to learn and innovate, given the available technology and know-how. Finally, the value maintenance function considers the motivation the actors in the system have in order to maintain and improve the health system. This includes the organizational culture, worker satisfaction, and so on. These four functions can be studied independently but their interactions and trade-offs must also be considered, allowing for a more dynamic representation of the system.

EU Open Method of Coordination (2000)

The Open Method of Coordination (OMC) was officially introduced in 2000 by the European Council in order to assist EU Member States in jointly progressing towards the goals laid out by the Lisbon Agenda[3]. The OMC is essentially a joint governance process, which encourages learning and collaboration between stakeholders in the European Union. The aim of the OMC is to encourage coordination of national policies by encouraging Member States to voluntarily work together towards shared goals while respecting their national diversity. According to Jassem (2004), it was devised as an instrument to share best practices and increase policy convergence in areas that are the primary responsibility of national governments but of concern across the EU as a whole, such as, long-term unemployment, the ageing population and social protection. While the OMC has been applied to key policy areas, we will focus only on its implementation within the area of health.

The OMC operates much like a performance framework by setting goals, which are measured through quantitative and qualitative indicators and benchmarks. The ultimate aim is to guide national and regional policies in specified areas by setting specific guidelines, timetables and targets, and to encourage mutual learning and the sharing of best practice throughout the process (WHO Regional Office for Europe, 2012). While the operation of the OMC differs across the policy areas to which it is applied, it generally works in the following four stages:

- agreement of key policy goals at the EU level;
- policy goals are translated into guidelines for national and regional policies;
- specific benchmarks and indicators to measure best practice are agreed upon;
- monitoring and evaluating results.

According to Article 152(5) of the European Convention, the responsibility for the organization and funding of health care and elderly care rests primarily with Member States. However, as Member States face similar concerns in health care, such as the ageing of their populations, there is scope for the OMC to be applied (Jassem, 2004). In 2001, a European Commission communication proposed three long-term policy objectives for EU health care systems: (1) ensuring access to care based on the principles of universal access, fairness and solidarity; (2) promoting high-quality care; and (3) guaranteeing the financial sustainability of health care (European Commission, 2005). A number of health indicators have been selected to measure country attainment with regards to these goals and are available through Eurostat.

Murray and Frenk (2000): WHO Framework

The health system framework developed by Murray and Frenk (2000) attempts to provide a clear conceptualization of health system performance in terms of health system functions and goals (Figure A2). This framework was then used in *WHR2000* to measure the health system performance of 191 Member States.

The first issue that Murray and Frenk (2000) consider is where the boundaries of the health system lie, an issue that has troubled policy-makers and scholars alike. Definitions of 'the health system' range from narrow approaches focusing on the medical care provided, to broader conceptualizations including all activities that can directly or indirectly be attributed to health (Figueras & McKee, 2012). Although health is influenced by many determinants beyond health services, using a broader definition that embraces factors, such as 'the social determinants of health', leaves no meaningful boundaries within which to clearly assign managerial responsibility and ensure accountability. On the other hand, a very narrow definition of health services is also problematic, as it can be too limiting, may cause fragmentation, and introduces analytic difficulties in attributing outcomes to the actions of health services. It can also appear to ignore the responsibility of medical professionals to engage in health promotion activities (Duran et al., 2012).

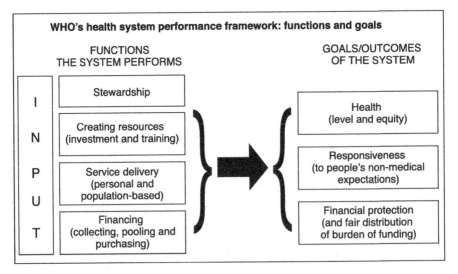

Figure A2 WHO (2000) framework

Source: WHO, 2007.

In order to overcome these issues, Murray and Frenk (2000) define the health system in terms of a 'health action';

> A health action is defined to be any set of activities whose primary intent is to improve or maintain health. And a health system includes the resources, actors and institutions related to the financing, regulation and provision of health actions.

This definition encompasses all organizations that include the contribution to health as a primary objective while omitting actions that may influence health but whose primary aim is not health-related. For example, policies targeted at reducing poverty levels will profoundly influence health; however, improved health is not their primary goal and so they are not part of the health system according to this definition.

In order to clarify the purpose of a health system, Murray and Frenk (2000) make the distinction between intrinsic and instrumental goals. A goal is defined as *intrinsic* if attainment of that goal is desirable in and of itself, but *instrumental* if it merely contributes to the attainment of an intrinsic goal (Anand et al., 2003). Each intrinsic goal should measure a different outcome, meaning that it must be independent of all other goals to some extent. It is therefore possible for the outcomes of that goal to change while holding the other intrinsic goals constant. The measurement of the attainment of intrinsic goals on a regular basis should be undertaken only if the health system influences the goal substantially enough to make it worth the costs of measurement and it is feasible to measure this impact.

The framework identifies three intrinsic goals:

- the improvement of health
- responsiveness
- fairness in financial contribution.

The primary goal of any health system is to improve population health. Without this initial motivation, societies would not choose to have health systems. When considering the health of the population, it is in principle important to measure health at different parts of the life-cycle, and to include the effects of morbidity and premature mortality.

Enhancing the responsiveness of the health system to the legitimate expectations of the population is the second defining goal of a health system. In this framework, responsiveness is separated into two components: respect for persons and client orientation. Respect for persons concerns the health system and health provider's respect for dignity, individual autonomy and confidentiality. Client orientation considers the population's right to prompt attention to health needs, basic amenities of health services, access to patient social support networks and a choice of institutions or individuals providing care. For the goals of both health attainment and responsiveness, it is important to consider not only the average level achievement but also the inequalities in the distribution across individuals in different social, economic, demographic or other groups.

The third intrinsic goal of a health system, as defined by this framework, is the fairness in financial contribution. The authors define financial contributions as fair when they incorporate financial risk-pooling so that households do not become impoverished or pay an excessive amount of their income to receive health care, and when the contributions reflect the difference in the disposable incomes of households. Note that, while efficiency and equity are not explicitly stated as being intrinsic goals of a health system, they are considered to be present amongst the goals: the average level attainment of each goal represents efficiency, while their distributions denote equity.

In assessing a health system, it is crucial to be able to understand the construction of that health system and what parts of the system contribute to the achievement of its intrinsic goals and overall performance. In order to provide such understanding, the framework identifies four basic functions:

- financing
- service provision
- resource generation
- stewardship.

The *financing* function deals with the collection of revenues to allocate for provider activities, including user charges. In practice, the organization, implementation and management of this function may have an important influence on performance. *Service provision* considers the organizational setting into which inputs and production processes are structured in order to deliver personal and non-personal health services. In addition to the institutions that finance and provide services, each health system has a sector that generates the inputs needed to provide these services, such as human resources, physical resources and knowledge. This function is called *resource generation*. Finally, there is the umbrella under which the direction of the health system is defined, the stewardship function. *Stewardship* involves setting, implementing and monitoring the rules of the health system (Murray & Frenk, 2000). Every health system struggles with deciding upon the best way to organize, implement and evaluate the organizations responsible for these functions.

In order to assess how good a health system is in terms of its performance, *WHR2000* used this framework to measure and rank the performance of 191 nations in respect of achieving the intrinsic goals mentioned above. The framework suggests a need to measure the average level and distribution of health improvement and responsiveness, as well as the distribution of financial contributions. These goals were operationalized as in Table A2.

WHO attempted to relate the health system architecture to performance by examining goal attainment in relation to expenditure on the health system after adjusting for variations in the level of social development. This measure of comparative performance, often referred to as efficiency or productivity, was the basis for the controversial rankings of individual health systems contained in the Appendices of the Report.

OECD 2001

Building upon their 1999 framework (Jee & Or, 1999), and openly incorporating the approach proposed by the WHO 2000 framework, the OECD published a new conceptual framework in 2001 (Hurst & Jee-Hughes, 2001). While

Table A2 WHO 2000 Index of Health System achievement

Improvement in the health of the population

Average level of population health	Disability-adjusted life expectancy (DALE)
Inequality in health outcomes	Index on equality of child survival

---

Responsiveness (reflecting respect for persons and client orientation)

Overall health system responsiveness	Assessed by a panel of key informants
Inequality in health system responsiveness	Assessed by a panel of key informants

---

Fairness in financial contribution

Fairness in financial contribution	Index based on the proportion of non-food expenditure spent on health care

---

Adapted from: WHO, 2000.

it included many features from the WHO framework, the OECD framework also made modifications. The OECD framework adopts a narrower definition of health system boundaries than that used by WHO. Its definition is limited to include only the boundaries of the performance of the health care system rather than to encompass public health activities or other wider issues.

The set of objectives defined in the OECD framework is also based upon the WHO 2000 framework but with some modifications (Table A3). When defining health system objectives, the OECD argues that access should be a *component* of responsiveness, unlike the WHO, which considers access to be a *determinant* of responsiveness. This allows the OECD framework to consider questions of equity of access. The OECD framework also adds the level of health expenditure

Table A3 OECD and WHO performance framework objectives and measurement dimensions

---

Framework objectives

WHO	OECD
• Health improvement	• Health improvement/outcomes
• Responsiveness to expectations	• Responsiveness and access
• Fairness in financial contributions	• Financial contribution/health expenditure

---

Measurement dimensions

WHO	OECD
• Level and distribution of health	• Health improvement/outcomes
• Level and distribution responsiveness	• Responsiveness
• Fairness in financing	• Equity
• Efficiency	• Macroeconomic and microeconomic efficiency

Adapted from: Hurst & Jee-Hughes, 2001.

as an objective, allowing it to address the issue of desirable health spending. This means that the three goals of the OECD framework are:

- health improvement and outcomes;
- responsiveness and access;
- financial contributions and health expenditure.

For each of these goals, there are 'two components of assessment': the average level and the distribution of each goal.

In a similar approach to the WHO, the OECD framework evaluates how good a health system is, its performance and the extent to which the system is meeting its objectives (Hurst & Jee-Hughes, 2001). While the OECD does not calculate the performance of national health systems, it does illustrate which of the key health indicators it collects from Member States and other international databases could be used for this purpose, by reviewing the different indicators of performance being collected, or proposed for collection at the time of the framework, in each of the dimensions proposed (Table A4). Indicators measured in Australia, Canada, the United Kingdom and the United States are also reviewed alongside the compilation of WHO and OECD indicators.

In order to relate health system architecture to performance, the OECD framework also includes a dimension of efficiency in its measurement, and similar to the WHO 2000 framework, this dimension is not an intrinsic goal as such but is instead reflected in attainment of the goals. However, in its framework the OECD separates efficiency into microeconomic efficiency and macroeconomic efficiency. The *microeconomic efficiency* dimension is very similar to WHO's efficiency concept and involves comparing the measured productivity of a health system to its maximum attainable productivity. Productivity is defined as the ratio of outputs to inputs (health outcome and responsiveness per dollar), a measure of technical efficiency. *Macroeconomic efficiency* relates to total spending on health, involving an examination of the benefit of health spending relative to other goods and services, a concept of allocative efficiency. The OECD framework does not envisage ranking health systems, and does not require any weighting or combination of the goals.

While this framework only reviewed possible indicators that could be collected for each dimension, as opposed to conducting a health system performance assessment exercise, Hurst & Jee-Hughes (2001) noted some of the limitations that arise when attempting to operationalize the framework. Due to its narrow definition of health system boundaries, the OECD framework is interested in measuring the improvement in health outcomes defined as changes in health status attributable to the activities of the health care system but not to wider factors. The authors note the difficultly in isolating the impact of health care from that of other determinants, and also that most indicators in this category are proxy indicators of outcomes that fall into one of two categories: health status measures, where there is reason to assume that mortality or morbidity is amenable to appropriate and timely medical care; and process measures, where utilization of care is believed to be related to positive outcomes. With respect to the indicators available for responsiveness, the OECD notes that the concepts included in the responsiveness dimension still vary widely among nations and international organizations. Finally, with regard to the measurement of

Table A4 Key indicators of performance

Health outcomes	
WHO	OECD
• DALE • Infant mortality	• Avoidable mortality by selected conditions • Infant mortality • Perinatal mortality • Low birth weight • Incidence of infectious diseases • Avoidable hospitalizations by selected conditions • Survival rates from cancer • In-hospital AMI mortality • Vaccination rates • Breast/cervical cancer screening

Responsiveness	
WHO	OECD
• Patient-rated dignity of treatment • Patient-rated autonomy and confidentiality • Patient-rated promptness of attention • Patient-rated quality of basic amenities • Patient-rated access to support networks during care • Patient-rated choice of care provider	• Waiting times

Equity	
WHO	OECD
n/a	Equity of patient-reported health status

Efficiency	
WHO	OECD
Composite measure of performance	n/a

Adapted from: Hurst & Jee-Hughes, 2001; OECD, 2009.

efficiency, aside from the WHO composite indicator of overall performance, there is a lack of system-wide efficiency indicators. In recognition of the lack of a suitable indicator, the authors left this area blank in an effort to emphasize the need to address the way we think about measuring efficiency.

Control Knobs Framework 2003

In their book, *Getting Health Reform Right*, Roberts et al. (2008) introduce their Control Knobs framework (Figure A3), a framework based on practical

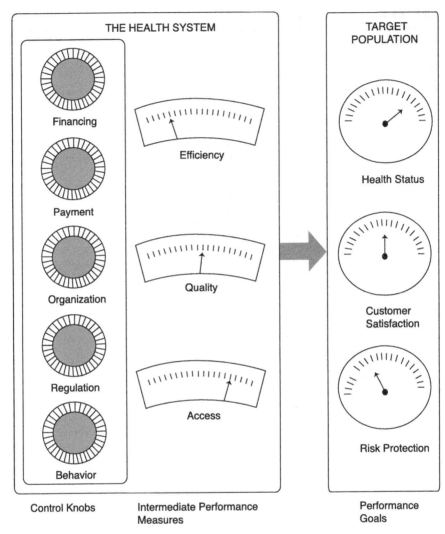

Figure A3 Control Knobs framework, 2004

Source: Roberts et al., 2008.

experience of designing, implementing and evaluating reforms. This framework conceptualizes the health system as "a set of relationships where the structural components (means) and their interactions are associated and connected to the goals the system desires to achieve (ends)". This framework describes the system 'control knobs' (health system financing, payment regulation, organization and behaviour) that policy-makers can use to achieve health system goals; and establishes a continuum between the interventions (control knobs), outcomes (intermediate performance measures) and objectives (performance goals) that allow policy-makers to consider whole system interactions. This framework has been used as the basis for the World Bank Health System Strengthening Program.

The authors argue that, in order to successfully understand the goals and objectives of health reforms, context matters. For this reason, it is essential to understand the societal and political preferences, or value system, of a country in which the framework is to be applied.

OECD Health Care Quality Indicators (HCQI) Framework 2006

The HCQI project was initiated in 2001 with the long-term objective of developing a set of indicators that could be used to investigate the quality of health care across countries, using comparable data (Mattke et al., 2006). In 2006, Arah and colleagues (2006) published the conceptual framework which defined 'quality of health care', placing it within a wider performance framework, which acknowledged the key healthy policy goals adopted by the OECD and its Member States (Figure A4). The authors adhere to the WHO definition of a health system in terms of health actions, and define 'health care' as the combined functioning of public health and personal health care services. Their 'health system' framework thus considers not only health care but also other activities that have a primary purpose of promoting, restoring or maintaining health. This framework has four interconnected tiers (connected in a fashion that denotes potential causal pathways), representing:

- *Health*: this tier denotes society's broader health as influenced by health care and non-health care factors;
- *Non-health care determinants of health*: this tier denotes the mostly society-wide, non-health care factors that also influence health;
- *Health care system performance*: the tier denotes the processes, inputs and outcomes of the health care system, as well as its efficiency and equity, recognizing that these may sometimes influence health care determinants. Note that the link between the third tier and the second is captured by primary care/prevention and health promotion; and
- *Health system design and context*: this denotes pertinent country and health system policy and delivery characteristics, which will influence the health system in terms of its costs, expenditure and utilization patterns, which must be considered in order to contextualize the findings of the health performance tier.

Within this health system framework, a certain section of the health care system performance tier (shaded in Figure A4) denotes the core quality dimensions to be measured in the HCQI project:

- effectiveness
- safety
- responsiveness/patient-centredness.

The four tiers of the health system framework allow health care to be placed within a broader conceptualization of a health system in addition to the economic, social and political context of its country. While acknowledging

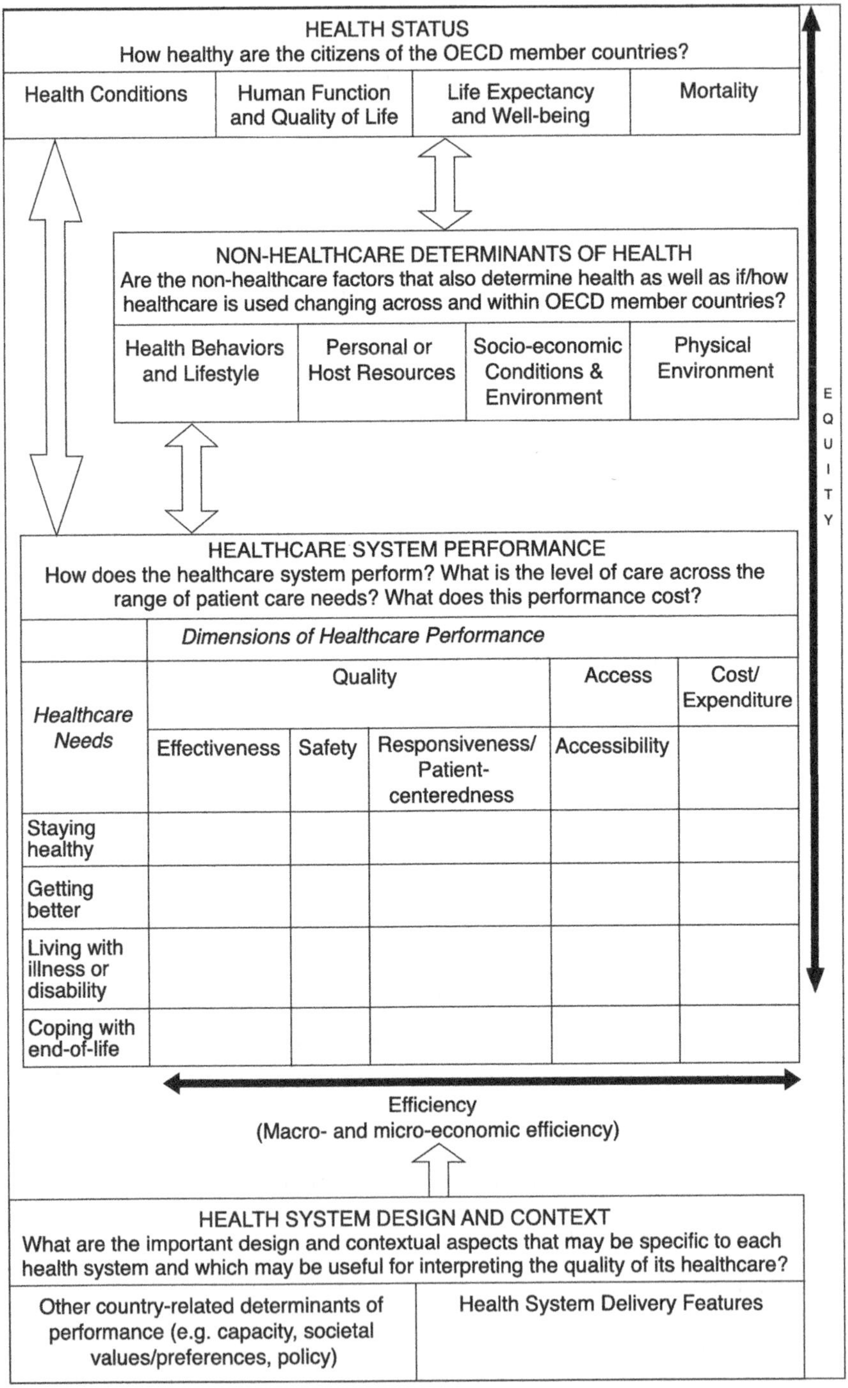

HEALTH STATUS			
How healthy are the citizens of the OECD member countries?			
Health Conditions	Human Function and Quality of Life	Life Expectancy and Well-being	Mortality

NON-HEALTHCARE DETERMINANTS OF HEALTH			
Are the non-healthcare factors that also determine health as well as if/how healthcare is used changing across and within OECD member countries?			
Health Behaviors and Lifestyle	Personal or Host Resources	Socio-economic Conditions & Environment	Physical Environment

HEALTHCARE SYSTEM PERFORMANCE
How does the healthcare system perform? What is the level of care across the range of patient care needs? What does this performance cost?

	Dimensions of Healthcare Performance				
Healthcare Needs	Quality			Access	Cost/ Expenditure
	Effectiveness	Safety	Responsiveness/ Patient-centeredness	Accessibility	
Staying healthy					
Getting better					
Living with illness or disability					
Coping with end-of-life					

Efficiency
(Macro- and micro-economic efficiency)

HEALTH SYSTEM DESIGN AND CONTEXT
What are the important design and contextual aspects that may be specific to each health system and which may be useful for interpreting the quality of its healthcare?

Other country-related determinants of performance (e.g. capacity, societal values/preferences, policy)	Health System Delivery Features

E Q U I T Y

Figure A4   OECD HCQI, 2006

Source: Arah et al., 2006.

that health care is only one of the wider determinants of health, this structure allows health care performance to be measured without being subsumed within the wider health system model. Arah et al. note that 'health care performance' refers to the "maintenance of an efficient and equitable system of health care without emphasizing an assessment of the non-health care determinants", while 'health performance' is a "much broader conceptual approach to measuring performance by explicitly using non-health care determinants, health care and contextual information to give a clearer picture of population health" (Arah et al., 2006). In terms of the framework, health care performance would be concerned only with the evaluation of the third tier, while health performance would be concerned with all four tiers.

The authors define three wider goals of health policy: (1) improving health; (2) efficiency; and (3) equity. They note that efficiency is subdivided into macroeconomic efficiency/sustainability (setting the right level for health expenditure) and microeconomic efficiency/value for money. Their conceptualization of equity is also twofold in that it applies both to the distribution of payments for health care across the population (fair financing), as well as to the distribution of access to health services across the population (fair access) (Arah et al., 2006).

Instead of 'functions', the OECD 2006 framework considers dimensions, defined as "definable, preferably measureable, attributes of the system that are related to its functioning to maintain, restore or improve health". The dimensions represented in the health care system framework are:

- effectiveness
- safety
- responsiveness/patient-centredness
- access
- cost/expenditure.

These are included because they are the core attributes of health care that increase the likelihood of desired outcomes. While not dimensions of the health care system tier, equity and efficiency are considered as mentioned above (Table A5).

Table A5 Dimensions in HCQI health care system framework

Effectiveness: The degree of achieving desirable outcomes, given the correct provision of evidence-based health care services to all who could benefit, but not to those who would not benefit.

Safety: The degree to which health care processes avoid, prevent and ameliorate adverse outcomes or injuries that stem from the processes of health care itself.

Responsiveness/patient-centredness: How a health care system treats people to meet their legitimate non-health expectations.

Accessibility: The ease with which health services are reached.

Cost/expenditure

Adapted from: Kelley & Hurst, 2006.

Commonwealth Fund Framework for a High Performance System 2006

The Commonwealth Fund is a private foundation, based in the United States, which aims to promote a high performance health care system through supporting independent research on health care practice and policy (http://www.commonwealthfund.org). In its efforts to improve performance, the Fund established the Commission on a High Performance Health System in 2005 (Davis, 2005). In its efforts to move the United States to a better health care system, the Commission seeks to identify public and private policies and practices that can lead to health system improvements.

One of the first activities undertaken by the Commission was to create a *Framework for a High Performance Health System for the United States* (Commonwealth Fund, 2006). In its framework a health care system is defined as:

> the ways in which health care services are financed, organized, and delivered to meet societal goals for health. It includes the people, institutions, and organizations that interact to meet the goals, as well as the processes and structures that guide these interactions.

Moreover, they identify a high performance health care system as one "that helps everyone, to the extent possible, lead long, healthy and productive lives". A high performance health care system has four main goals: high-quality, safe care; access to care for all people; efficient, high-value care; system capacity to improve (Figure A5). Each of these four goals is made up of four to five criteria, upon which indicators can be mapped (Table A6).

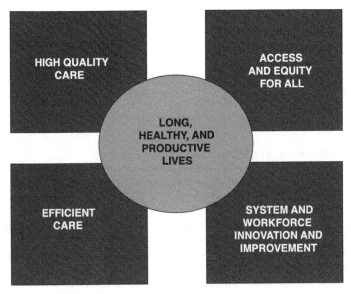

Figure A5   Commonwealth Fund framework, 2006

Source: Commonwealth Fund, 2006.

Table A6 Four goals of a high performance health care system

High-quality safe care

- Patients get health care that is known to be effective – as needed – for treatment, prevention or palliation.
- Health care provided is safe and delivered in a manner that achieves high reliability in care processes and minimizes medical errors.
- Health care is coordinated over time.
- Care is patient-centred: provided in a timely way with compassion; effective communication; and excellent service. Patients are informed and active participants in their care.

Access to care for all people

- There is universal participation.
- Everyone has available to them a minimum level of financial protection, as well as established benefits.
- Care is affordable, from the perspective of both the patient and the nation.
- Care is provided equitably according to medical need, regardless of race/ethnicity, insurance status, income, age, sex, or geographical location.

Efficient, high-value care

- Care delivery and insurance administration are efficient.
- Care is delivered at the right time and in the right setting.
- There is a system whereby new technologies, devices, producers, laboratory testing and pharmaceuticals can be evaluated for both effectiveness and value, including defined processes for their introduction, surveillance, retesting and re-evaluation over time.

System capacity to improve

- There is significant investment in innovation and research.
- There is an interoperable information infrastructure that supports: integration and continuity of care; transparency of information on the price and quality of care; and accountability.
- The educational system adequately prepares the next generation of health care providers and leaders, and the nation develops a stable, competent workforce committed to providing ill Americans with patient-centred, high-quality care.
- The health system responds quickly, at both the individual and population levels, to major health threats and disasters.
- There is a culture of improvement and professional satisfaction among health care professionals.
- There is an appropriate balance between autonomy and accountability.

Adapted from: Commonwealth Fund, 2006.

WHO Building Blocks 2007

In 2007, WHO published its *Framework for Action*, with the aim of "clarifying and strengthening WHO's role in health systems in a changing world" (WHO, 2007). In this publication, the 2000 framework was modified to incorporate some of the feedback received after its publication (Figure A6).

THE WHO HEALTH SYSTEM FRAMEWORK

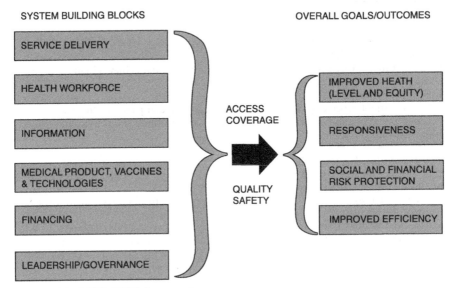

Figure A6 WHO (2007) framework

Source: WHO, 2007.

As part of this role, the 2007 framework begins by seeking to establish a common understanding of what constitutes a health system; what its defining goals are; and what activities are included in health system strengthening. The boundary of the health system and the intrinsic goals identified are the same as those laid out in the 2000 report. However, there is a stronger emphasis on the functions, or instrumental goals, than in the 2000 framework and these have been renamed and regrouped into the six 'building blocks' of the health system (Table A7). Through the identification of these building blocks, WHO is able not only to define the desirable attributes of a health system but also to provide a way to identify where gaps in attributes exist. The 2007 framework emphasizes the necessity of measuring not only the intrinsic goals of the system but also the six building blocks.

While there are six distinct building blocks, the interactions between these blocks are essential for the health system to achieve its overarching goals. Changes in one area will have repercussions in another, and so the distinct parts of the system must function together in order to be effective. The report notes that, while there has been progress in creating a common language to describe the component parts of a health system and the actions necessary to promote effectiveness, there remains work still to be done. Standardized tools and methods need to be developed to facilitate this process in all countries, and this is a fundamental role of WHO. The *Framework for Action* identifies a key priority in this process to be agreeing a set of indicators that can capture the performance of a health system over time and also relative to other systems. A common understanding will make it easier for action to strengthen individual systems to be taken.

Table A7 The six building blocks of a health system

Service delivery

Good health services deliver effective, safe, quality personal and non-personal health interventions to those who need them, when and where needed, with a minimum waste of resources.

Health workforce

A well-performing health workforce is one that works in ways that are responsive, fair and efficient, to achieve the best health outcomes possible, given available resources and circumstances.

Information

A well-functioning information system is one that ensures the production, analysis, dissemination and use of reliable and timely information on health determinants, health systems performance and health status.

Medical products, vaccines and technologies

A well-functioning health system ensures equitable access to essential medical products, vaccines and technologies of assured quality, safety, efficacy and cost–effectiveness, and their scientifically sound and cost–effective use.

Financing

A good health financing system raises adequate funds for health, in ways that ensure people can use needed services and are protected from financial catastrophe or impoverishment associated with having to pay for them.

Leadership and governance (stewardship)

Leadership and governance involves ensuring strategic policy frameworks exist and are combined with effective oversight, coalition-building, the provision of appropriate regulation and incentives, attention to system-design and accountability.

Source: WHO, 2007.

Systems thinking (Atun & Menabde, 2008)

The 'systems thinking' frameworks attempt to create a framework that identifies important inter-relationships and repeated events, so that it is a dynamic framework rather than focusing on a static snapshot of health system structures. Atun and Menabde (2008) expand on existing international frameworks in that they take into account the wider context within which a health system functions (Figure A7). The context identified by systems thinking includes the demographic, economic, political, legal and regulatory, epidemiological, sociodemographic, environmental and technological contexts, referred to as DEPLESET. In order to better understand the interactions between health system elements and the DEPLESET factors, the authors refer to "health system

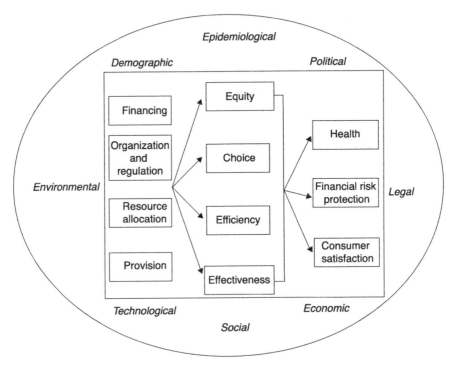

Figure A7 Atun framework, 2008

Source: Atun & Menadbe, 2008.

behaviour". The systems framework identifies four levers available to policy-makers when managing a health system:

- stewardship and organizational arrangements;
- financing;
- resource allocation and provider payment systems;
- service provision.

There are four intermediate goals identified in the framework (equity; efficiency (technical and allocative); effectiveness; and choice) and three ultimate goals (health improvement; financial risk protection; consumer satisfaction). The systems framework has been extended to develop a Systemic Rapid Assessment (SYSRA) toolkit, which allows simultaneous and systematic examination of the broader context, the health care system and the features of health programmes (such as communicable disease control programmes).

IHP Framework 2008

The International Health Partnership and Related Initiatives (IHP+), led by WHO and the World Bank, introduced a common framework to evaluate the

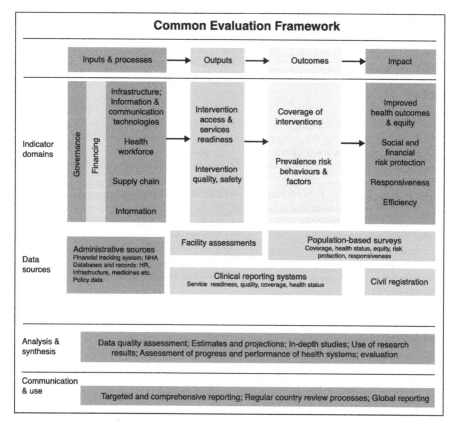

Figure A8 IHP framework, 2008

Source: IHP, 2008.

performance of international initiatives and partnerships, while maintaining country relevance (Figure A8).

The framework is made up of a sequence of components, ranging from inputs and processes to outputs, outcomes and impact (IHP, 2008), defined as:

- *Inputs and processes*: this refers to domestic and international inputs, including funding, improved planning and harmonization practices.
- *Outputs*: this part of the sequence represents the expected outputs of health reforms or interventions.
- *Outcomes*: increased outputs are expected to lead to better outcomes, such as coverage and responsiveness.
- *Impact*: better outcomes are ultimately expected to lead to a better impact, such as improved health. The impact will be influenced by the efficacy of the interventions.

In the IHP (2008) document there is more emphasis on how to map the monitoring and evaluation actions to the framework, rather than to define the boundaries, functions, goals or domains. While this framework is less useful as a heuristic than some of the other theoretical frameworks, it is better tailored to data considerations and may be more helpful when considering how to evaluate a reform process and identifying areas for which indicators need to be selected.

Notes

1 We would like to acknowledge the WHO Regional Office for Europe, Division of Health Systems and Public Health, which commissioned an earlier draft of this work, as well as the comments received at the WHO Technical Experts Meeting on Health System Performance Assessment in Barcelona (January 2010) and at a later authors' workshop hosted by the European Observatory (January 2011).
2 These categories apply to both national and international frameworks, but as our report focuses only on international frameworks, it will include only the relevant categories. For further information, see Hsiao & Sidat (2008) or Shakarishvili (2009).
3 The Lisbon Agenda (also known as the Lisbon Strategy or Lisbon Process) was introduced in 2000 by the European Council and laid out the broad objectives for the EU Member States for the next decade. The key objective of the agenda was to make Europe the most competitive and the most dynamic knowledge-based economy in the world by 2010.

References

Aday, L.A. et al. (1993) *Evaluating the Medical Care System: Effectiveness, efficiency, and equity*, 1st edn. Chicago: Health Administration Press.

Aday, L.A. et al. (1998) *Evaluating the Health Care System: Effectiveness, efficiency, and equity*, 2nd edn. Chicago: Health Administration Press.

Aday, L.A. et al. (1999) A framework for assessing the effectiveness, efficiency and equity of behavioural health care, *American Journal of Managed Care*, 5(Special issue): SP25–44.

Aday, L.A. et al. (2004) *Evaluating the Healthcare System: Effectiveness, efficiency, and equity*, 3rd edn. Chicago: Health Administration Press.

Anand, S. et al. (2003) Report of the Scientific Peer Review Group on health systems performance assessment, in C.J.L. Murray and D.B. Evans (eds) *Health Systems Performance Assessment: Debates, methods and empiricism*. Geneva: World Health Organization.

Arah, O.A. et al. (2003) Conceptual frameworks for health systems performance: a quest for effectiveness, quality, and improvement, *International Journal for Quality in Health Care*, 15(5): 377–98.

Arah, O.A. et al. (2006) A conceptual framework for the OECD Health Care Quality Indicators project, *International Journal for Quality in Health Care*, 18(Suppl): 5–13.

Atun, R. and Menabde, N. (2008) Health systems and systems thinking, in R. Coker, R. Atun and M. McKee (eds) *Health systems and the challenge of communicable diseases: Experiences from Europe and Latin America*. Buckingham: Open University Press (European Observatory on Health Systems and Policies Series).

CIHI (1999) *National Consensus Conference on Population Health Indicators: Final report*. Ottowa: Canadian Institute for Health Information (https://secure.cihi.ca/free_products/phi.pdf, accessed 25 September 2012).

Commonwealth Fund (2006) *Framework for a high performance health system for the United States*. New York: The Commonwealth Fund.

Contandriopoulos, A.P., Trottier, L.H. and Champagne, F. (2008) Improving performance: a key issue for Quebec's health and social services centres, *Infoletter*, 5(2): 2–6.

Davis, K. (2005) Toward a high performance health system: The Commonwealth Fund's new commission, *Health Affairs (Millwood)*, 24(5): 1356–60.

Duran, A. et al. (2012) Understanding health systems: scope, functions and objectives, in J. Figueras and M. McKee (eds) *Health Systems, Health, Wealth and Societal Well-being: Assessing the case for investing in health systems*. Maidenhead: McGraw-Hill Education (European Observatory on Health Systems and Policies Series).

European Commission (2005) *Working together, working better: A new framework for the open coordination of social protection and inclusion policies in the European Union*. Communication from the Commission to the Council, the European Parliament, the European Economic and Social Committee and the Committee of the Regions.

Figueras, J. and McKee, M. (eds) (2012) *Health Systems, Health, Wealth and Societal Well-being: Assessing the case for investing in health systems*. Maidenhead: McGraw-Hill Education (European Observatory on Health Systems and Policies Series).

Frenk, J. (2010) The World Health Report 2000: expanding the horizon of health system performance, *Health Policy and Planning*, 25: 343–5.

Gauld, R. et al. (2011) Scorecards for health system performance assessment: the New Zealand example, *Health Policy*, 103(2): 200–8.

Harbers, M.M. et al. (2008) *Dare to compare! Benchmarking Dutch health with the European Community Health Indicators (ECHI)*. Bilthoven: National Institute for Public Health and the Environment.

Hsiao, W.H. (2003) *What is a health system? Why should we care?* Cambridge, MA: Harvard School of Public Health.

Hsiao, W.H. and Sidat, B. (2008) *Health systems: Concepts and deterministic models of performance*. Background paper prepared for the Workshop on Research Agendas on Global Health Systems, Harvard University, 3–5 December 2008.

Hurst, J. and Jee-Hughes, M. (2001) *Performance measurement and performance management in OECD health systems*. Paris: Organisation for Economic Co-operation and Development Publishing (OECD Labour Market and Social Policy Occasional Paper, no. 47).

IHP (2008) *Monitoring performance and evaluating progress in the scale-up for better health: A proposed common framework*. Document prepared by the monitoring and evaluating working group of the International Health Partnership and Related Initiatives (IHP+), led by the WHO and the World Bank.

IOM (2001) *Crossing the Quality Chasm: A new health system for the 21st century*. Washington, DC: The National Academies Press (Institute of Medicine).

Jassem, A. (2004) *EPHA briefing for members: An introduction to the open method of coordination* (http://www.epha.org/IMG/pdf/EPHA_briefing_on_OMC_AJ_20050216final.pdf, accessed 8 October 2012).

Jee, M. and Or, Z. (1999) *Health outcomes in OECD countries: A framework of health indicators for outcome-oriented policymaking*. Paris: Organisation for Economic Co-operation and Development Publishing (OECD Labour Market and Social Policy Occasional Paper, no. 36).

Kelley, E. and Hurst, J. (2006) *Health Care Quality Indicators project: Conceptual framework paper*. Paris: Organisation for Economic Co-operation and Development Publishing (OECD Health Working Paper, no. 23).

Klassen, A. et al. (2009) Performance measurement and improvement frameworks in health, education and social services systems: a systematic review, *International Journal for Quality in Health Care*, 22: 44–69.

Mattke, S. et al. (2006) *Health Care Quality Indicators project: initial indicators report*. Paris: Organisation for Economic Co-operation and Development Publishing (OECD Health Working Paper, no. 22).

Murray, C.J.L. and Frenk, J. (2000) A framework for assessing the performance of health systems, *Bulletin of the World Health Organization*, 78(6): 717–30.

Naylor, C.D., Iron, K. and Handa, K. (2002) Measuring health system performance: Problems and opportunities in the era of assessment and accountability, in P.C. Smith (2002) *"Measuring up" – Improving health systems performance in OECD countries*. Paris: Organisation for Economic Co-operation and Development.

OECD (2009) *Health at a Glance 2009*. Paris: Organisation for Economic Co-operation and Development.

Parsons, T. (1951) *The social system*. New York: The Free Press.

Parsons, T. (1977) *Social systems and the evolution of action theory*. New York: The Free Press.

Roberts, M.J. et al. (2008) *Getting health reform right: A guide to improving performance and equity*. Oxford: Oxford University Press.

Shakarishvili, G. (2009) *Building on health systems frameworks for developing a common approach to health systems strengthening*. Background document for the World Bank, the Global Fund and the GAVI Alliance Technical Workshop on Health System Strengthening, Washington, DC, 25–27 June 2009.

Sicotte, C. et al. (1998) A conceptual framework for the analysis of health care organizations performance, *Health Services Management Research*, 11(1): 24–48.

WHO (1946) *Constitution of the World Health Organization* (http://apps.who.int/gb/bd/PDF/bd47/EN/constitution-en.pdf, accessed 16 October 2012).

WHO (1986) *Ottawa Charter for Health Promotion*. First International Conference on Health Promotion, 17–21 November 1986, Ottawa, Canada.

WHO (2000) *World Health Report 2000. Health systems: improving performance*. Geneva: World Health Organization.

WHO (2007) *Everybody's business: Strengthening health systems to improve health outcomes. WHO's framework for action*. Geneva: World Health Organization Document Production Services.

WHO (2008) *A framework to monitor and evaluate implementation*. Geneva: World Health Organization Document Production Services (http://www.who.int/dietphysicalactivity/M&E-ENG-09.pdf, accessed 3 June 2012).

WHO Regional Office for Europe (2012) *Case studies on health system performance assessment*. Copenhagen: World Health Organization Regional Office for Europe (http://ec.europa.eu/invest-in-research/coordination/coordination01_en.htm, accessed 3 June 2012).

chapter three

International Comparisons of Health Systems[1]

Irene Papanicolas and Peter C. Smith

3.1 Introduction

International comparison of health system performance can exert a major influence on national policy-makers. It offers the potential for the evaluation of national performance and policies; an empirical base on which to design reform; and a way in which to promote accountability and engage the public. The response to the World Health Report 2000 (*WHR2000*) gave an indication of the potential power of such comparison, but also highlighted some severe methodological difficulties that arise when seeking to make it operational (WHO, 2000). This chapter seeks to draw out some general lessons that have emerged to date from efforts to compare health systems. Throughout, we concentrate on health *system* comparison, discussing more detailed international comparison only when it sheds light on the comparative performance of health systems.

While offering meaningful insights into the performance of national health systems, approaches to international performance assessments and the benchmarking of health systems face numerous challenges. Despite major advances that have been made in data collection and analysis, there are still big gaps in health performance data and limitations in existing methodologies. Furthermore, differences in terminology, coding and culture limit the amount of data that are suitable for direct comparison. Finally, interpretation is far from straightforward given the complex and multidimensional nature of health systems.

In recent decades, various international organizations have worked on addressing these issues in order to create a body of work that would provide a sound empirical basis for a comparative understanding of the differences between health systems (Nolte et al., 2008). WHO and the OECD have been instrumental in collecting comparable data across a range of countries, as well as producing reports to provide analysis and interpretations of these data. In addition, the European Observatory on Health Systems and Policies carries out structured descriptions of health systems in their Health Systems in Transition (HiT) reports. Finally, the EU has also been very active in not only collecting data but also in funding large-scale research projects to promote advances in the collection and analysis of data for performance assessment. This chapter aims to review some of the main health system comparative performance efforts to date, with the aim of drawing out key lessons and challenges.

The chapter begins by summarizing the key data collection and comparative initiatives undertaken by international organizations. It then briefly summarizes a number of academic research studies that seek to compare aspects of health system performance. Next, it offers an assessment of these initiatives and then concludes with a discussion of the key issues to be drawn for international comparison.

3.2 Existing health system performance assessment initiatives

The main health system comparative performance efforts implemented to date include many data collection efforts that have followed the frameworks reviewed in Chapter 2, such as:

- The WHO's *WHR2000* and its 2007 update *Framework for Action*;
- The OECD's *Health System Performance Framework*, and its subsequent *Health Care Quality Indicators* project;
- The *European Community Health Indicators* project, part of the Commission's *Programme of Action in the Field of Public Health*; and
- The Commonwealth Fund's *Framework for a High Performance Health System*, developed originally for the United States, but now being applied to an increasing number of developed nations (Commonwealth Fund, 2006).

In this chapter, the ongoing efforts in data collection being undertaken by some of the main international organizations working in this area, such as the WHO, OECD and EU, will be considered, as well as other ongoing international comparison initiatives in Europe, such as:

- The Health Consumer Powerhouse (based in Sweden) has produced a *Euro Health Consumer Index* since 2005;
- The Nordic Council is seeking to take a coordinated approach towards measuring progress in health and social well-being across the Nordic countries.

We describe these in turn.

The World Health Organization

WHO first presented a systematic framework for health system performance assessment in *WHR2000*, building on the work of Murray and Frenk (2000). This framework was subsequently updated in its 2007 publication *Everybody's*

Business: Strengthening health systems to improve health outcomes. WHO's Framework for Action, which built upon the 2000 report by taking into account the key debates it had provoked (WHO, 2007). In 2008, the WHO European Region, with other international partners and the Member States, signed the Tallinn Charter (WHO, 2008) at the WHO European Ministerial Conference on Health Systems in Tallinn, Estonia. The Charter provided a strategic framework for strengthening health systems and promoting transparency and accountability through the measurement of performance and exchange of experiences. It included a commitment to promote "transparency and accountability for health system performance, to produce measurable results".

A key decision in any analysis of health system performance is the definition of the 'system' under observation. WHO considers that the health system ". . . comprises all organizations, institutions and resources devoted to producing actions whose primary intent is to improve health." This definition goes beyond the narrow considerations of health care to embrace preventative services and public health. However, it stops short of embracing the broader social and environmental determinants of health. The focus is therefore principally on those issues that are usually considered to be the responsibilities of the health ministry.

WHR2000 identified five key intrinsic goals that are relevant to any health system and proposed operational methods for their measurement. It then sought to estimate the relative performance of systems by examining goal attainment in relation to expenditure on the health system, after adjusting for variations in the level of social development. This measure of comparative performance, often referred to as efficiency or productivity, was the basis for the controversial rankings of individual health systems contained in the Appendices of the Report.

The five intrinsic goals proposed in *WHR2000* were:

1. Population health, as captured by disability-adjusted life expectancy (DALE);
2. Variations in population health, as measured by an index of equality of child survival;
3. The responsiveness of the health system, as measured by indicators of respect for persons and client orientation;
4. Variations in responsiveness of the health system;
5. Fairness in financial protection: the extent to which citizens are protected from impoverishment associated with health care.

Goals 1 and 2 indicated concerns with both the level and distribution of life expectancy within the population, while goals 3 and 4 indicated concerns with both the level and equality of responsiveness. The fifth goal was inherently equity focused.

The report sought to measure attainment of these goals for 191 member countries, a considerable practical challenge, which was achieved with varying levels of success. The five measures were combined into a single composite measure of attainment for each country. Using econometric techniques applied to five years' data, countries were then ranked according to their level of attainment after adjusting for: (a) the country's level of expenditure on health services; and (b) the country's level of social development, as indicated by average years of schooling per person. The debate unleashed by *WHR2000* is summarized in the report of the Scientific Peer Review Group (Anand et al., 2003).

The report proposed four basic functions that contribute to the achievement of health system performance:

- financing (how the necessary revenues are raised);
- service provision (how inputs and production processes are structured);
- resource generation (including human resources, physical resources and knowledge); and
- stewardship (setting, implementing and monitoring the operation of the health system).

These were clarified (but not materially amended) in the 2007 report as follows:

- service delivery;
- health workforce;
- information;
- medical products, vaccines and technologies;
- financing; and
- leadership and governance (formerly stewardship).

The intention was that governments should focus on strengthening these functions in order to improve the performance of their health systems, as measured by the intrinsic goals.

Since 2000, WHO has developed partnerships with other organizations and institutions with the overarching aim of collecting comparable data and the harmonization of health statistics. Table 3.1 summarizes some of the main efforts. However, there remain criticisms that WHO data are still limited in scope and quality, especially for developing countries.

Organisation for Economic Co-operation and Development

The OECD has maintained a series of *OECD Health Data* for its member countries dating from the 1960s. Since 1980 it has developed an analytic capacity in health and health care, with its first report on health, *Measuring Health Care 1960–1983: Expenditure, Costs and Performance* and the first paper edition of the OECD *Health Database,* published in 1985. The OECD has provided key work aimed at improving the comparability of health data, especially in the areas of health expenditure and financing and more recently health care quality. In the year 2000, the OECD released the manual, *A System of Health Accounts* (SHA) which serves as the basis for organizing national health system expenditure (OECD, 2000). The original manual was recently updated and a second edition was released jointly by the OECD, WHO and Eurostat in 2011. Work is also continuing on the development of health-specific purchasing power parity (PPP) measures, a crucial element in any international comparison of spending or efficiency.

In 2001, the OECD Health Project was launched with the aim of addressing key policy challenges and improving the performance of OECD health systems.

Table 3.1 Main data collection efforts of WHO

WHO statistical databases

- *Global Health Observatory (GHO) (incorporates the former WHO Statistical Information System (WHOSIS))*: the GHO theme pages provide data and analyses on global health priorities, including data on mortality, World Health Report data, progress on health-related Millennium Development Goals, basic health indicators and the incidence of infectious diseases.
- *Health metrics network.*
- *European Health for All database (HFA-DB)*: data on about 600 health indicators and basic demographic, socioeconomic, lifestyle and environment-related indicators.
- *Mortality indicators by 67 causes of death, age and sex (HFA-MDB)*: data on about 25,000 mortality-based indicators by age and sex.
- *European Detailed Mortality Database (DMDB)*: mortality data by ICD code and five-year age groups.
- *European Hospital Morbidity Database (HMDB)*: morbidity and hospital activity patterns in countries by diagnosis, age and sex.
- *Centralized Information System for Infectious Diseases (CISID)*: data gathered through surveillance of communicable diseases and data on country immunization coverage and recent outbreaks in Europe.

Health policy information (WHO Europe)

- *Health system profiles (HiTs)* (European Observatory on Health Systems and Policies): country-level information on the organization and structure of the health care system.
- *Health evidence network*: synthesis of best available evidence by health topic to be used by policy-makers to guide policy.
- *Alcohol control database*: information on alcohol policies with links to alcohol consumption and related harm in the European Health for All database.
- *Nutrition policy database*: policy documents, dietary guidelines and lists of institutions for policy implementation and stakeholders in Europe. Also contains information on surveillance and micronutrient-deficiency interventions.
- *Prison health database*: will develop an overview of health in prisons and the organization, practice and quality control for prisoners in the European region.
- *Tobacco control database*: data on smoking prevalence and various aspects of tobacco control policy in Europe. Also contains information on tobacco control legislation.

Survey data

- *World Health Survey*: comprehensive baseline information on the health of populations and on the outcomes associated with the investment in health systems; baseline evidence on the way health systems are currently functioning; and ability to monitor inputs, functions and outcomes.

Performance assessment tools

- *World Health Report 2000.*
- *Performance Assessment Tool for Hospitals (PATH)*: European effort to support hospitals in defining quality improvement strategies by: (1) identifying areas for further scrutiny; and (2) sharing best practices.

One of the earliest contributions to this effect was the publication of a conceptual framework for health system performance (Hurst & Jee-Hughes, 2001). The framework drew on the work of WHO, and was intended to serve as a basis for developing a common set of health indicators. Arah et al. (2003) classify the OECD indicators into 10 main data fields: health status, health care resources, health care utilization, expenditure on health, financing and remuneration, social protection, pharmaceutical market, non-medical determinants of health, demographic references and economic references.

The OECD framework reports performance on four main dimensions:

- health improvement/outcomes;
- responsiveness;
- equity (of health outcomes, access and financing); and
- efficiency.

Efficiency in this framework is embodied in terms of microeconomic efficiency and macroeconomic efficiency. The microeconomic efficiency dimension is very similar to WHO's efficiency concept and involves comparing the measured productivity of a health system to its maximum attainable productivity. Productivity is defined as the ratio of outputs to inputs (health outcome and responsiveness per dollar), a measure of technical efficiency. Macroeconomic efficiency relates to total spending on health, involving an examination of the benefit of health spending relative to other goods and services, a concept of allocative efficiency. The OECD framework does not envisage rankings of health systems, and does not require any weighting or combination of the goals.

Since the publication of the OECD framework in 2001, the OECD has embarked on further health performance measurement projects. The OECD Health project (2001–2004) focused on measuring and analysing the performance of Member States' health care systems in order to assist decision-makers in their formulation of evidence-based policies (OECD, 2004). The key components of performance that were measured in this project were:

- technical quality of medical care;
- income-related equity of access to health care;
- waiting times for non-emergency surgery.

In addition, the project described and analysed the institutional and incentive arrangements existing in the health systems of the Member States in the areas of:

- monitoring and improving quality of care;
- human resources;
- access;
- long-term care;
- technological diffusion;
- decision making.

The OECD Health Care Quality Indicators (HCQI) project was initiated in 2001 with the long-term objective of developing a set of indicators that could be used to investigate quality of health care across countries using comparable data (Mattke et al., 2006). Quality is defined as "the degree to which health services for individuals and populations increase the likelihood of desired health outcomes and are consistent with current professional knowledge". Indicators should be definable, preferable measurable and actionable attributes of the system that are related to its functioning to maintain, restore or improve health (Kelley & Hurst, 2006).

The core quality dimensions the OECD chose to focus on (effectiveness, safety and responsiveness) were selected from a variety of dimensions found in the conceptual frameworks of various Member States (Box 3.1). The quality indicators consist mainly of process and outcome measures for the most important disease, risk and client groups at the population level, and their preventative, curing or caring interventions.

The set of indicators available to date has been constrained by availability

Box 3.1   Dimensions of quality of care

Effectiveness: The degree of achieving desirable outcomes, given the correct provision of evidence-based health care services to all who could benefit, but not to those who would not benefit.

Safety: The degree to which health care processes avoid, prevent and ameliorate adverse outcomes or injuries that stem from the processes of health care itself.

Responsiveness: How a health care system treats people to meet their legitimate non-health expectations.

Accessibility: The ease with which health services are reached.

Equity: The extent to which a system deals fairly with all concerned.

Efficiency: The system's optimal use of available resources to yield maximum benefits or results.

Acceptability: Conformity to the realistic wishes, desires and expectations of health care users and their families.

Appropriateness: The degree to which provided health care is relevant to the clinical needs, given the current best evidence.

Competence or capability: The degree to which health system personnel have the training and abilities to assess, treat and communicate with their clients.

Continuity: The extent to which health care for specified users, over time, is coordinated across providers and institutions.

Timeliness: The degree to which patients are able to obtain care promptly.

Adapted from: Kelley & Hurst, 2006.

and comparability, but continuing work is seeking to broaden the scope and reliability of the data. The items available in 2011 are summarized in Table 3.2 below. A summary of progress and commentary on some aspects of international comparison are provided in the biennial publication *Health at a Glance* (OECD, 2009).

Table 3.2 Existing OECD health care quality indicators

Care for chronic conditions

Outcome	**Process**
• Hospital admission rate for asthma (age 15+) • Hospital admission rate for COPD (age 15+) • Uncontrolled diabetes hospital admission rate (age 15+)	

Care for acute exacerbation of chronic conditions

Outcome	**Process**
• In-hospital acute myocardial infarction case-fatality rates • In-hospital ischaemic/haemorrhagic stroke case-fatality rates	

Patient safety

Outcome	**Process**
• Foreign body left in during procedure • Accidental puncture or laceration • Postoperative pulmonary embolism or deep vein thrombosis • Postoperative sepsis	• Obstetric trauma, vaginal delivery with instrument • Obstetric trauma, vaginal delivery without instrument

Care for mental disorders

Outcome	**Process**
• Schizophrenia readmissions to the same hospital • Bipolar disorder readmissions to the same hospital	

Cancer care

Outcome	**Process**
• Five-year relative survival rate for colorectal cancer • Colorectal cancer mortality • Five-year relative survival rate for breast cancer • Breast cancer mortality • Five-year relative survival rate for cervical cancer • Cervical cancer mortality	• Mammography screening • Cervical cancer screening

Source: OECD, 2011.

The European Union

The European Commission recognizes that "high quality health services are a priority issue for European citizens". While the Commission has no specific framework for health system performance assessment, it does undertake some health system performance measurement. The *Health Monitoring Programme* (1997–2002) funded programmes aimed at instituting community health monitoring systems in Member States. Following this, the 2003–2008 *Programme of Community Action in the Field of Public Health* produced comparable information on health and health-related behaviour, diseases and health systems within the Member States through a set of European Community Health Indicators (ECHI-1), which was later updated (ECHI-2) (European Commission, 2004). The ECHI shortlist includes more than 80 indicators that are a priority for data harmonization among EU Member States, as summarized in Table 3.3.

This work has been extended under the *European Community Health Indicators Monitoring* (ECHIM) project, which continues to develop and improve health indicators as well as to implement health monitoring in the EU and all its Member States in order to achieve good coverage. One of the main outputs of this project has been detailed documentation sheets for the 88 shortlisted indicators of the previous ECHI projects. These sheets provide details on the construction of each indicator as well as information on the extent of data availability and periodicity.

Table 3.3 Main categories for the ECHI indicator set

Demographic and socioeconomic situation
• Population measures • Socioeconomic measures
Health status
• Mortality measures • Morbidity, disease-specific measures • Generic health status measures • Composite health status measures
Determinants of health
• Personal and biological factor measures • Health behaviour measures • Living and working condition measures
Health systems
• Prevention, health protection and health promotion measures • Health care resource measures • Health expenditure and financing measures • Health care quality/performance measures

The Dutch National Institute for Public Health and the Environment (RIVM) recently benchmarked the EU Member States using the ECHI indicator shortlist, in order to assess the performance of the Dutch health system (Harbers et al., 2008). The report found that the Netherlands ranked very high in certain indicators but was quite a poor performer on others. The report raises for all ECHI indicators the question of whether the data available are truly comparable. In practice, there is still some diversity in data collection mechanisms between Member States, as well as the quality and availability of the data.

The EU has collaborated with the OECD and the WHO Regional Office for Europe to produce the *International Compendium of Health Indicators* (ICHI), first in 1999 and then again in 2005, as a step towards the harmonization of data. The ICHI-2 is a web-based application, which contains the health indicators used by WHO Europe (Health for All), the OECD (Health Data) and Eurostat (Cronos) in their websites. The database provides the indicator definitions for each database, allowing a quick comparison through one system.

The EU has also sought to harmonize the data collection of social and health-related topics in its individual level surveys. Part of this effort has consisted of the creation of the *European Community Household Panel* (ECHP) survey and its successor, the *EU Statistics on Income and Living Conditions* (EU-SILC) survey, as well as the inclusion of special health modules in the *Eurobarometer* surveys. Other developments include the *Survey of Health, Ageing and Retirement in Europe* (SHARE), which collects panel data on individuals of age 50 and over, and the *European Core Health Interview Survey* (ECHIS). Not all of these surveys were designed with the aim of collecting information on health indicators (e.g. ECHP and EU-SILC) and this accounts for the more limited health information included in them.

The Institute of Public Health in Belgium has created an inventory of health surveys administered at both national and international levels in the EU, the European region, Australia, Canada and the United States (funded by DG SANCO). This database outlines the different surveys available, the indicators included in the surveys, and the methodologies used to compile them. The variation across countries highlights the need for improved harmonization.

Within the framework of the EU Commission's Health Monitoring Programme, the National Federation of Regional Health Observatories, France (FNORS) established the Indicateurs Santé Régionaux d'Europe (ISARE) project to focus on the health of regions within the EU. An initial project (ISARE 1), carried out in the years 1999–2001, aimed to identify (in the then 15 countries of the EU) the sub-national level, which was most appropriate for the production and comparison of indicators (the ISARE health regions). The project then assessed the data availability at these sub-national levels. The second project (ISARE 2), carried out in 2002–2004, aimed to test the feasibility of gathering data at these regional levels. The project concluded that, despite variations between the regions, the exchange of health indicators is feasible. The third project (ISARE 3), carried out in 2005–2007, extended the research to new countries to examine the different ways of effective data presentation and dissemination.

Finally, the EU is also instrumental in funding many projects in health that aim to collect better data or use existing data to learn more about national and international health system performance. There are many funding programmes in health, with major initiatives such as the Sixth and Seventh Framework Programmes of DG-Research, as well as funding from DG SANCO and the EU Public Health Programme. Table 3.4 below illustrates some examples of work that has been funded in this area.

The Commonwealth Fund

The Commonwealth Fund, a private foundation based in New York, has established a Commission on a High Performance Health System. One of its activities has been to create a *Framework for a High Performance Health System for the United States*. The health care system is defined as: "the ways in which health care services are financed, organized, and delivered to meet societal goals for health. It includes the people, institutions, and organizations that interact to meet the goals, as well as the processes and structures that guide these interactions." A high performance health care system is one "that helps everyone, to the extent possible, lead long, healthy and productive lives". A high performance health care system has four main goals:

- high-quality, safe care;
- access to care for all people;
- efficient, high-value care; and
- system capacity to improve.

Note that this framework focuses very much on health care, and there is no explicit consideration of prevention, public health, or the broader determinants of health.

Through the Commission on a High Performance Health System (created in 2005) the Commonwealth Fund has developed a *National Scorecard on U.S. Health System Performance* to assess how well the US health system is performing as a whole, relative to what is achievable, through 37 indicators (Davis, 2005). It aims to assess and monitor the key dimensions of performance (health outcomes, access, quality, equity and efficiency) in relation to benchmarks and over time. The benchmarks are set according to the levels achieved internationally or within the United States, with a maximum score of 100.

In addition, *The Commonwealth Fund State Scorecard* uses a selection of key indicators (32 in 2007, 38 in 2009) to measure the system performance of US states in five dimensions: access; prevention and treatment; potentially avoidable use of hospitals and costs of care; equity; and healthy lives (McCarthy et al., 2009). Where possible, indicators were selected to be comparable to those used in the *National Scorecard*. The State Scorecard ranks states from best to worst on each of the 38 indicators, and also on overall performance (estimated by a composite measure created from the average ranking in each of the five dimensions).

Since 1998, the Commonwealth Fund has also run their *International Health Policy Survey*. Initially this included Australia, Canada, New Zealand, the United Kingdom and the United States, but over time more countries have been added to the survey. By its last round in 2011, six more countries had been added (France, Germany, the Netherlands, Norway, Sweden and Switzerland).

Table 3.4 Examples of EU funded projects in comparative health system performance research

Project name (EU funding programme)	Project aims
HealthBasket (FP6)	• To collect and describe how different countries define the services provided within the system by analysing both the structure and contents of benefit 'catalogues' (or 'baskets') as well as the process of defining these benefit catalogues. • To explore the possibilities of building a European taxonomy of benefits, based on that analysis and other relevant classifications, to enable a common language for cost comparisons. • To review methodologies used to assess costs and prices of services across countries and to identify 'best practice' in the analysis of costs at the micro-level with the scope of international comparability. • To assess cost variations between and within countries, using a selection of 'case vignettes' representing needs for care in both inpatient and outpatient settings. *Source*: EHMA (2012)
EuroDRG (FP7)	• To understand the differences and similarities of the objectives, purposes and methodologies underlying the case payment systems for hospitals in 10 European countries. • To identify pan-European issues in hospital case payment by conducting cost analysis across European countries, with special emphasis placed on: (1) identifying ways to calculate these payments in an adequate fashion; (2) examining hospital efficiency within and across European countries; and (3) identifying factors that affect the relationship between the costs and quality of inpatient care. • To develop and implement the first Europe-wide hospital benchmarking system as a means of identifying common issues and systemic factors that will be crucial when designing successful policies for the slowly emerging pan-European hospital market. *Source*: EuroDRG (2012)
EuroHOPE (FP7)	• To develop methods to measure outcome and costs of care for specific diseases that can be used for routine evaluation of care in the treatment pathway. • To develop methods to measure quality, access, outcomes and cost of care that can be used for routine evaluation and monitoring of performance. • To develop methods for international comparative health service research using health data. • To investigate the relationship between outcomes and costs between European countries, regions and providers. *Source*: EuroHOPE (2012)

Project name (EU funding programme)	Project aims
EuroREACH (FP7)	To develop a toolbox of guidance on international comparisons research which: • identifies information sources of patient-level, disease-based data; • offers guidance on key data challenges such as data access, linkage and comparability; • highlights gaps in existing data to encourage data collection in under-represented areas. *Source*: EuroREACH (2012)
ECAB (FP7)	• To facilitate a process whereby Europe's citizens can make informed choices about whether to seek health care in another Member State, and if they so choose, to ensure that the administrative and clinical processes are straightforward and ensure continuity of care. • ECAB firstly examines five aspects of health care delivery where it will be necessary for procedures to be compatible if patients are to be assured that the care they receive is safe, of adequate quality, and capable of providing continuity where some parts of the overall care process are provided in different Member States. These are: provisions with regard to the continuing quality of health professionals; treatment pathways; content and scope of medical records; medical prescribing; public reporting of quality; and long-term care, including media reporting. • Secondly, it looks at three areas where there is already cross-border collaboration to identify practical issues that have arisen, and how they have or have not been addressed. These areas of practice are collaborations between hospitals in border areas, telemedicine, and dentistry. *Source*: ECAB (2012)
PROMeTHEUS (FP7)	To better understand the organizational, contextual and personal factors of health professional mobility, mapping international, national and managerial responses that seek to manage it better. *Source*: WHO Regional Office for Europe (2012)
BIRO (DG SANCO)	• To provide an enhanced capacity to combat diabetes, through improved monitoring of risk factors directly related to the disease, including: obesity, impairment, social exclusion, and the much higher risk of adverse effects among aged subjects. • To support policy-making through the systematic evaluation of different strategies for health care and prevention based on a scheme that is generally valid for all chronic diseases. *Source*: BIRO (2012)

(Continued)

Table 3.4 Examples of EU funded projects in comparative health system performance research *(Continued)*

Project name (EU funding programme)	Project aims
EUCID (DG SANCO)	To collect data on morbidity, mortality and risk factors connected to diabetes, as well as on complications and quality of care, together amounting to 35 indicators, from 19 countries. *Source*: EUCID (2008)
ECHO (FP7)	To bring together national hospital databases of several European countries and make them easily accessible to policy-makers and researchers for policy information and improvement. *Source*: ECHO (2001)
AMIEHS (Public Health Programme)	To develop a 'new' list of indicators (causes of death) for which mortality rates are likely to reflect variations in the effectiveness of health care, with health care being limited to primary care, hospital care and personalized health services. *Source*: AMIEHS (2012)
RN4Cast (FP7)	• To determine how hospital nurse staffing, skill mix, educational composition, and quality of the nurse work environment impact on hospital mortality, failure to rescue, quality of care and patient satisfaction. • To produce actionable recommendations to improve nursing care and patient outcomes at the individual hospital level and to inform national policies that could improve care outcomes by strategic investments in nursing. *Source*: RN4CAST (2012)
EURHOBOP (Public Health Programme)	To provide the European Community with valid standardized and adjusted benchmarking tools that permit European hospitals to monitor their outcomes in key procedures used in coronary artery disease. *Source*: Eurhobop (2012)
EUPrimeCare (FP7)	To provide evidence through a set of research methods and tools of the links between quality of care and its cost in primary care in Europe. *Source*: EUprimecare (2012)
EPIC	To investigate the relationships between diet, nutritional status, lifestyle and environmental factors and the incidence of cancer and other chronic diseases. EPIC is a large study of diet and health having recruited over half a million (520 000) people in 10 European countries: Denmark, France, Germany, Greece, Italy, The Netherlands, Norway, Spain, Sweden and the United Kingdom. *Source*: EPIC (2012)

Health Consumer Powerhouse

The Health Consumer Powerhouse (HCP) is a private health care analyst and information provider registered in Sweden. It focuses on consumer empowerment and patients' rights. In 2004, the HCP published an index comparing the responses of Swedish county councils to consumer care. The success of this indicator caused the Swedish authorities to develop their own set of indicators for comparative purposes. This ranking was then transferred to the European level in 2005 when the *Euro Health Consumer Index* was published. The index is now published annually. It uses a number of indicators to assess the extent to which health systems are 'user friendly' (Table 3.5). The 2009 index evaluated a total of 38 indicators within six evaluation areas:

- patient rights and information;
- e-health;
- waiting times for treatment;
- outcomes;
- range and reach of services provided; and
- pharmaceutical.

The individual indicators are combined within each evaluation area, and then overall to create a total score between 0–1000. Countries are ranked according to their overall score. The information sources for the indicators vary, with some data (such as those for informal payments) being collected by the HCP themselves through patient surveys, and others being sourced from existing datasets or surveys compiled by other organizations, such as the WHO, OECD and EU. Since 2008, the HCP has also published the *Euro-Canada Health Consumer Index*, which extended the European index to include Canada.

In order to take account of the different financial resources available to different countries, the 2009 *Euro Health Consumer Index* created the 'Bang-For-Buck adjusted score (BFB)', which adjusts for annual health care spending. This index divides the basic EHCI summary scores by the square root of health care spending per capita in PPP dollars (from the WHO HFA database), seeking to standardize for differences in scale.

Table 3.5 Evaluation areas and indicators of the Euro Health Consumer Index (2009)

Patient rights and information

Indicators:

- Health care law based on patients' rights.
- Patient organizations involved in decision-making.
- No-fault malpractice insurance.
- Right to second opinion.
- Access to own medical record.
- Register of legit doctors.
- Web or 24/7 telephone health care information with interactivity.
- Cross-border care-seeking financed from home.
- Provider catalogue with quality ranking.

(Continued)

Table 3.5 Evaluation areas and indicators of the Euro Health Consumer Index (2009) *(Continued)*

e-Health

Indicators:

- EPR penetration.
- e-transfer of medical data between health professionals.
- Are lab test results communicated direct to patients via e-health solutions?
- Do patients have access to online booking of appointments?
- Online access to check how much doctors/clinics have charged insurers.
- e-prescriptions.

Waiting time for treatment

Indicators:

- Family doctor same day access.
- Direct access to specialist.
- Major non-acute operations in under 90 days.
- Cancer therapy in under 21 days.
- CT scan in less than 7 days.

Outcomes

Indicators:

- Heart infarction case fatality.
- Infant deaths.
- Ratio of cancer deaths to incidence.
- Preventable years of life lost.
- MRSA infections.
- Rate of decline of suicide.
- Percentage of diabetics with high HbA1c levels (greater than 7%).

Range and reach of services provided

Indicators:

- Cataract operations per 100 000 age 65+.
- Infant four-disease vaccination.
- Kidney transplants per million.
- Is dental care included in the public health care offering?
- Rate of mammography.
- Informal payments to doctors.

Pharmaceuticals

Indicators:

- Rx subsidy.
- Layman-adapted pharmacopeia.
- Novel cancer drugs deployment rate.
- Access to new drugs (time to subsidy).

Adapted from: HCP, 2009c.

Alongside the general *Euro Health Consumer Index*, the HCP has also published indices on diabetes (HCP, 2008a), heart disease (HCP, 2008b), HIV (HCP, 2009a) and patient empowerment (HCP, 2009b). For each of these indices, evaluation areas and indicators were compiled to best represent the patient situations across European health care systems (Table 3.6). Summary measures were calculated for each evaluation area and the overall system in the same way as for the general index.

The Nordic Collaboration

The Nordic Council is the official inter-parliamentary body in the Nordic Region. It was formed in 1952 between the governments of Denmark, Finland, Iceland, Norway and Sweden, as well as the three autonomous territories: the

Table 3.6 Evaluation areas of HCP specialized indices

Euro consumer diabetes index (2008)

Evaluation areas:

- Information, consumer rights, choice (5 indicators).
- Generosity in provision of care (3 indicators).
- Prevention (8 indicators).
- Access to procedures (6 indicators).
- Outcomes (4 indicators).

Euro consumer heart index (2008)

Evaluation areas:

- Information, consumer rights, choice (4 indicators).
- Access (4 indicators).
- Prevention (8 indicators).
- Procedures (7 indicators).
- Outcomes (5 indicators).

Euro HIV index (2009)

Evaluation areas:

- Involvement and rights (7 indicators).
- Access (6 indicators).
- Prevention (9 indicators).
- Outcomes (6 indicators).

European empowerment index (2009)

Evaluation areas:

- Patients' rights (10 indicators).
- Information (5 indicators).
- Health technology assessment (1 indicator).
- Financial incentives (3 indicators).

Adapted from: HCP, 2008a, 2008b, 2009a, 2009b.

Faroe Islands, Greenland and Åland. The Council focuses on seven areas of cooperation, including that of welfare and gender equality, which includes a health component. The main areas targeted are public health and general well-being, with an explicit effort made to reduce inequalities in health and to spread knowledge about healthy lifestyles. The cooperation project for health involves several Nordic institutions involved in the social and health affairs domain, including the Nordic Medico-Statistical Committee (NOMESKO), which publishes a comparison of medical statistics between the Nordic countries.

The Northern Dimension Partnership in Public Health and Social Wellbeing (NDPHS) is a cooperative effort of thirteen governments and nine international organizations, which aims to take joint action to tackle challenges in health and social well-being in the Northern Dimension Area. One of the main activities of the NDPHS is to collect and disseminate information. While no overarching conceptual framework exists, the NDPHS does publish an annual workplan that outlines the key objectives for the year, plus final targets and specific actions that should be undertaken to achieve these. At the end of the year, an annual progress report is published, which describes the achievements.

The National Institute for Health and Welfare (formerly STAKES), a Finnish expert agency, the key functions of which are research, development and statistics, initiated a Nordic hospital comparison study group (NHCSG) as a collaborative effort between health statistics and research groups in the Nordic area. This aims to provide relevant and comparable performance measures for hospital care in four Nordic countries. This work, which began in 2006, will be undertaken in three phases:

- comparing productivity and technical efficiency indicators of costs and processes;
- explaining the differences in the indicators collected; and
- examining whether quality and outcome indicators explain variations in hospital efficiency, to determine whether there is a trade-off between efficiency and quality of care.

3.3 Other research

A number of approaches have also been tested for cross-country comparisons at a finer level of detail than the aggregate system level. For example, several comparisons of hospital performance have been reported (Hollingsworth and Peacock, 2008). However, a fundamental problem with studies at the hospital level is that they usually cannot control adequately for differences in case-mix. Furthermore, regulatory, accounting and institutional variations make international comparison especially difficult. An episode-specific approach might therefore be a better alternative. This approach is based on the assumption that data pertaining to specific health conditions will illuminate interconnected aspects (such as financing and utilization of medical technologies) responsible for health systems performance (Häkkinen and Joumard, 2007).

In addition, a number of approaches to comparing costs and outcomes for specific diseases or care episodes have been developed, such as the McKinsey study (McKinsey Global Institute, 1996), the OECD ageing-related disease (ARD) project (OECD, 2003) and the Technological Change in Health Care (TECH) Global Research Network (McClellan & Kessler, 2002). The McKinsey study gathered data on four diseases relating to three countries at aggregate national level from secondary sources such as literature reviews. The OECD ARD project explored the availability of necessary and comparable information on three diseases in OECD countries, but also did not gather any primary micro-level data. The TECH network study was the first to collect micro-level data from a number of countries. This project was able to obtain data on utilization, comorbidity, mortality and demographic characteristics for patients with acute myocardial infarction (AMI) from seven countries. However, the main emphasis of the project was on documenting technological change rather than focusing on performance.

From the individual treatment perspective, the European Commission funded the *HealthBasket* project (Table 3.4), which sought to compare the costs of 10 common treatments across nine European countries (Busse, Schreyögg & Smith, 2008). The motivation for this study was the concern that the interpretation of health care cost comparisons is difficult because it is not usually clear what causes reported cost variations. In particular, the delivery of a seemingly identical service may vary across countries due to variations in: (1) the definition of the start and end of a service (e.g. whether rehabilitation following a hip replacement is part of the hospital treatment or seen as a separate service with its own tariff); (2) the technology used (especially regarding the use of innovative or expensive technologies, e.g. cemented hip replacement vs more costly uncemented hip replacement); and (3) the accounting treatment of associated services (e.g. whether anaesthesia is included in the service 'surgical procedure' or counted and charged separately).

Even for a comparable service, different factors might be included in the cost calculations (e.g. how overheads are treated, whether volume-variable, 'fixed', amortization or investment costs are included, or whether any available subsidies, such as from local authorities, are made explicit). Any observed variations in costs might then be explained through the differences in accounting treatments. Finally, an important source of variation within Europe is the variation in input prices, especially workforce pay (e.g. doctor and nursing time), which differs significantly across borders. The analytic challenge is to make all this information available, so that one can then explore the underlying reasons for treatment and cost variations. Ultimately, the ambition is to determine whether differences in inputs and processes translate into differences in outcomes, although these did not form part of the current study.

The *HealthBASKET* project developed, tested and used an approach termed 'case vignettes' to explore variations in resource use and costs. The case vignettes depicted 'typical' patients, including specified age, gender and relevant comorbidity (see Box 3.2). Vignettes were developed for both inpatient and outpatient, primary and secondary, elective and emergency settings. For each vignette, a questionnaire was developed to collect detailed information on the services that a patient similar to the one described in the vignette would have received, as well as the costs associated with the services provided.

Box 3.2 Overview of the ten vignettes

Vignette 1:	Appendectomy; male aged 14–25; inpatient; emergency (Schreyögg, 2007)
Vignette 2:	Normal delivery; female aged 25–34; inpatient; elective (Bellanger & Or, 2007)
Vignette 3:	Hip replacement; female aged 65–75; inpatient; elective (Stargardt, 2007)
Vignette 4:	Cataract; male aged 70–75; outpatient; elective (Fattore & Torbica, 2007)
Vignette 5:	Stroke; female aged 60–70; inpatient; emergency (Epstein et al., 2007)
Vignette 6:	Acute myocardial infarction; male aged 50–60; inpatient; emergency (Tiemann, 2007)
Vignette 7:	Cough; male aged ~2; outpatient; emergency
Vignette 8:	Colonoscopy; male aged 55–70; outpatient; elective
Vignette 9:	Tooth filling; child aged ~12; outpatient; emergency (Tan et al., 2007)
Vignette 10:	Physiotherapy; male aged 25–35; outpatient; elective

An example is the following vignette for colonoscopy:

Male, 55–70 years old, with positive Faecal Occult Blood test is referred to an internist/ gastroenterologist's office/hospital out-patient department for diagnostic colonoscopy.

Start of vignette: patient presents for the first time in office/outpatient department. Please include all visits including the one where the colonoscopy is performed (i.e. most likely two), specify explicitly if and which sedatives, e.g. benzodiazepines (flumazenil), fluids etc. are used/prescribed.

Cases with polypectomy during colonoscopy, pathological examinations and follow-up visits are excluded.

The use of the vignette methodology proved to be feasible and well accepted. While it 'standardizes' patients – thereby avoiding the necessity to risk-adjust – it is sensitive to differences in treatment patterns and can be used for cross-provider and cross-country comparisons. The researchers concluded that the method represents a good triangulation between qualitative and quantitative methods, and constitutes a promising basis for future research (Busse, Schreyögg & Smith, 2008). An example of the results (for the appendectomy vignette) is given in Figure 3.1.

The vignette approach has, however, some methodological limitations. First, the simple vignettes cannot reflect the clinical reality with complete accuracy. Furthermore, the relatively small samples of both providers and patients recruited led to quite large confidence intervals for the estimates in some countries. Countries, and providers within countries, differed in their ability to provide data according to the required methodology. Some structural differences between countries were identified. For example, hospital providers

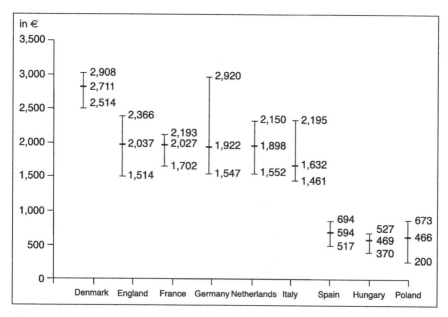

Figure 3.1 Summary of variations in costs of appendectomy

Source: Schreyögg, 2008.

in some countries do not own their assets, and international accounting standards regarding the cost of capital have not always been fully implemented. Furthermore, administrative differences between countries included: legal barriers to accessing patient data; variation in the willingness to disclose data; variation in the quality of information systems between countries and providers; variation in the number of providers contributing data to each vignette in each country and the numbers of patients sampled by each provider; differences in the accounting rules used to allocate indirect and overhead costs to services; and challenges in currency conversion.

The *HealthBasket* project therefore offers some illumination on how a micro-comparison of health system performance might be undertaken, but also on the challenges that such a study would encounter. In particular, it highlights the immense difficulty of securing universal access to data and compliance with measurement rules. At present, weaknesses in information systems and a lack of uniformity in accounting practices make the approach quite research-intensive. However, the approach could become more widely useful if current informational weaknesses can be remedied. The research is being followed up through a new EuroDRG study that is exploring the scope for improved alignment of classification systems and costing methodologies across Europe.

An alternative approach using vignettes was adopted in the *World Health Survey* (*WHS*), an initiative launched by WHO in 2001, aimed at strengthening national capacity to monitor critical health outputs and outcomes through the fielding of a valid, reliable and comparable household survey instrument (see Üstün et al., 2003). Seventy countries participated in the *WHS 2002–2003*, which consisted of a combination of 90-minute in-household interviews (53 countries), 30-minute face-to-face interviews (13 countries) and computer-assisted telephone interviews (4 countries). All surveys were drawn from nationally representative frames with known probability, resulting in sample sizes of between 600 and 10,000 respondents across the countries surveyed. Samples have undergone extensive quality assurance procedures, including the testing of the psychometric properties of the responsiveness instrument (for example, see Valentine et al., 2009).

The *WHS* used the method of 'anchoring vignettes', which has been promoted as a means of controlling for systematic differences in preferences and norms when responding to survey questions (for example, see Salomon et al., 2004). Vignettes represent hypothetical descriptions of fixed levels of a performance concept, such as health status or responsiveness. Some examples are given in Box 3.3. The intention is to use responses to a uniform set of fixed vignettes to adjust for systematic variation in reporting behaviour across individuals and countries. This information can be used to adjust the self-reported data of a respondent's own contact with health services. For cross-country comparative analysis, responses can be rescaled to a chosen benchmark country, thereby seeking to adjust for systematic differences between countries in cultural norms and expectations.

A number of studies have applied the vignette approach and made use of what has been termed the hierarchical ordered probit (HOPIT) model to adjust self-reported data for systematic differences in respondents' use of threshold

Box 3.3 Examples of vignette questions used in the WHS

Respectful treatment

[Anya] took her baby for a vaccination. The nurse said hello but did not ask for [Anya's] or the baby's name. The nurse also examined [Anya] and made her remove her shirt in the waiting room.

Q1: How would you rate her experience of being greeted and talked to respectfully?

Q2: How would you rate the way her privacy was respected during the physical examinations and treatments?

Communication

[Rose] cannot write or read. She went to the doctor because she was feeling dizzy. The doctor didn't have time to answer her questions or to explain anything. He sent her away with a piece of paper without telling her what it said.

Q1: How would you rate her experience of how clearly health care providers explained things to her?

Q2: How would you rate her experience of getting enough time to ask questions about her health problem or treatment?

Confidentiality

[Simon] was speaking to his doctor about an embarrassing problem. There was a friend and a neighbour of his in the crowded waiting room and because of the noise the doctor had to shout when telling [Simon] about the treatment he needed.

Q1: How would you rate the way the health services ensured [Simon] could talk privately to health care providers?
Q2: How would you rate the way [Simon's] personal information was kept confidential?

Quality of basic amenities

[Wing] had his own room in the hospital and shared a bathroom with two others. The room and bathroom were cleaned frequently and had fresh air.

Q1: How would you rate the cleanliness of the rooms inside the facility, including toilets?
Q2: How would you rate the amount of space [Wing] had?

Source: Rice, Robone & Smith, 2012.

---

values. The method has mostly been applied to self-reported data on health status (for example, see Iburg et al., 2002; Murray et al., 2003; Tandon et al., 2003; King et al., 2004; Bago d'Uva et al., 2008). More recently, there have been attempts to extend the methodology to health systems responsiveness (Valentine et al., 2003; Puentes Rosas et al., 2006; Rice, Robone & Smith, 2011). Although still experimental, such methods offer promising new avenues to develop comparable performance data in hitherto problematic areas such as responsiveness.

3.4 Assessment of initiatives to date

The initiatives outlined above offer 10 years' experience of seeking to compare the performance of health systems. In this section we summarize what they have taught us, the debates that they have stimulated, and the unresolved issues they have raised.

In assessing progress, it is perhaps first worth returning to the *WHR2000*. The controversy provoked by that report stimulated a wide-ranging debate that embraces general issues applicable to all efforts at international comparison. The debate is discussed in the report of the Scientific Peer Review Group (Anand et al., 2003), which grouped criticisms under four headings:

• Matters of principle: should comparison of health system performance be undertaken at all and, if so, by whom?

- The model of production: did the *WHR2000* use an appropriate underlying model of the health system?
- Measurement issues: were the metrics used in the *WHR2000* fit for purpose?
- Econometric issues: were the econometric tools used in the report appropriate and were they correctly deployed?

The criticisms are summarized in Table 3.7.

Many of the matters of principle raised by critics of the *WHR2000* related to the legitimacy of an international agency choosing objectives for the health system and applying value weights to those objectives through the construction of the composite measure of attainment. It was argued that these are properly matters for national governments. These are powerful arguments that – at the very least – imply a need for caution in constructing the composite measure. The values placed on different health system objectives are ultimately a personal judgement and, in practice, individuals vary quite markedly in their preferences. National accountability processes are in place to reconcile such

Table 3.7 Criticisms of the *World Health Report 2000*

Matters of principle

- The methods used by WHO involve numerous value judgements that are properly the domain of sovereign national governments and not an international agency.
- A focus on efficiency may send a confused message when set alongside the objective of improving health outcomes.
- The determinants of health system performance are too complex to be reducible to a tractable statistical model.
- Statistical models traditionally focus on estimating the relationship between a stimulus (inputs) and a response (in this case, attainment) but not on the residual for an individual observation.
- There will always be significant measurement error and incomplete model specification.
- The uncertainty analysis used by WHO does not fully consider modelling errors that are potentially important sources of uncertainty.
- Econometric methods used to estimate efficiency are too complex to be helpful.
- There are numerous unresolved issues surrounding the methodology of productivity analysis.

The model of production

- The health production function may not be identical between nations, so use of a single model is inappropriate.
- The WHO approach uses an inappropriate theoretical model of the production process it seeks to capture.
- Outcomes are determined by both the level and distribution of income and other environmental factors.
- The methods used in *WHR2000* do not adequately model the 'reasons' why a given level of efficiency is observed.
- The chosen model does not recognize the important time lags that exist in producing health outcomes.
- The need to calculate a 'minimum' level of health attainment in the absence of a health system is contested.

Measurement issues

- The treatment of missing data is inadequate.
- The components of the efficiency model refer to different definitions of the health system.
- The composite measure of output is highly contested and embraces numerous assumptions and value judgements.
- Relative prices of inputs differ between nations.
- The measures of cost rely on inadequate PPP-adjusted estimates of expenditure.
- Years of education is an inadequate proxy for external influences on health system performance.
- The methodology and data used to measure the 'minimum' are contested.

Econometric issues

- The use of the fixed-effects panel data estimator is inappropriate, given the very low degree of variation from one year to the next in most observations.
- The models used presume a fixed level of efficiency across the entire four-year period examined.
- All fixed-effect variations are attributed to inefficiency.
- The methods do not adequately treat the important contribution of income to the production of health.
- Formal model selection techniques should be employed in choosing the preferred functional form for the model.
- More details are required on whether the chosen model passes the usual model misspecification statistical tests.
- There is evidence of a structural difference between developed and less-developed countries.

Adapted from: Anand et al., 2003.

variations, and there is certainly a question mark over the extent to which an international agency should seek to impose a uniform set of values.

The other main arguments of principle directed at the *WHR2000* related to whether the endeavour was feasible or helpful to national governments. Many commentators argued that the methodology was too complex and opaque to explain the published ranking of a health system. It was also argued that no useful action could be taken as a result of the published tables. It was certainly the case that the rankings could only be used as a basis for further more detailed analysis, and that considerable analytic capacity was needed to understand the reasons for a specific ranking.

The debates about the model used by WHO centred on a number of issues, including whether time lags in producing health outcomes had been properly modelled. In particular, health outcomes are the results of years of health system endeavour and cannot in their entirety be attributed to current or recent actions. In the same vein, there was concern that health outcomes were in part the result of numerous determinants outside the health system that were not properly captured by the model. These continue to be unresolved issues that need careful attention in international comparison. It was also questioned whether it was appropriate to use a single model for countries at all levels of development. If only countries with similar social and other environmental determinants of health are compared, then it is possible that some of these concerns will diminish.

WHO encountered numerous measurement difficulties in seeking to make its model operational. The required data were not available in many countries, and there were broader concerns about reliability and comparability, exacerbated by different data collection and accounting treatments across countries. The use of statistical methods to infer missing observations was questioned. The treatment of missing, incomplete and unreliable data continues to be a major issue for international comparison.

There was also discussion of whether appropriate metrics were being used. The use of key informants to assess levels and equity of responsiveness was an obvious cause for concern. However, there was also a debate about whether the appropriate concepts of equity (of health, responsiveness and financial contribution) were being measured. The use of the composite measure of health system attainment came under sustained scrutiny. It relied on value weights that were secured from an unrepresentative sample of respondents, and the methodology used to construct the composite measure was considered unsatisfactory by many commentators.

Making the WHO model operational required the use of advanced econometric methods. These came under intense scrutiny and the subsequent debate exposed the generally underdeveloped state of methodology for measuring comparative efficiency. Methodological concerns are compounded by the use of international data, often collected according to different protocols with differing levels of reliability.

Upon the anniversary of the publication of the *WHR2000*, Julio Frenk (2010) outlined some of the key lessons he has drawn from the experience. He highlighted specific concerns of national governments with regard to the nature of information being used by third party entities, such as WHO, in holding their governments to account, including:

- WHO should report whatever figures governments produce without correcting them;
- WHO should only use official sources of data;
- WHO should not introduce composite summary measures that most people cannot understand;
- WHO should not compare countries with each other because this can embarrass some governments;
- The data are of such poor quality that composite measures are invalid;
- WHO should not estimate missing data; and
- It is reductionist to use a single number to characterize health system performance.

The key issue emerging from such criticisms is that, whilst some of the analysis undertaken by WHO in the 2000 Report was technically questionable, the compensating benefits of the initiative have been manifest. They include: increased clarity about the need to hold governments to account for their stewardship of the health system; the importance of performance measurement as a prerequisite of such accountability; a concerted search for better data; and the recognition that evaluation should play a central role in health system reform. As highlighted by McKee (2010):

Perhaps the greatest achievement of the 2000 World Health Report was to place health systems performance on the political agenda. While some of the countries that fared poorly in the rankings simply ignored them, others commissioned research to discover reasons for their poor performance. They also asked questions of those providing health services. More generally, there are now a number of examples where seemingly poor performance compared with other countries has stimulated new policies, such as the once poor cancer survival in the United Kingdom (Abdel-Rahman et al., 2009). It is now much more difficult for a politician to dismiss comparative data on performance; perhaps this is the report's greatest legacy.

The OECD has sought to develop health system comparison in a more incremental style, based on consensus and relying on the use of widely available metrics. Veillard et al. (2009) summarize the experience, and identify the following key issues that need to be considered in establishing and monitoring cross-country performance:

- *Specifying indicators using internationally standardized definitions.* Without agreed specification, comparison is immensely complicated, and hitherto the lack of uniformity in many metrics has been notable.
- *Controlling for differences in population structures across countries.* The attainment of many health outcomes is highly dependent on the demographic structure and underlying morbidity of the populations under scrutiny. Helpful comparison can usually be achieved only after proper adjustment for differences that are beyond the control of the health system.
- *Adjusting for differences in the ability of information systems to track individual patients.* Proper calculation of many indices used for comparison (such as cancer survival rates) requires tracking patients over a period of time. National systems vary markedly in their ability to do this successfully.
- *Controlling variability of data sources.* In the same vein, there is a need to ensure that the various information sources that must be combined to construct many indicators (such as vaccination rates) are fit for purpose, and any shortcomings properly understood.
- *Identifying nationally representative data.* Data for many indicators are often available only for subsets of the population, such as selected regions or voluntary registers. Judgements must then be made about their national representativeness.
- *Determining retrospective completeness of the time series.* Many health outcomes can be properly assessed only after a considerable lapse of time. The extent to which national datasets permit proper assessment of the dynamics of health outcomes varies considerably.

Experience to date has highlighted not only the information requirements for international comparison. The need for relevant analytic capacity to understand and explain comparative data has also become manifest. Weaknesses in this area were a frequent theme from the commentary on *WHR2000*, and the detailed analytic requirements for international comparison are evident from the footnotes and caveats that accompany the OECD quality data.

Only through careful, context-specific comparison, with explanation of the reasons for variations, can comparative performance data support an intelligent benchmarking function, as frequently deployed in the corporate sector. The Commonwealth Fund *High Performing Health System* initiative has sought to promote this principle, especially at the state level. However, at the international level, it becomes more challenging to provide persuasive evidence because of the fundamental differences in the organization, governance and financing of national health systems. For example, considerable debate surrounds the inclusion of the indicator 'direct access to specialists' in the HCP annual *European Consumer Health Index*, where countries with gatekeeping systems are penalized in the performance assessment. While the HCP maintains that all gatekeeping impedes access without cost-saving, critics argue that countries should not be penalized for organizational differences in their systems (HCP, 2012).

Finally, adapting Klazinga, Fischer & ten Asbroek (2012), it is possible to summarize the requirements for persuasive health system benchmarking as follows: (1) to focus on the needs of policy-makers; (2) to respond to those needs with adaptability, flexibility and timeliness; (3) to standardize and compare the underlying data; (d) to use the appropriate presentational devices, such as report cards and graphics; and (e) to provide a careful commentary on the limitations of the comparisons being made.

3.5 Key issues for international comparison

In this section we draw out what we believe to be the key issues for the future development of international comparisons of health systems. These have been grouped under six headings, which summarize the main cross-cutting issues identified in this chapter.

Whole system or fragmentary comparison?

There is a clear tension between seeking to offer a 'single number' measure of whole health system performance and a series of fragmentary metrics that offer insights into the performance of parts of the health system. More specifically, the arguments for developing a composite indicator of performance (as distinct from separate consideration of the partial performance indicators) are that it:

- places system performance at the centre of the political debate;
- can offer a rounded assessment of system performance;
- enables judgements to be made on system efficiency;
- facilitates communication with ordinary citizens and promotes accountability;
- indicates which systems represent the beacons of best performance;

- indicates which systems represent the priority for improvement efforts;
- can stimulate the search for better data and better analytic efforts; and
- in contrast to piecemeal performance measures, which usually imply a specific means to securing improvement, offers national policy-makers the freedom to determine their own means of securing improvement.

Against this, the use of composite indicators (in preference to piecemeal scrutiny of partial performance measures) can give rise to serious difficulties:

- by aggregating individual measures of performance, a composite indicator may disguise serious failings in some parts of some systems;
- as measures of performance become more aggregate, it becomes increasingly difficult to know to what poor performance should be attributed, and therefore what remedial action to take;
- a composite measure that seeks to be comprehensive in its coverage may have to rely on very feeble or opaque data in some dimensions of performance (so, how should missing or questionable data be handled?);
- a composite measure which ignores dimensions of performance that are difficult to measure may distort the behaviour of policy-makers in undesirable ways;
- the weights used in a composite indicator reflect a single set of preferences, yet all the evidence suggests that there exists great diversity in preferences amongst policy-makers and ordinary citizens.

The experience of *WHR2000* and the subsequent debate suggest that – at this stage of measurement and methodological development – it is premature to advocate widespread use of composite measures of attainment. There was a persuasive argument in favour of WHO adopting that approach in 2000, in order to capture the attention of policy-makers and researchers, and to accelerate the debate about health system performance. However, now that the need to compare performance is established, and the associated research agenda is being addressed, the usefulness of a comparison of 'whole system' performance is open to question. In short, any global ranking of health systems is likely to be readily challenged; its usefulness for policy action will be limited; and it may distract the attention of policy-makers from the more detailed work of seeking out and remedying the parts of their system that require attention.

Development of appropriate metrics

Almost all performance metrics are summary measures that to some extent disguise many of the nuances of performance that they are seeking to capture. For example, the widely accepted indicator of life expectancy at birth may disguise quite large differences in performance for different age groups, and the ease of attaining a specific level of life expectancy depends (among many other things) on the demographic structure of the population under scrutiny. Performance measures by their nature are therefore contestable and all exhibit shortcomings of some sort.

However, this does not imply that the search for more and better metrics is futile. Rather, it argues for careful commentaries on the data and better understanding of the reasons for variations. For example, while life expectancy is on its own of limited use in assessing health system performance, work is progressing on the development of measures of avoidable mortality that may prove to be more sensitive indicators of the contribution of health systems to life expectancy (see Chapter 5). From an international comparative perspective, the crucial requirement is that such metrics should enjoy widespread acceptance and are defined in unambiguous terms that are consistent with most countries' data collection systems.

Whilst there has been steady progress in some clinical areas (such as cancer survival rates), there are many domains of health system performance where there is a need for international agreement on concepts and refinement of metrics. Most notably, responsiveness measures (such as waiting times and patient satisfaction) are in the early stages of development (see Chapter 9). There are numerous dimensions of health system responsiveness, and so far there has been little consensus on how to summarize and present the various concepts for the purposes of international comparison.

Similarly, although equity (of health or access to health services) is a well-established goal, there continues to be fundamental debate about how this might be conceptualized and measured (see Chapter 7). Equity is also linked to the fundamental goal of financial protection from the consequences of ill health, the measurement of which is underdeveloped. To date, analytic effort has concentrated on the incidence of catastrophic spending, but it is recognized that such metrics show only part of the story relating to financial protection.

The OECD quality indicators initiative has exposed the unsatisfactory development of performance indicators suitable for international comparative purposes. Many apparently relevant indicators had to be rejected for the time being because of a lack of uniformity in current specification and data collection methods. The initiative has also brought to light major gaps in the existing data collection efforts (Chapter 11).

In summary, there is clearly a major agenda to be addressed in agreeing a conceptual framework for collecting comparative information, agreeing on the domains that require measures, and specifying and agreeing those measures. Although some work can be pursued by expert collaborations (such as the *Eurocare* cancer network), it is likely that in order to be sustainable and comprehensive much of the work will have to be undertaken under the auspices of a relevant international partnership or agency.

Attribution

One of the most fundamental requirements for almost all meaningful comparisons is to determine whether observed variations can be attributed to the entities under scrutiny (the health systems) or are the result of uncontrollable external influences, such as a nation's diet. To this end, it is usually necessary to adjust for variations in the demographic, social, cultural and economic circumstances of nations. Many analyses make rudimentary adjustments for variation in demographic profiles, but more advanced progress in this area has been very limited.

A variety of statistical approaches have been used to address causality and attribution bias, such as propensity scores, instrumental variables or hierarchical models. Particular care should be taken when examining just a single snapshot (cross-section) of comparative performance. The use of time series can offer more secure inferences, but places greater demands on data availability.

A typical statistical approach is exemplified by an OECD analysis of variations in life expectancy between its Member States. A statistical model of life expectancy at birth is developed in which potential explanatory variables include measures of a nation's health care spending, educational attainment, gross domestic product, air pollution levels, alcohol and tobacco consumption, and diet (Joumard et al., 2008). The residual from this model is intended to indicate the level of efficiency of the health system. That is, after adjusting for a range of possible influences on health outcomes (including health care spending), any remaining variation is attributed to the efforts of the health system. WHO attempted a similar task for *WHR2000*, when just years of schooling were eventually used as the index of all external influences on attainment.

These examples illustrate the complexity of the attribution task. The objective is to isolate the element of measured performance that is attributable to the health system. Therefore, all external influences on (say) health outcome should, in principle, be modelled. Clearly, what is deemed an acceptable 'excuse' for poor performance must be considered to lie outside the influence of the health system, so a clear definition of what comprises the health system is an essential prerequisite for any risk adjustment. For example, does the existing prevalence of human immunodeficiency virus (HIV)/AIDS lie within or outside the control of the health system? If the former, then in principle no adjustment for it should be made when comparing health outcomes such as life expectancy.

A key decision is therefore: what is the entity under scrutiny accountable for? In the short run, for example, a health system has to deal with the epidemiological patterns and risky behaviours that it inherits. This implies a major need for risk adjustment when comparing with other health systems. In the longer run, one might expect the health system to be accountable for improving epidemiological patterns and health-related behaviour. The need for risk adjustment then becomes less critical, as the health system should be held accountable for many of the underlying causes of the measured outcomes.

Dynamic effects – current measures of future performance

Outcomes (such as mortality) are often the product of the inputs of previous years, and will not necessarily be a reflection of the performance of the current health system. Conversely, current inputs may contribute in part to future attainment. A naive comparison of current levels of attainment might ignore the *trajectory* of the health system, for example, attributing good current performance to current efforts, rather than (say) preventative programmes in the past. It is therefore, in principle, vital that any comparison of such outcomes takes into account these time lags – the comparison should be dynamic.

Issues that could be taken into account in assessing the trajectory of the health system might include: investment in physical and human capital; investment in disease prevention and health promotion; financial sustainability; governance; and trends in population risk factors. However, whilst acknowledging the importance of such issues is straightforward, it is methodologically extremely challenging to propose a convincing model that properly integrates dynamic issues into health system comparison. Rather, it is likely to be the case that – in the immediate future – health system sustainability should be measured by a series of indicators of future performance.

One example is the notion of 'effective coverage'. Shengelia et al. (2005) define effective coverage as "the fraction of maximum possible health gain an individual with a health care need can expect to receive from the health system". Effective coverage has three main theoretical underpinnings: access; utilization; and effectiveness (Shengelia et al., 2005). *Access* refers to the availability, accessibility, affordability and acceptability of health services. *Utilization* serves as a proxy for demand for health services, given access. *Effectiveness* is a function of several variables such as: efficacy of health care; the extent to which health interventions are available; inputs (quality and quantity of resources); quality assurance mechanisms; patient compliance and health behaviour; and external factors (i.e. socioeconomic and environmental factors). As an indicator, effective coverage can identify the effectiveness of current health system activities and the areas where more investment should be made in the future. It is a potentially important indicator in HSPA as it is directly linked to the health system, and can serve as an important contemporary measure of future performance.

In general, concepts such as effective coverage, risk factors and investment in human resources offer contemporary indicators of the structure and processes of health services, rather than the future outcomes they seek to achieve. This is inevitable, given the time lags involved and the need to offer a judgement on current performance. However, the risk of using structure and process indicators is that health systems are encouraged to adopt ritual responses to health problems that do not maximize the improvement in eventual outcomes. It is therefore essential that any contemporary indicators are reliably linked, through research evidence, to future performance.

Treatment of efficiency – overarching goal or just one dimension?

Measurement of productivity is a fundamental requirement for securing the accountability of providers to their payers, and for ensuring that health system resources are spent wisely. However, the areas of efficiency and productivity are perhaps the most challenging measurement area of all (see Chapter 10). Under some conceptualizations (as in *WHR2000*), it is the fundamental health system performance measure that links resources used to measures of effectiveness. Under an alternative viewpoint, it can be considered as merely one aspect of performance in a specific domain, indicating the extent to which resources deployed secure the expected levels of outcome.

The measurement of productivity can take many forms, from the cost–effectiveness of individual treatments or practitioners, to whole system productivity. Whatever level of analysis is used, a fundamental challenge is the need to attribute both the consumption of resources (costs) and the outcomes achieved (benefits) to the entities under scrutiny. The diverse methods used include: direct measurement of the costs and benefits of treatment; complex econometric models that yield measures of comparative efficiency; and attempts to introduce health system outcomes into the national accounts. The experience of *WHR2000* illustrates how difficult this task is at the macro level. Moreover, the accounting challenges of identifying resources consumed become progressively more acute as one moves to finer levels of detail, such as the meso-level (e.g. provider organizations), the clinical department, the practitioner, or – most challenging of all – the individual patient or citizen. There is a serious lack of consensus on the conceptualization of effectiveness, efficiency and productivity which must be resolved if progress is to be made.

The key question for health system comparison is whether to adopt 'efficiency' as the overarching goal of the health system, within which all comparison is to be embedded, or whether to adopt a more limited goal of offering fragmentary indicators of productivity, for example, in the form of unit costs of individual services. The advantages of the former are that it offers a coherent intellectual framework, and that many of the inputs to the health system (such as manpower) are easier to measure at the whole system level. The disadvantage is that whole system measures offer little diagnostic information on where inefficiencies are arising.

In practice, it may be most appropriate to seek to make progress in both directions. The macro indicators of performance are necessary, because of the different ways in which services can be delivered and the need to focus on whole system attainment, while the meso- and micro-indicators are needed to assess the performance of individual components of the health system.

However, the challenges of developing micro-level productivity measures should not be underestimated. The *HealthBasket* project showed that it was in principle feasible to develop measures of comparative resource use and costs of 10 common treatments across international settings. However, the study required substantial research input, and the study team was cautious in its conclusions about the feasibility of extending the work at that time. In particular, the study highlighted the need to harmonize international accounting practices and the data collection methodologies.

The other major requirement for many international comparisons of efficiency is for some sort of currency conversion. When relative input prices (such as for human resources) vary markedly between countries, it may be the case that radically different patterns of service delivery may be optimal. The conventional approach to currency conversion is to use a general PPP index. However, existing PPP metrics refer to general goods and services, and there is a clear need to develop health-specific PPP methodology along the lines currently pursed by the OECD (Huber, 2006).

Careful commentary on the limitations of the comparison

International comparison of health systems is undoubtedly an extremely powerful policy tool, and an increasingly wide range of comparative metrics is becoming available. These offer immense potential for stimulating health system improvements. However, the methodology of international comparison is at a developmental stage. Policy-makers therefore need to be made aware of both the strengths and limitations of health system comparison. Yet, hitherto, the presentation of comparisons has not always been especially helpful for policy-makers. Neither the bald presentation of league tables nor a detailed narrative of caveats is likely to guide them towards appropriate responses.

An important consideration is that many of the indicators used for international comparison contain implicit value judgements that must be brought to the attention of policy-makers. Most fundamentally, the concepts of health outcomes, disability weights, responsiveness and equity implicitly assume a certain set of values as to what constitutes the objectives of the health system, and what their relative importance is, and policy-makers at the very least need to be aware that certain value judgements have been made in the decision-making process of how indicators are selected, measured and presented.

Two types of risk arise from poor presentation of comparisons: uncritical acceptance of results and potentially costly and inappropriate reforms of the health system; or rejection of the comparisons as inadequate, and a consequent lost opportunity to reform. In either case, the key issue is the need to focus on the policy-maker's action and to ensure that it is well-informed, acknowledges the inevitable uncertainty and is proportionate.

For this to be achieved, it will usually be necessary to present indicators of health system environmental factors, functions and capacity alongside performance measures. These will assist in explaining the reported performance, and suggesting policy responses. More generally, there will always be a need to triangulate performance measure initiatives with supporting information and commentary.

In summary, the key requirements to address the needs of policy-makers are likely to be: appropriate methods of summarizing complex information; a narrative that picks out the key issues and uncertainties; a diagnosis of why the reported variations are arising; and the implications for policy action. It is nevertheless important to note that the comparisons might inform but should never be the overriding criterion for recommending policy action. National policies, values and priorities will always be prime amongst policy-makers' considerations.

Note

1 This chapter is largely based on a report prepared for the WHO Regional Office for Europe, as part of its follow-up to the Tallinn Charter on Health Systems. We would like to acknowledge the help of Ann-Lise Guisset, Manfred Huber and Jeremy Veillard.

References

Abdel-Rahman, M. et al. (2009) What if cancer survival in Britain were the same as in Europe: how many deaths are avoidable? *British Journal of Cancer*, 101(Suppl 2): S115–24.

AMIEHS (2012) *Avoidable Mortality in the European Union: Towards better indicators for the effectiveness of health systems*. Rotterdam: Avoidable Mortality in European Health Systems (http://amiehs.lshtm.ac.uk/, accessed 25 September 2012).

Anand, S. et al. (2003) Report of the Scientific Peer Review Group on health systems performance assessment, in C.J.L. Murray and D.B. Evans (eds) *Health Systems Performance Assessment: Debates, methods and empiricism*. Geneva: World Health Organization.

Arah, O.A. et al. (2003) Conceptual frameworks for health systems performance: A quest for effectiveness, quality, and improvement, *International Journal for Quality in Health Care*, 15: 377–98.

Bago d'Uva, T. et al. (2008) Does reporting heterogeneity bias the measurement of health disparities? *Health Economics*, 17(3): 351–75.

Bellanger, M.M. and Or, Z. (2008) What can we learn from a cross-country comparison of the costs of child delivery? *Health Economics*, 17(Suppl 1):S47–57.

BIRO (2012) *Best Information through Regional Outcomes: building a shared European diabetes information system*. Perugia: BIRO Coordination Centre (http://www.biro-project.eu/, accessed 26 September 2012).

Busse, R., Schreyögg, J. and Smith, P. (2008) Variability in health care treatment costs amongst nine EU countries – results from the *HealthBASKET* project, *Health Economics*, 17(Suppl 1): S1–8.

Commonwealth Fund (2006) *Framework for a high performance health system for the United States*. New York: The Commonwealth Fund.

Davis, K. (2005) Toward a high performance health system: The Commonwealth Fund's new commission, *Health Affairs (Millwood)*, 24(5): 1356–60.

ECAB (2012) *ECAB Project Overview*. London: LSE Health and Social Care (Evaluating Care Across Borders) (http://www2.lse.ac.uk/LSEHealthAndSocialCare/research/LSEHealth/7th%20Framework%20Programme%20Projects/ECAB%20Project%20Overview.aspx, accessed 26 September 2012).

ECHO (2001) *What is the ECHO Project?* Zaragoza: European Collaboration for Healthcare Optimization (http://www.echo–health.eu/, accessed 26 September 2012).

EHMA (2012) *HealthBasket*. Brussels: European Health Management Association (http://www.ehma.org/index.php?q=node/81, accessed 26 September 2012).

EPIC (2012) *European Prospective Investigation into Cancer and Nutrition (EPIC)*. Lyon: International Agency for Research on Cancer (http://epic.iarc.fr/, accessed 26 September 2012).

Epstein, D., Mason, A. and Manca, A. (2008) The hospital costs of care for stroke in nine European countries, *Health Economics*, 17(Suppl 1): S21–31.

EUCID (2008) *Final report: European Core Indicators in Diabetes project* (http://ec.europa.eu/health/ph_projects/2005/action1/docs/action1_2005_frep_11_en.pdf, accessed 16 October 2012).

EUprimecare (2012) *Quality and Cost of Primary Care in Europe*. Madrid: EUprimecare (http://www.euprimecare.eu/, accessed 26 September 2012).

EuroDRG (2012) *EuroDRG Project: Diagnosis-related groups in Europe: Towards efficiency and quality*. Berlin: EuroDRG (http://www.eurodrg.eu/, accessed 26 September 2012).

Eurhobop (2012) *European Hospital Benchmarking by Outcomes in acute coronary syndrome processes*. Barcelona: EURHOBOP (http://www.eurhobop.eu/, accessed 26 September 2012).

EuroHOPE (2012) *What is the EuroHOPE project?* Helsinki: EuroHOPE (http://www. eurohope.info/, accessed 26 September 2012).

European Commission (2004) *Strategy on European Community Health Indicators (ECHI): The 'short list'.* Network of Competent Authorities on Health Information, Luxembourg, 5–6 July 2004.

EuroREACH (2012) *EuroREACH: Improved access to health care data through cross-country comparisons.* Vienna: European Centre for Social Welfare Policy and Research (http:// www.euroreach.net/, accessed 26 September 2012).

Fattore, G. and Torbica, A. (2007) Cost and reimbursement of cataract surgery in Europe: a cross-country comparison, *Health Economics*, 17(Suppl 1): S71–82.

Frenk, J. (2010) The World Health Report 2000: Expanding the horizon of health system performance, *Health Policy and Planning*, 25(5): 343–5.

Häkkinen, U. and Joumard, I. (2007) *Cross-country analysis of efficiency in OECD health care sectors: options for research.* Paris: Organisation for Economic Co-operation and Development (OECD Economics Department Working Paper, no. 554.

Harbers, M.M. et al. (2008) *Dare to compare! Benchmarking Dutch health with the European Community Health Indicators (ECHI).* Bilthoven: National Institute for Public Health and the Environment.

HCP (2008a) *Euro Consumer Diabetes Index report.* Brussels: Health Consumer Powerhouse.

HCP (2008b) *Euro Consumer Heart Index report.* Brussels: Health Consumer Powerhouse.

HCP (2009a) *Euro HIV index 2009 report.* Brussels: Health Consumer Powerhouse.

HCP (2009b) *The empowerment of the European patient.* Brussels: Health Consumer Powerhouse.

HCP (2009c) *Euro Health Consumer Index 2009 report.* Brussels: Health Consumer Powerhouse.

HCP (2012) *Euro Health Consumer Index report.* Brussels: Health Consumer Powerhouse.

Hollingsworth, B. and Peacock, S. (2008) *Efficiency measurement in health and health care.* London: Routledge.

Huber, M. (2006) *International comparisons of prices and volumes in health care among OECD countries.* Vienna: European Centre for Social Welfare Policy and Research.

Hurst, J. and Jee-Hughes, M. (2001) *Performance measurement and performance management in OECD health systems.* Paris: Organisation for Economic Co-operation and Development Publishing (OECD Labour Market and Social Policy Occasional Paper, no. 47).

Iburg, K.M. et al. (2002) Cross-country comparability of physician-assessed and self-reported measures of health, in C.J. Murray et al. (eds) *Summary measures of population health: Concepts, ethics, measurement and applications.* Geneva: The World Health Organization.

Joumard, I. et al. (2008) *Health status determinants: lifestyle, environment, health care resources and efficiency.* Paris: Organisation for Economic Co-operation and Development (OECD Economics Department Working Paper, no. 627).

Kelley, E. and Hurst, J. (2006) *Health Care Quality Indicators project: Conceptual framework paper.* Paris: Organisation for Economic Co-operation and Development Publishing (OECD Health Working Paper, no. 23).

King, G. et al. (2004) Enhancing the validity and cross-cultural comparability of measurement in survey research, *American Political Science Review*, 98(1): 191–207.

Klazinga, N., Fischer, C. and ten Asbroek, A. (2012) Health services research related to performance indicators and benchmarking in Europe, *Journal of Health Services Research and Policy*, 16(Suppl 2): 38–47.

Mattke, S. et al. (2006) *Health Care Quality Indicators project: Initial indicators report.* Paris: Organisation for Economic Co-operation and Development Publishing (OECD Health Working Paper, no. 22).

McCarthy, D. et al. (2009) *Aiming higher: Results from a State Scorecard on Health System Performance 2009*. New York: The Commonwealth Fund.

McClellan, M.B. and Kessler, D.P. (eds) (2002) *Technological change in health care: A global analysis of heart attack*. Ann Arbor, MI: University of Michigan Press.

McKee, M. (2010) The World Health Report 2000: 10 years on, *Health Policy and Planning*, 25(5): 346–8.

McKinsey Global Institute (1996) *Health Care Productivity*. Los Angeles, CA: McKinsey Health Care Practice (http://www.mckinsey.com/insights/mgi/research/productivity_ competitiveness_and_growth/health_care_productivity, accessed 24 September 2012).

Murray, C.J.L. and Frenk, J. (2000) A framework for assessing the performance of health systems, *Bulletin of the World Health Organization*, 78: 717–30.

Murray, C.J.L. et al. (2003) Empirical evaluation of the anchoring vignettes approach in health surveys, in C.J.L. Murray and D.B. Evans (eds) *Health Systems Performance Assessment: Debates, methods and empiricism*. Geneva: World Health Organization.

Nolte, E. et al. (2008) Learning from other countries: an on-call facility for health care policy, *Journal of Health Services Policy and Research*, 13(Suppl 2): 58–64 (http://jhsrp. rsmjournals.com/content/13/suppl_2/58.short, accessed 24 September 2012).

OECD (2000) *A System of Health Accounts*. Paris: Organisation for Economic Co-operation and Development Publishing (http://www.oecd.org/health/healthpoliciesand-data/1841456.pdf, accessed 25 September 2012).

OECD (2003) Stroke treatment and care: a comparison of approaches in OECD countries, in *A Disease-based Comparison of Health Systems: What is best and at what cost?* Paris: Organisation for Economic Co-operation and Development Publishing.

OECD (2004) *Towards high-performing health systems*. Paris: Organisation for Economic Co-operation and Development Publishing.

OECD (2009) *Health at a Glance 2009*. Paris: Organisation for Economic Co-operation and Development.

OECD (2011) *Health at a Glance 2011*. Paris: Organisation for Economic Co-operation and Development.

Puentes Rosas, E., Gomez Dantes, O. and Garrido Latorre, F. (2006) Trato a los usarios en los servicios publicos de salud en Mexico [The treatment received by public health services users in Mexico], *Rev Panam Salud Publica*, 19(6): 394–402.

Rice, N., Robone, S. and Smith, P.C. (2011) Analysis of the validity of the vignette approach to correct for heterogeneity in reporting health system responsiveness, *European Journal of Health Economics*, 12(2): 141–62.

Rice, N., Robone, S. and Smith, P.C. (2012) Vignettes and health systems responsiveness in cross-country comparative analyses, *Journal of the Royal Statistical Society*, 175(Part 2): 337–69.

RN4CAST (2012) *Registered Nurse Forecasting (RN4CAST) study* (http://www.rn4cast.eu/, 26 September 2012).

Salomon, J., Tandon, A., Murray, C.J.L. and World Health Survey Pilot Study Collaborating Group (2004) Comparability of self-rated health: cross sectional multi-country survey using anchoring vignettes, *BMJ*, 328(7434): 258.

Schreyögg, J. (2008) A micro-costing approach to estimating hospital costs for appendectomy in a cross-European context, *Health Economics*, 17(Suppl): S59–69.

Schreyögg, J. et al. (2008) Cross-country comparisons of costs: the use of episode-specific transitive purchasing power parities with standardised cost categories, *Health Economics*, 17(Suppl 1):S95–103.

Shengelia, B. et al. (2005) Access, utilization, quality, and effective coverage: an integrated conceptual framework and measurement strategy, *Social Science and Medicine*, 61(1): 97–109.

Stargardt, T. (2008) Health service costs in Europe: cost and reimbursement of primary hip replacement in nine countries, *Health Economics*, 17(Suppl 1): S9–20.

Tan, S.S., Redekop, W.K. and Rutten, F.F.H. (2008) Costs and prices of single dental fillings in Europe: a micro-costing study, *Health Economics*, 17(Suppl 1): S83–S93.

Tandon, A. et al. (2003) Statistical models for enhancing cross-population comparability, in C.J.L. Murray and D.B. Evans (eds) *Health Systems Performance Assessment: Debates, methods and empiricism*. Geneva: World Health Organization.

Tiemann, O. (2008) Variations in hospitalization costs for acute myocardial infarction – a comparison across Europe, *Health Economics*, 17(Suppl 1): S33–45.

Üstün, T.B. et al. (2003) The World Health Surveys, in C.J.L. Murray and D.B. Evans (eds) *Health Systems Performance Assessment: Debates, methods and empiricism*. Geneva: World Health Organization.

Valentine, N.B. et al. (2003) Patient experiences with health services: population surveys from 16 OECD countries, in C.J.L. Murray and D.B. Evans (eds) *Health Systems Performance Assessment: Debates, methods and empiricism*. Geneva: World Health Organization.

Valentine, N.B. et al. (2009) Health systems responsiveness: a measure of the acceptability of health care processes and systems from the user's perspective, in P.C. Smith et al. (eds) *Performance measurement for health system improvement: Experiences, challenges and prospects*. Cambridge: Cambridge University Press.

Veillard, J. et al. (2009) International health system comparisons: from measurement challenge to management tool, in P.C. Smith et al. (eds) *Performance measurement for health system improvement*. Cambridge: Cambridge University Press.

WHO (2000) *World Health Report 2000. Health systems: improving performance*. Geneva: World Health Organization.

WHO (2007) *Everybody's business: Strengthening health systems to improve health outcomes. WHO's framework for action*. Geneva: World Health Organization.

WHO Regional Office for Europe (2008) *The Tallinn Charter: Health systems for health and wealth*. Copenhagen: World Health Organization Regional Office for Europe.

WHO Regional Office for Europe (2012) *PROMeTHEUS – Health PROfessional Mobility in THe European Union Study*. Copenhagen: World Health Organization Regional Office for Europe (http://www.euro.who.int/en/who-we-are/partners/observatory/activities/research-studies-and-projects/prometheus, accessed 26 September 2012).

chapter four

Benchmarking: Lessons and Implications for Health Systems[1]

Andy Neely

4.1 Introducing benchmarking: scope and definitions

There is widespread evidence that benchmarking has proved remarkably popular (Francis & Holloway, 2007). The origins of benchmarking are usually traced back to work by Xerox in the 1980s, popularized by Robert Camp in his book *Benchmarking: The search for industry best practices that lead to superior performance* (Camp, 1989). Data suggest that between 60–90% of organizations have engaged in benchmarking activities, a figure that has remained remarkably constant for over a decade (Adebanjo & Mann, 2008). For example, a CBI survey in the late 1990s put the number of UK companies involved in benchmarking at 85% (CBI, 1997), while a Bain and Company survey of the most popular management tools and techniques put the number of organizations using benchmarking at 73% in 2005 (Rigby & Bilodeau, 2005).

Traditionally, benchmarking is defined as "the search for industry best practices that lead to superior performance" (Camp, 1989). Of course, there are variants on this definition. The American Productivity and Quality Centre (APQC) define benchmarking as "the process of improving performance through continuous identification, understanding and adapting outstanding practices and processes found inside and outside the organization and implementing the results" (APQCI, 1999), while the European Foundation for Quality Management (EFQM) defines benchmarking as "the process of systematically comparing your own organizational structure, processes and performance against those of good practice organizations globally, with a view to achieving business excellence" (EFQM, 2010). Fischer provides a particularly succinct definition of benchmarking. He explains that benchmarking can create "a series of performance measures – standards known as benchmarks". Through these "a person can identify the best in class among those doing a particular task.

Then, the best practices are analysed and adapted for use by others wanting to improve their own way of doing things" (Fischer, 1994).

Implicit in Fischer's definition is a distinction between benchmarking as a process and benchmarks as targets or yardsticks. This theme of benchmarks, as opposed to benchmarking, is echoed in other definitions:

> The term benchmarking describes the overall process by which a company compares its performance with that of other companies, then learns how the strongest-performance companies achieve their results. Benchmarking is really a discovery process – discovering what truly strong performance is in a particular area of interest, which companies are getting the best results, and how they are doing so.
>
> Given this focus, companies usually seek to achieve three objectives with their benchmarking efforts: assess their current performance relative to other companies, discover and understand new ideas and methods to improve business processes and practices, and identify aggressive, yet achievable, future performance targets (Goldwasser, 1995).

Many of the standard benchmarking definitions use classic private sector language. There are, of course, definitions that have been tailored to the public sector. The UK's Cabinet Office, for example, describes benchmarking:

> as an efficiency tool ... based on the principle of measuring the performance of one organization against a standard, whether absolute or relative to other organizations. It can be used to: (i) assess performance objectively; (ii) expose areas where improvement is needed; (iii) identify other organizations with processes resulting in superior performance, with a view to their adoption; and (iv) test whether the improvement programmes have been successful. Benchmarking can be effective at all levels of operations, from the conduct of individual processes, such as invoice handling, to the operational performance of organizations with tens of thousands of staff, such as a welfare benefits delivery agency (Cowper & Samuels, 1996).

As well as the distinction between benchmarking and benchmarks, it is important to recognize the difference between benchmarking performance and benchmarking practice. Performance benchmarking concentrates on establishing performance standards (the benchmarks). Practice benchmarking is concerned with establishing the reasons why organizations achieve the level of performance that they do.

Most commentators appear to agree that benchmarking practice may be more beneficial than benchmarking performance, but benchmarking performance remains much more common than benchmarking practice. Data drawn from a variety of surveys and other sources support this assertion (see, for example, Hinton, Francis & Holloway, 2000). A study in New Zealand found that, while 48% of firms conducted benchmarking, only 2% were involved in practice benchmarking (Knuckey et al., 2000). Camp quotes the former chairman of Xerox as saying:

> the primary objective of benchmarking is understanding exemplary business practices. Four things count in benchmarking: the process on which you

focus, the organizations you visit, the best practices you find and the changes you institute. Target-setting is secondary (Camp, 1993).

4.2 Benchmarking performance and practice

The distinction between benchmarking performance and benchmarking practice is important for three reasons. First, as already mentioned, benchmarking practice is likely to be more beneficial in the long run, especially if the objective of the benchmarking process is to identify potentially beneficial organizational changes. Second, benchmarking practice treats benchmarking as a process of learning or discovery. Many commentators have pointed out that when measurement processes (including benchmarking) are used as control processes rather than learning processes they can have dysfunctional consequences (Neely & Al-Najjar, 2006). When those subjected to benchmarking think that their performance is going to be made public and compared with others, there are strong incentives for the individuals concerned to paint their own organizations in the best possible light, even if this means gaming the performance data (Smith, 1995). Third, benchmarking practice legitimizes organizational comparisons outside the norm. When Xerox wanted to improve their distribution processes they compared themselves to L.L. Bean, a mail order company. Clearly, the mail order company was not expert in producing reprographic equipment, but L.L. Bean had excellent distribution processes and it was these that Xerox wished to focus on. Comparing the organizational performance of Xerox and L.L. Bean would have been meaningless as both organizations operated in different industries, offered different products and services, and worked in different contexts. Comparing at the level of the distribution process, however, made much more sense as both organizations operated distribution processes to deliver goods and services to their customers.

Too often, particularly in the public sector, this distinction between benchmarking performance and benchmarking practice is lost. Indeed, many commentators use the language of benchmarking almost interchangeably with the language of performance – they talk about benchmarks, targets, yardsticks and performance measures as if they were all the same construct. Room (2005), for example, uses the phrase "benchmark indicators" throughout his report on progress towards the Lisbon Treaty (Room, 2005) and Wait opens her 2004 report on benchmarking by stating:

> the past decade has witnessed an explosion in the development of indicators and targets in healthcare. These data are used for comparative performance assessment within countries as well as international health system comparisons (Wait, 2004).

Clearly the individual statements these authors make are valid. There has been "an explosion in the development of indicators and targets in healthcare", but these indicators and targets are used primarily for comparison and accountability, not necessarily for benchmarking in the pure sense of "the search for industry best practices that lead to superior performance".

Why has this happened? Why is it that organizations appear to focus more on benchmarking performance rather than practice? The first reason is pragmatic. It is often easier – quicker and cheaper – to benchmark performance rather than practice. Benchmarking practice requires a much more careful investigation. If practices are to be compared, one has to explore in depth the ways in which particular activities are carried out in organizations. The level of access and the time required can be prohibitive, especially if the organization being benchmarked is identified as best in class and therefore perceives that they have little to learn from those doing the benchmarking.

Beyond the resourcing question, there are also other benefits to benchmarking performance. Particularly when there is no obvious market mechanism, benchmarking and comparing performance allows assessment to be made about the relative efficiency and effectiveness of different organizational units. Clearly, there are challenges of organizational comparability. Are health services that are offered in highly populated areas really comparable with those offered in more rural locations? Can the dietary and exercise habits of different populations be controlled for so that the organizational units being compared are competing on a level playing field? However, assuming these challenges can be overcome, then knowing what return on investment is being achieved by different hospitals and/or doctor's surgeries is valuable information. Being able to highlight to hospital A that hospital B conducts three times as many operations with the same level of resource is extremely useful. So the value of benchmarking performance should not be underestimated, but of course the question that hospital A should ask in the example mentioned above is how can hospital B conduct three times as many operations with the same level of resource? What can we learn from hospital B and what should we do differently? In order to answer that question, hospital A needs to understand hospital B's practices – hence the value of benchmarking practice.

4.3 A fundamental question: why benchmark?

Ultimately, the first question that has to be asked is 'Why benchmark?' Only when this question has been addressed is it possible to establish which form of benchmarking is most appropriate. Various authors have offered benchmarking frameworks, categorizing different forms of benchmarking. The classic distinction between benchmarking performance and benchmarking practice features in these frameworks (Trosa & Williams, 1996), but then additional forms of benchmarking are also introduced (Francis & Holloway, 2007). Camp, in his original work, for example, distinguishes between internal, competitive, functional and generic benchmarking (Camp, 1989). Internal benchmarking involves comparison between similar operations within the same organization. In competitive benchmarking the comparator organizations are the best direct competitors. Functional benchmarking is the comparison of similar processes within functions, but can involve organizations from the same or different industries. Finally, generic benchmarking involves the comparison of innovative and exemplar work processes.

A useful public sector distinction is made by Trosa and Williams who add standards benchmarking to the categories of results (performance) benchmarking and process (practice) benchmarking. Standards benchmarking involves the "setting of performance standards which an effective organization can be expected to achieve" (Trosa & Williams, 1996).

This range of options highlights the importance of first addressing the question why we are benchmarking. If the aim is to establish performance standards or yardsticks then performance benchmarking with the aim of establishing standards is appropriate. If the aim is to compare organizational units for the purposes of public information or accountability, then performance benchmarking is appropriate. If, however, the aim is to drive performance improvement, then practice benchmarking is more relevant. Deciding which of these three generic purposes of benchmarking is most important – (1) establishing standards; (2) enabling comparison and accountability; or (3) driving performance improvement – should be the first step in any benchmarking activity.

The reason the answer to this question is so important is that it has implications for the subsequent process of benchmarking. If, for example, the aim of the benchmarking activity is to establish standards, then particular care and attention has to be paid to the comparability of the organizational units that will be subject to the subsequent targets. If, on the other hand, the aim of the benchmarking activity is to enable comparison and accountability, it will be necessary to build checks and audits into the benchmarking process to ensure high-quality and valid data are being gathered. The reputational – and sometimes financial – stakes for the organizations and individuals involved are high and hence the likelihood of gaming the performance data increases. So there is a greater need to include checks and audits. Finally, if the purpose is to drive organizational change, then it may be more appropriate for the organization itself to undertake the benchmarking. This has the advantage of exposing people within the organization to new ideas and ways of working, showing them the art of the possible. Additionally, if the purpose is to stimulate organizational change, then one needs to consider how the outcomes of the benchmarking process can be adapted and adopted for the organization concerned. Rarely can one organization simply copy the practices used by another. Organizational practices are highly context dependent, often evolving over long periods of time. So, in seeking to drive performance improvement through benchmarking, a great deal of attention needs to be devoted to the change process itself. Table 4.1 expands on these themes, illustrating how the benchmarking process needs to be modified depending on the aims of the benchmarking activity.

4.4 The benefits of benchmarking

So what are the benefits of benchmarking? Through a survey of 231 government executives from 10 countries, Howard and Kilmartin (2006) identified the following reasons why governments benchmark:

1. To improve their ability to use standard metrics.
2. To assess performance objectively.

Table 4.1 Implications of benchmarking purpose for benchmarking activity

Purpose of benchmarking	To drive performance improvement	To enable comparison and accountability	To establish standards
What type of benchmarking?	Practice benchmarking	Performance benchmarking	Performance benchmarking
Who should conduct the benchmarking activity?	Self-assessment conducted by members of the organization.	Independent agency to ensure data validity.	Independent agency to ensure target validity.
How should they conduct the benchmarking activity?	When seeking to use benchmarking to drive performance improvement, it is necessary first to decide which organizational processes you are interested in improving. Often this form of benchmarking works best when applied at the level of a specific organizational process, hence the need to consider this at the outset. Second, members of the benchmarking organization have to map how they currently conduct the process they are interested in benchmarking. Third, they have to identify appropriate benchmarking partners and conduct the necessary site visits. The aim of the site visits is to establish what is different about the way the benchmarked organization conducts the process of interest. Once the site visits have been completed, the benchmarking team need to revisit their own organization's processes, deciding if and how they can be improved. Finally, the change process begins.	Initially, effort should be devoted to defining which dimensions of performance will be tracked. Clarity of measure definition and data source is essential if the results are to be valued. Second, the question of how to deal with multiple inputs and outputs has to be considered. Popular methods include data envelopment analysis and stochastic frontier analysis.	Focus on establishing which metrics matter, then search for best-in-class performers. Capture data on how well they are performing and use these data to inform targets.
How long will the benchmarking activity take?	As the description of the benchmarking process suggests, practice benchmarking to drive organizational improvement is often the most involved.	Often this form of benchmarking involves the collection and analysis of new primary data – hence it can be time-consuming.	This form of benchmarking is often the fastest and cheapest, especially when appropriate external agencies are used as they will already have access to value data.

What resources will be required?	Resources will be required to identify which metrics matter, to establish best-in-class performers, and to develop and communicate appropriate targets.	Often performance benchmarking for comparability and accountability purposes is resource-intensive, especially when new primary data have to be collected. Particularly resource-intensive parts of the process include: (i) identifying and defining metrics; (ii) primary data collection; and (iii) analysis and comparison. Each of these steps requires the involvement of skilled performance analysts.	Resources will be required throughout the benchmarking process. Many organizations establish formal and dedicated benchmarking teams to manage the benchmarking process. Given that this form of benchmarking involves organizational change, it is also essential to involve those who will be affected by the change as well as those who might block it.
What challenges will be encountered?	The key challenges will be identifying a limited, yet robust, set of metrics to focus on and establishing targets that are sufficiently stretching, but seen as achievable, especially if best-in-class comparators are drawn from other sectors.	Data availability is often the major issue in performance benchmarking for the purposes of comparability and accountability. Organizations often measure the same constructs in slightly different ways. Indeed, it is common to find different methods of measurement for the same construct in the same organization. Hence, significant time and effort needs to be devoted to ensuring consistency and comparability of data.	In practice benchmarking the biggest challenge is making the change stick. The length of the process can be problematic – as benchmarking practice is a time-consuming process the organization's priorities can shift before the process is complete. As with all change processes, the key is focus and remaining dedicated to the task.

3. To prioritize improvement opportunities.
4. To identify what offers the greatest potential return on investment.
5. To identify other organizations' superior performance processes with an eye to adopting them.
6. To test whether improvement programmes were successful (Howard & Kilmartin, 2006).

Tangible benefits reported by their survey respondents included: one-third reporting efficiency and productivity gains; one-quarter reporting measured cost improvement; and one organization that claimed to have saved $28 million in a single year.

Numerous benefits of benchmarking are proposed in the academic literature (Zairi & Al-Mashari, 2005). These can be classified in terms of:

1. Learning and innovation:
    (i) learning from others and not reinventing the wheel – if someone else has already solved the problem why waste time trying to solve it yourself?
    (ii) finding innovative and unusual solutions – 'out of the box' thinking;
    (iii) process improvement – benchmarking forces organizations to review their own processes, which can result in the identification of new opportunities;
    (iv) creating a culture of learning.

2. Accelerating change:
    (i) things can be done more quickly by adopting methods that have been tried and tested in other organizations;
    (ii) change can be enacted more quickly by convincing sceptics that things can be done differently – they see it with their own eyes;
    (iii) creating a sense of urgency – when performance gaps are revealed;
    (iv) increasing the likelihood of change and implementation, especially when the process owner is involved in benchmarking.

3. Focusing externally:
    (i) watching the competition and customers;
    (ii) encouraging the organization to look outside and learn from others;
    (iii) proactive monitoring of competition to head off new threats;
    (iv) focusing on what customers value and how to deliver it.

4. Overcoming inertia and a sense of complacency:
    (i) by showing people how good others are;
    (ii) setting stretch goals to encourage performance improvements;
    (iii) overcoming the syndrome of 'not invented here' – a commonly used benchmarking call to arms is "steal with pride".

Of course, not all organizations or benchmarking initiatives realize all of these benefits. Indeed, as well as discussing benefits, the academic literature also explores the challenges of benchmarking. These include challenges associated with data gathering; resistance to change; and resource constraints (Howard & Kilmartin, 2006).

In terms of data gathering, it is clear that many organizations find it difficult to identify other organizations with whom they can benchmark. Often, the problem is one of comparability, whether this be of organization, organizational context, or even something as prosaic as comparability of data. Organizations define and structure their processes in different ways. They choose to collect different forms of data and often work to different definitions of measure; hence, finding comparable data proves to be problematic (Guven-Uslu & Conrad, 2008).

Even if benchmarking proves possible and potentially valuable changes are identified, all the normal challenges of change management come into play. Organizations can rarely just adopt the practices used by another organization. Organizational practices tend to be highly context dependent and often evolve over significant periods of time. They cannot simply be transplanted from one setting to another (Antonacopoulou et al., 2011). It is partly for this reason that many academic commentators question the notion of best practice, arguing instead for *promising* practice (Lesure et al., 2004). At a practical level, an important contribution is that of Smith (1997), who introduces the 90–10 rule. Smith's argument is that many organizations spend 90% of their time on benchmarking and only 10% on thinking about the ensuing change process. He suggests that this ratio should be reversed, with far more effort being devoted to questions of how to make organizational change stick following benchmarking activities (Smith, 1997).

The third set of challenges – those to do with resourcing – cover both the absolute level of resourcing, as well as the question of skills. In absolute terms, benchmarking, particularly benchmarking practice, takes time and effort. Often organizations do not have the spare resources or capacity to devote to benchmarking. Even when they do, there is the question of skill and capability. There is a world of difference between visiting other organizations – somewhat disparagingly called industrial tourism – and actually seeing what other organizations are doing (Hutton & Zairi, 1995). In order to really see, and perhaps more importantly to understand, what organizations are doing takes a great deal of skill and experience. The influential differences between organizational practices are rarely easy to see. Indeed, often the influential organizational practices are deeply ingrained and can be tacit, maybe not even known to those who practise them in the organization. Hence, it takes a great deal of skill and experience to see beyond the surface and to really identify the practices that have the potential to be beneficial.

4.5 Deriving value from benchmarking

Given these challenges, it is not surprising that some organizations report that they struggle to derive value from benchmarking (Zairi & Al-Mashari, 2005). One consequence is a stream of work that seeks to explore how best to derive value from benchmarking activities. Zairi and Al-Mashari (2005) present a useful summary of this, suggesting that good practices for successful benchmarking include:

1. Senior management's strong support for the benchmarking activity. Research by the American Productivity and Quality Centre (APQC) finds that when

senior managers vigorously support benchmarking, organizations achieve operational benefits and see higher financial returns (APQC, 1995).
2. Developing a culture that actively seeks out new ideas from different sources. Often these ideas need to be adapted rather than adopted (Ammons, 1999).
3. Producing a robust business case before implementing any findings from a benchmarking study.
4. Following up on benchmarking activities by evaluating the operational and financial consequences of any changes implemented.
5. Insisting on a formal methodology for benchmarking, covering the three main elements of benchmarking – comparative analysis, new process design and implementation (Zairi, 1996).
6. Instituting a strict code of conduct, such as those suggested by APQC or EFQM. Such codes of conduct cover legal issues, as well as confidentiality, use of information and preparation.
7. Clarifying the objectives of the study at the outset: "what needs to be accomplished, which questions must be asked, which areas should be looked at" (Feltus, 1994).
8. Understanding your own processes – choosing the right benchmarking partner requires you to understand your own process first (APQC, 1995).

A particularly important theme that runs through Zairi's list, and indeed through much of the other literature, is that benchmarking is a change process. As with all change processes, engaging people in the process is essential (Goldwasser, 1995). As Goldwasser says:

benchmarking most effectively leads to bottom-line improvements if it goes beyond information exchange to include one more crucial objective: to build desire, motivation and commitment among key individuals and groups to implement significant change. It is this additional objective that changes the benchmarking effort from a learning exercise to a vehicle for change. It causes benchmarking to be managed not as an end, but as a means to an end.

4.6 Shortcomings of benchmarking

Not all of the literature is positive about benchmarking. A common criticism, especially when benchmarking against competitors, is that benchmarking only enables organizations to catch up. Copying what others do, rather than innovating for yourself, is unlikely to lead to breakthrough improvements in performance (Dervitsiotis, 2000).

Survey data suggest that organizations find benchmarking difficult to do effectively. Research by Howard and Kilmartin, for example, finds that only 22% of organizations rate themselves as very effective at benchmarking and, while 70% of organizations expected to see improvements in customer satisfaction as a result of benchmarking, only 5% claim to have seen measurable benefits (Howard & Kilmartin, 2006).

A particularly important line of critique of benchmarking lies in the literature on unintended consequences. Here, authors argue that benchmarking, especially when used as a control process, can result in organizations becoming defensive and playing the numbers game. Bowerman and Ball (2000), for example, describe benchmarking in the public sector as a defensive activity. Benchmarking becomes a process of demonstrating organizational performance. Data are collected and shared, but the organizations involved know that the game is to make themselves look good in the league tables (Bowerman & Ball, 2000).

In a particularly robust critique of benchmarking, De Bruijn and colleagues argue that benchmarking (De Bruijn et al., 2004):

1. Blocks innovation – simply copying the ideas of others does not stimulate creativity.
2. Blocks ambition – benchmarking encourages organizations to maximize their outputs and minimize their inputs. While this can be productive, there are examples where organizations seek to be selective about their inputs in an attempt to maximize their outputs. Schools and hospitals provide examples of this: schools selectively choose pupils who are likely to do well in exams because they are measured in terms of exam success, while hospitals choose patients who are more likely to survive, or patients choose hospitals with better reputations. In heart disease, for example, the difficult cases go to a small select group of hospitals, hence their survival statistics suffer, but this is because they are dealing with difficult cases in the first place.
3. Corrodes professionalism – there is a rich stream of literature on the appropriateness of different types of control systems for different roles. In roles where outputs cannot be easily observed and there is a high dependency on professional judgement, falling back on the easy to measure might be demotivating and undermine the importance of subjective professional judgement. Indeed, a study by Iaquito shows that organizations that have tried to make an effort to meet the requirements of benchmarking eventually achieve a lower performance because non-definable aspects of performance are neglected (Iaquito, 1999).
4. Corrodes system responsibility – if benchmarking results in league tables and public comparisons, the organizations subjected to these comparisons can end up competing with one another rather than sharing information. The result is that nobody takes responsibility for the system and for sharing lessons that might be beneficial to society as a whole. Fiske and Ladd (2000) illustrate this phenomenon with data on schools and show how benchmarking encouraged schools to compete rather than collaborate with one another (Fiske & Ladd, 2000).

4.7 Ensuring benchmarking has a positive impact

So how valid are these criticisms and how do we ensure that benchmarking has a positive impact? In terms of the validity of the criticisms, it is worth noting that they are based on a narrow definition of benchmarking – in essence, the critics see, with good reason, benchmarking performance as being the primary activity. The critics have good reason to take this view. As already discussed, research data show that more organizations end up benchmarking performance

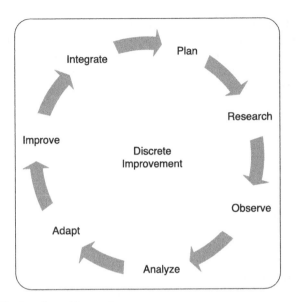

Figure 4.1 The benchmarking cycle

Source: Zairi & Ahmed, 1999.

than benchmarking practice, but this does not need to be the case. To get value from benchmarking, we need to move beyond benchmarking performance to benchmarking practice. We need to recognize that the benchmarking process is one that extends beyond the benchmarking activity itself into a change process (Francis & Holloway, 2007). Authors who have studied the benchmarking processes used in different organizations identify a reasonably consistent set of steps in successful benchmarking projects. Yellow Pages, which won the EFQM Award in 1999, has a 12-step benchmarking process, which includes: (i) ensure management commitment; (ii) process selection; (iii) select your target; (iv) process mapping; (v) start partnership selection; (vi) successful selection; (vii) preparation for the site visit; (viii) the site visit; (ix) identify practical solutions and plan actions; (x) implement; (xi) keep in touch; (xii) continuous improvement (Simpson & Kondouli, 2000). At a more aggregate level, these 12 steps are summarized in the benchmarking cycle (Zairi & Ahmed, 1999), shown in Figure 4.1.

4.8 Implications for health system benchmarking

For health system benchmarking the implications are clear. First, health benchmarks should focus on practice as well as performance. Second, they should not be used simply to evaluate and compare performance. Third, the benchmarks need to be grounded in a broader change process. Fourth, the benchmarking process itself needs to be well structured and planned, and designed to engage people in making change in their organizations. Fifth, the designers of health benchmarking systems need to consider very carefully the link between resource allocation and benchmark performance if they are to avoid dysfunctional behaviour.

Note

1 This report has been prepared for the WHO Regional Office for Europe, as part of a project on health system performance assessment, directed by Professor Peter Smith at Imperial College.

References

Adebanjo, D. and Mann, R. (2008) Sustainability of benchmarking networks: a case-based analysis, *Total Quality Management and Business Excellence*, 19(1): 107–22.

Ammons, D. (1999) A proper mentality for benchmarking, *Public Administration Review*, 59(2): 105–9.

Antonacopoulou et al. (2011) The challenge of delivering impact: making waves through the ODC debate, *Journal of Applied Behavioral Science*, 47(1): 33–52 (http://jab.sagepub.com/content/47/1/33.short, accessed 16 October 2012).

APQC (1995) *Benchmarking: Leveraging 'best practice' strategies* – a White Paper for senior management, based on *Organizing and managing benchmarking* – final report. Houston, TX: The International Benchmarking Clearing House of the American Productivity and Quality Centre.

APQCI (1999) *What is Benchmarking?* Houston, TX: American Productivity and Quality Centre (http://www.apqc.org/knowledge-base/documents/what-benchmarking, accessed 9 June 2012).

Benchmarking Exchange (2001) Do you benchmark? A short poll: Benchmarking update, *Global Benchmarking Newsbrief* (www.benchnet.com).

Bowerman, M. and Ball, A. (2000) Great expectations: benchmarking for best value, *Public Money & Management*, 20(2): 21–6.

Camp, R. (1989) *Benchmarking: The search for industry best practices that lead to superior performance*. Milwaukee, WI: ASQ Quality Press.

Camp, R. (1993) A bible for benchmarking, *Financial Executive*, July, 9(4).

CBI (1997) *Fit for the future: How competitive is UK manufacturing?* London: Confederation of British Industry.

Cowper, J. and Samuels, M. (1996) *Performance benchmarking in the public sector: the United Kingdom experience*. London: Next Steps Team, Office of Public Services, Cabinet Office.

De Bruijn, H., van Wendel de Joode, R. and van der Voort, H. (2004) Potentials and risks of benchmarking, *Journal of Environmental Assessment Policy and Management*, 6(3): 289–309.

Dervitsiotis, K.N. (2000) Benchmarking and business paradigm shifts, *Total Quality Management*, 11(4/5/6): S641–6.

EFQM (formerly European Foundation for Quality Management) (2012) (www.efqm.org, accessed 29 September 2012).

Feltus, A. (1994) Exploding the myths of benchmarking. *American Productivity and Quality Centre articles*. Houston, TX: American Productivity and Quality Centre.

Fischer, R.J. (1994) An overview of performance measurement, *Public Management*, 76(9): S2–8.

Fiske, E.B. and Ladd, H.F. (2000) *When Schools Compete. A Cautionary Tale*. Washington, DC: Brookings Institution Press.

Francis, G. and Holloway, J. (2007) What have we learned? Themes from the literature on best-practice benchmarking, *International Journal of Management Reviews*, 9(3): 171–89.

Goldwasser, C. (1995) Benchmarking: people make the process, *Management Review*, 84(6): 39–45.

Guven-Uslu, P. and Conrad, L. (2008) Uses of management accounting information for benchmarking in NHS Trusts, *Public Money and Management*, 28(4): 239–46.

Hinton, M., Francis, G. and Holloway, J. (2000) Best practice benchmarking in the UK, *Benchmarking: An International Journal*, 7(1): 52–61.

Howard, M. and Kilmartin, B. (2006) *Assessment of benchmarking within government organizations*. New York: Accenture.

Hutton, R. and Zairi, M. (1995) Effective benchmarking through a prioritization methodology, *Total Quality Management*, 6(4): 399–411.

Iaquito, A.L. (1999) Can winners be losers? The case of the Deming Prize for quality and performance among large Japanese manufacturing firms, *Managerial Auditing Journal*, 14(1/2): 28–35.

Knuckey, S. et al. (2002) *Firm foundations 2002: a study of New Zealand business practices and performance*. Wellington: Ministry for Economic Development.

Lesure, M.J. et al. (2004) Adoption of administrative innovations: a systematic review of the evidence, *International Journal of Management Review*, 5/6: 169–90.

Neely, A.D. and Al-Najjar, M. (2006) Management learning not management control: the true role of performance measurement, *California Management Review*, 48(3): 101–14.

Rigby, D. and Bilodeau, B. (2005) *Management Tools and Trends 2005*. Boston: Bain & Company.

Room, G. (2005) Policy benchmarking in the European Union, *Policy Studies*, 26(2): 117–32.

Simpson, M. and Kondouli, D. (2000) A practical approach to benchmarking in three service industries, *Total Quality Management*, 11(4–6): 623–30.

Smith, P.C. (1995) On the unintended consequences of publishing performance data in the public sector, *International Journal of Public Administration*, 18(2): 277–310.

Smith, S. (1997) Benchmarking: lessons for disciplined improvement, *IIE Solutions*, 29(19): 40–5.

Trosa, S. and Williams, S. (1996) Benchmarking in public sector performance management, in OECD, *Performance Management in Government*. Paris: Organisation for Economic Co-operation and Development (OECD Occasional Papers, no. 9).

Wait, S. (2004) *Benchmarking: a policy analysis*. London: The Nuffield Trust.

Zairi, M. (1996) A strategy for improvement, *The Benchmark*, May, 21–6.

Zairi, M. and Al-Mashari, M. (2005) The role of benchmarking in best practice management and knowledge sharing, *Journal of Computer Information Systems*, 45(4): 14–31.

Zairi, M. and Ahmed, P.K. (1999) Benchmarking maturity as we approach the millennium? *Total Quality Management*, 10(4/5): 810–16.

chapter five

Comparing Population Health

Marina Karanikolos, Bernadette Khoshaba, Ellen Nolte and Martin McKee

5.1 Why measure population health outcomes?

The 2000 World Health Report (*WHR2000*) identified three fundamental goals for a health system: improving the health of the population it serves; responding to the reasonable expectations of that population; and collecting funds to do so in a way that is fair (WHO, 2000). In this chapter, we focus on the first of these: improving population health. Before doing so, however, we summarize briefly the work that has taken place on this issue so far.

The authors of the *WHR2000* faced a challenge. They were required to estimate performance for all 191 of the WHO Member States, of which only about 60 had any data on causes of death. Consequently, the only measure of population health outcomes available to them was mortality, and even then it was necessary to produce estimates for many countries, based on empirical relationships with other measures, such as economic status (McKee, 2010). This determined their chosen definition of the health system, which they decided would include "all activities, whose primary purpose is to promote, restore and maintain health". The actual indicator used was disability-adjusted life years, which incorporated a measure of morbidity, but again this was estimated for most countries.

This approach was the only one possible given the need to include so many countries. Although controversial, it has served as a basis for many of the subsequent developments in assessing health systems performance. It was also consistent with a considerable body of previous research on the performance of countries worldwide that had also used mortality-based measures of health outcome (although more often infant and under-five mortality), which are available from *Demographic and Health Surveys* for many countries without vital registration systems.

Other research has focused on high-income countries where more data are available, creating the potential for more sophisticated analyses that take advantage of the availability of information on deaths by cause to develop indicators that more closely relate to the delivery of health care as opposed to broader social and economic factors (Arah et al., 2006). One use of these data is to measure avoidable mortality, defined as deaths that should not occur in the presence of timely and effective care (Nolte & McKee, 2004).

Although avoidable mortality is clearly an advance on all-cause mortality, it too has a number of limitations, in particular, attribution of outcomes to particular policies or interventions, as will be discussed later. It is also limited in its definition of avoidable deaths, as it tends to limit them to deaths occurring below a specified age (now typically 75), thus denying the contribution of health care to reducing mortality at older ages. This is in large part because of the difficulty of assigning a single cause of death for those dying at old age while suffering from multiple disorders. Its focus on mortality also disregards the role of health care in reducing disability and discomfort.

Other work takes advantage of data on the process of care and the outcomes of specific interventions, mostly drawn from the growing volume of administrative data in some countries. An example is the OECD's HCQI project (Kelley & Hurst, 2006).

We begin this chapter by exploring the differing definitions of a health system. We then describe contemporary usage of population health measures; the strengths and limitations of existing measures; and the methodological challenges to employing them to assess health systems performance. We conclude by exploring potential areas for further research and, specifically, the scope for using the concept of avoidable mortality and tracer conditions, both of which offer a set of complementary mechanisms to compare health systems across countries and over time. Finally, we discuss what they cannot tell us about health systems and the potential unintended consequences of using them.

5.2 What is a health system?

The scope of what constitutes a 'health system' in a given setting varies. There are many activities contributing – directly or indirectly – to improving the population's health that, in different countries, may or may not be included in what is considered to be the health system. For example, it is not always clear how much a health system can be held responsible for promoting healthy lifestyles and reducing the prevalence of risk factors in the general population. Policies that affect population health are often outside the direct control of the health system, such as tobacco and alcohol policies. In addition, the boundary with other sectors within a country can be indistinct. This is typically a problem with social care, with boundaries often being determined by diverse administrative arrangements. There are also differences in how areas such as medical education and research are dealt with in comparisons, although work on National Health Accounts seeks to address these issues.

A further complication relates to the population covered by a given system. This may be determined by financial and/or organizational arrangements exemplified by multiple systems that vary in ownership. One example is the US health system, which represents a composite of multiple subsystems, comprising a mix of overlapping public and private elements, variously covering those in employment, older people (Medicare), those at the lower or no income scale (Medicaid), military personnel (Veterans Affairs), and others. Even in countries with nearly universal coverage, privately funded subsystems are common; for example, in the United Kingdom, about 10% of the British population have private insurance to supplement their coverage by the NHS (OECD, 2004).

Elsewhere, administrative territorial divisions within countries may also challenge the definition of what should be considered to be the health system. For example, following political devolution for the constituent countries of the United Kingdom in 1999, responsibility for the NHS in Northern Ireland, Scotland and Wales was transferred to subnational governments, while the Department of Health retained oversight of the NHS in England. This has led to increasingly diverging health systems in the four countries, while the Department of Health remains responsible for UK-wide health matters, such as the control of infectious diseases, and for representing UK health policy in international and European fora.

These issues add to the complexity of comparing health systems performance internationally and help to explain why *WHR2000* adopted a broad definition of a health system, which includes "all activities and structures that impact or determine health in its broadest sense within a given society" (WHO, 2000). Arah et al. (2006) more specifically distinguished between the health system and health care system, with the former closely resembling the one adopted by *WHR2000*. In contrast, the *health care* system is defined as the "combined functioning of public health and personal health care services" that are under the "direct control of identifiable agents, especially ministries of health" (Arah et al., 2006) (see Chapter 2 for more details). A related issue concerns the boundaries with sectors such as social care, which are often determined by diverse administrative arrangements and thus may or may not be included in the definition of the health (care) system.

To some extent, the definition of the health (care) system will depend on the question being asked. While it is important to recognize the various distinctions, it is equally important to realize that, in practice, concepts are likely to mean different things to different actors and that the precise boundaries of health (care) systems remain difficult to define, although it is important to keep in mind issues relating to sectoral boundaries, ownership and geography.

5.3 Broader determinants of population health

Variation in health outcomes such as mortality is often used to explain the success or failure of health systems. However, the reasons for diversity in health patterns between and within populations are multifaceted, reflecting a complex interplay of factors, ranging from underlying economic and political circumstances to more proximal risk factors, such as lifestyle-related determinants of health, with health care also playing a role, as identified by the health field concept advanced by Lalonde (Lalonde, 1974).

Irrespective of how narrow (or broad) our definition of a health system is, it is essential to begin with an understanding of the range of influences on population health. Figure 5.1 (WHO, 2009), which is itself a greatly simplified representation of reality, indicates the complexity of interactions among different factors that contribute to the onset of, and ultimate mortality from, just one condition: ischaemic heart disease (IHD).

Some of these factors are clearly beyond the control of the health system, such as age and levels of income and education, although arguably health systems might indirectly exert influence to minimize the health impact of such factors through active engagement with other sectors in society with a more immediate impact on socioeconomic factors in particular. Similarly, changes in common behavioural risk factors for ill health, such as smoking, alcohol use and poor diet, through population-wide strategies tends to be outside the immediate control of health systems as they require close interaction and cooperation with other sectors (economy, education, etc.), although measures to address lifestyle factors such as smoking are usually, but not inevitably, initiated by

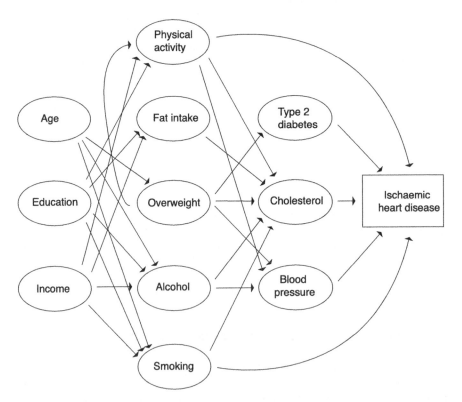

Figure 5.1 Major factors leading to ischaemic heart disease

Adapted from: WHO, 2009.

the health sector. Health professionals can also advocate for increases in taxes on cigarettes, or a ban on smoking in public places. It is equally possible to identify both individual and population-based measures to tackle the other intermediate risk factors identified in Figure 5.1.

Crucially, the health system, however broadly defined, cannot tackle these risk factors on its own; nor can it be held accountable for failure to reduce the resulting deaths that arise from a lack of action. This does not, however, absolve governments as a whole from responsibility, and it is possible to translate this model of disease causation into indicators of overall government performance on health. This is analogous to the way that commentators judge governments on their ability to achieve growth in gross national product (GNP); they are not expected to create growth directly by, for example, nationalizing manufacturing and services, but they are expected to create the conditions within which economic growth can take place. From this perspective, it is entirely appropriate to hold governments accountable for improvements in aggregate measures of health, such as life expectancy at birth, as well as for their implementation, or failure thereof, of evidence-based policies to reduce deaths from preventable causes and their corresponding risk factors. An obvious example of the latter is a ban on smoking in public places, which many European governments have introduced successfully, with rapid reductions in cardiovascular disease. However, this does not mean that a government must do everything itself. As the example in Box 5.1 shows, there is an important role for civil society, although ultimately, where others do not take action, governments must step in to advise, regulate or legislate where appropriate.

The implication of this brief discussion is that governments should be held to account for progress in the overall health of their populations, in exactly

Box 5.1   Sudden infant death syndrome prevention in the UK

In the United Kingdom, a national campaign to prevent sudden infant death syndrome (SIDS) was launched in 1991 by a voluntary organization, the Foundation for the Study of Infant Deaths, as a result of the Avon study. After attracting wide media publicity, the government responded by issuing a policy statement to health professionals, followed by a national leaflet accompanied by television and press advertising (McKee et al., 1996). Prior to this formal campaign, the Foundation for the Study of Infant Deaths had issued a press release about the Avon research (Fleming et al., 1990) showing the ninefold increase in the probability of prone sleeping among sudden infant deaths. This attracted considerable media attention and, together with the publication of research from the UK and other countries, some health professionals began to advise a change in sleeping position before the official campaign (Scott et al., 1993). A combination of several factors (accumulation of research, active voluntary group, media coverage and capacity to review health policy) resulted in an almost threefold decrease in deaths attributed to SIDS in the UK between 1990 and 1991 (FSID, 2011).

the same way as they are judged on economic progress. This must, however, be informed by an understanding of the locus of authority; there is little point in holding a national government to account for failure to implement policies that are, constitutionally, the responsibility of regional authorities.

In the next section we explore the strengths and weaknesses of various measures of population health as potential indicators of health system performance.

5.4 Common measures of population health

The most commonly used measures of population health, such as total mortality, life expectancy, premature or infant mortality, years of life lost, DALYs, capture generic information on population health. Although informative, these measures are unable to distinguish between the health care input and the contribution of other activities to population health status. This was circumvented by the adoption of a broad definition of a health system in *WHR2000* (WHO, 2000). However, as noted above, this is not a satisfactory solution.

We begin, however, by reviewing the mortality-based measures most commonly used in assessing population health. These measures have been categorized into two groups: generic and disease/age-specific indicators. This is followed by a brief overview of morbidity and summary measures, and their current and potential use for international comparisons. Table 5.1 summarizes the most common measures of population health (including broader determinants of health and risk factors), and demonstrates examples of indicators, their key methodological issues and potential policy uses.

Generic indicators

Generic indicators are used to summarize the total mortality experience in a given population over a specific period of time. The most common examples are life expectancy and age-standardized death rates (SDRs). Other indicators include less informative crude mortality rates and standardized mortality ratios (SMRs). Their greatest advantage is the availability and relative reliability of data (at least in high-income countries), as well as ease of calculation and analysis. However, the absence of data on cause of death constrains the scope to infer the contribution of health care. These indicators do not show the direct link between health system performance and population health, as they are often crude and depend on numerous other factors (Anell & Willis, 2000). As these indicators mask contributions of specific causes of death and risk factors, caution is needed when seeking to attribute observed changes to health care.

Age/disease-specific indicators

Infant mortality rate (the number of deaths in children within the first year of life per 1000 live births) is often used as an indicator of quality of health

Table 5.1 Common measures of population health

Measurement category	Indicators (examples)	Data and methodological issues	Policy uses
Mortality	Generic mortality-based indicators: – age-standardized death rates – life expectancy	• Broad indicator of health • Mask contributions of specific causes • Exclude morbidity • Need further disaggregation by age and cause	These are broad indicators of health service delivery and achievement of desired population health outcomes. While some reflect generic population health status (SDRs, life expectancy, DALYs), others (perinatal mortality, cause-specific mortality, survival, amenable mortality) allow more detailed analysis of specific outcomes of the quality of health care. Selected mortality-based indicators combined with supplementary techniques (such as tracer methodology) allow the exploration of the individual aspects of health service delivery process and highlight potential gaps and weaknesses.
	Age-specific mortality indicators: – infant, perinatal mortality	• Susceptible to variations in recording and reporting practices • Rely on precise definitions not always adhered to in practice (perinatal mortality) • Are influenced by factors outside of health system (infant mortality) • Are based on small numbers • Complex interpretation of underlying causes	
	Cause-specific mortality indicators: – age-standardized mortality from specific causes – IHD, cancer, etc.)	• Data quality and coding • Capture influence of broader health determinants • Need to be interpreted in context of risk factor and disease prevalence, and policies in other sectors	
	5-year survival: – cancer	• Variations in coverage and diagnostic practices • Lead-time bias • Need to account for staging • Has to be viewed alongside mortality and incidence rates	
	Summary measures: HALE, DALYs, YLL*	• Controversial methodology (age and disability weightings)	
	Amenable mortality	• Aggregate measure requiring further disaggregation • Variations in list of amenable causes and age limits • Time lags for outcomes of specific interventions	

(Continued)

Table 5.1 Common measures of population health (*Continued*)

Measurement category	Indicators (examples)	Data and methodological issues	Policy uses
Morbidity	General health: – health surveys data	• Reporting bias • Non-specific to healthcare interventions	At present, morbidity data are of limited use in assessing the contribution of health care to population health (see data and methodological issues), but there are great emerging initiatives to develop registries for specific conditions that focus on health outcomes and service delivery aspects.
	Incidence: – notifications	• Variations in notification requirements and diagnostic practices	
	Prevalence: – registries	• Coverage • Representativeness	
	Health service utilization: – hospital statistics	• Data quality (completeness, coding, recording) • Coverage (often excludes private sector) • Representativeness (only shows population who accessed health service)	
Risk factors	Demographic, socioeconomic, behavioural, environmental, etc.	• Completeness and comparability of data • Not always possible to measure exposure (environmental risks) • Are not under direct control of a health system	These are predictors of future population health, rather than an indicator of health system performance, as many risk factors are a product of wider intersectoral policies.

DALYs: disability-adjusted life years; HALE: health-adjusted life expectancy; SDR: standardized death rates; YLL: years of life lost.

care. Worldwide, this is more widely available than all-age mortality (and thus life expectancy) as it is often taken from surveys (especially *Demographic and Health Surveys*). However, it is a poor measure of the contribution of health care as it combines neonatal and post-neonatal deaths, which have quite different causes. In the first four weeks of life mortality is more sensitive to the quality of medical care, while post-neonatal mortality is more strongly associated with socioeconomic factors (Leon, Vågerö & Olausson, 1992), and does not necessarily reflect the overall health system performance (Mathers, Salomon & Murray, 2003).The perinatal mortality rate (the number of stillbirths and deaths in the first week of life per 1000 live and stillbirths) is also frequently used as an indicator of health systems performance. Problems affecting comparisons include: the varying application of the definition of a live birth (although supposedly standardized), especially at low birth weights; the increase in multiple births (which are at greater risk) as a consequence of new treatments for infertility; the need to consider differences in patterns of birth weight; the very small numbers of deaths now occurring in high-income countries (making rates unstable in small populations); and variation in the application of prenatal screening for congenital anomalies (often linked to policies on abortion) (Richardus et al., 1998; Garne et al., 2001; van der Pal-de Bruin et al., 2002), although one study suggested that the last of these had been of limited importance in a longitudinal study of perinatal mortality in Italy (Scioscia et al., 2007). The interpretation of apparent differences among countries and over time is therefore problematic (Nolte & McKee, 2004).

Turning to older ages, age-standardized mortality rates by cause are easy to calculate and reliable data are available for all high- and many middle-income countries. However, despite the existence of a standardized system of disease classification (the International Classification of Disease (ICD)), some caution is required in both longitudinal and cross-sectional studies. First, there may be differences in interpretation of coding rules, especially those involving the treatment of multiple causes. These can change during the course of an ICD version. Second, although the classification is revised regularly, there may be interim changes, such as the introduction of codes for human immunodeficiency virus (HIV) disease during the 1980s when ICD-9 was used in most countries. Finally, different countries switch to new versions at different times and there may be differences in the effects of change among countries, making it necessary to undertake bridge coding exercises whereby a set of death certificates are coded using both old and new versions and then compared. Other issues include completeness of registration of deaths and, more often, of the population denominator, a growing problem with more mobile populations.

An example of a disorder that has been examined as an indicator of health care quality is IHD, one of the most frequent causes of premature mortality in industrialized countries (Nolte, Bain & McKee, 2009). It has been estimated that about 40–50% of the total reduction in IHD in Western countries can be attributed to improvements in specific medical interventions (Beaglehole, 1986; Kesteloot, Sans & Kromhout, 2006) with the remaining decline attributed to the decrease in prevalence of risk factors, such as smoking, high cholesterol and hypertension (some of which can also be attributed to medical intervention) (Bots & Grobbee, 1996; Ford et al., 2007). However, cross-national comparisons of mortality rates from IHD have to be interpreted in the context of policies in other sectors (such as agriculture, which influences traditional dietary patterns) and of cultural differences (in diet, for example), which influence the levels of prevalence and risk factors in specific populations (Box 5.2). Thus, the complex epidemiology of IHD means that this indicator on its own may not necessarily identify weaknesses in health care, but may also capture other environmental and socioeconomic factors. Persisting high levels of mortality from IHD usually indicate systematic problems that cover the entire course of the disease – from primary prevention and health promotion to treatment.

In those cases where there are data on incidence and mortality, it is possible to calculate disease-specific survival. This is the average length of time that individuals survive following diagnosis. Survival rates are most frequently applied to cancer and have been influential in international and longitudinal

Box 5.2 Explaining differences in mortality trends from IHD

We have previously shown how the contribution of health care to changes in deaths from IHD remains contested and can be difficult to ascertain (Nolte, Bain & McKee, 2009). This can be illustrated by comparing research from the German Democratic Republic and Poland, both of which experienced substantial, and similar, declines in mortality in the 1990s (Nolte et al., 2002).

In Poland, this improvement has been largely attributed to changes in diet, with increasing intake of fresh fruit and vegetables, and reduced consumption of animal fat (Zatonski, McMicheal & Powles, 1998). The authors of that study judged the contribution of health care to be negligible. In contrast, the WHO MONICA project found a considerable increase in the intensity of treatment of acute coronary events in Poland between 1986–89 and the early 1990s (Tunstall-Pedoe et al., 2000). Yet a further complication is that a much higher proportion of deaths from IHD in Poland are sudden, compared with western European countries, so limiting the scope for health care to make a difference in the acute stage. This is a phenomenon that has also been noted in the neighbouring Baltic States and Russian Federation (Uusküla, Lamp & Väli, 1998; Tunstall-Pedoe et al., 1999) and has been related to binge drinking (McKee et al., 2001).

The eastern part of Germany also experienced a substantial decline in mortality from IHD but here research has focused more on health care. There is evidence of intensified treatment of cardiovascular disease during the 1990s (for example, an increase in cardiac surgery of 530% between 1993 and 1997 (Brenner, Altenhofen & Boqumil, 2000). Although this may not necessarily translate into improved survival (Marques-Vidal et al., 1997), there has been a (non-significant) increase in the prevalence of those with a history of myocardial infarction among east Germans aged 25–69 years between 1990–92 and 1997–98 which, given the accompanying decline in mortality from IHD, suggests that there has been improved survival (Wiesner, Grimm & Bittner, 1999).

comparisons. However, there are a number of issues that must be taken into account. First, coverage by cancer registries is limited in many countries, either geographically (covering only certain regions in much of Europe (Coleman et al., 2008)) or in other ways (the American Surveillance Epidemiology and End Results (SEER) system systematically under-represents the African-American population with their poorer outcomes (Mariotto, Capocaccia & Verdecchia, 2002)). Second, calculation of survival is critically dependent on consistent approaches to diagnosis. Countries with extensive screening activities will inevitably detect cases earlier but, if this confers no survival benefit (as with prostate cancer), the survival will seem longer although the time of death is unchanged (lead time bias) (Desai et al., 2010). Countries with weak linkage systems may have a high proportion of Death Certificate Only cases, in which first registration takes place at death. This may artefactually shorten recorded survival. Ideally, stage at diagnosis is recorded to facilitate adjustment for some of these factors, but such data are often unavailable. Nonetheless, cancer survival data, if interpreted suitably cautiously, can offer insights into various aspects of cancer service quality: timeliness, technical competence and adherence to protocols (Jack et al., 2003).

International comparisons of cancer survival have shown substantial differences in performance among European countries (Verdecchia et al., 2007), suggesting variations in quality of care. However, this poses the question of why. Thus, it has been suggested that historically relatively poor cancer survival rates in the United Kingdom and Denmark may be because the gate-keeping function of primary care delays access to specialist investigation (Crawford, 2010) but also that there may be high levels of stoicism among the population, leading to late presentation (Anderson & Murtagh, 2007). This issue is not, however, resolved.

Dickman and Adami (2006) noted that, "in order to evaluate progress against cancer one must simultaneously interpret trends in incidence, mortality and survival" as none of the three measures is fully interpretable without knowledge of the other two. An example of combining this information is a recent study by Coleman et al. (2011), which shows how rapid improvements in survival following breast cancer in the United Kingdom, despite increasing incidence, are associated with an overall reduction in mortality (Figure 5.2).

Measuring morbidity

One of the principle limitations of the measures discussed above is their focus on mortality. One attempt to circumvent this was the work of Bunker, Frazier & Mosteller (1994) that assessed the "magnitude of relief in treated patients" with a range of conditions (unipolar depression, osteoarthritis, terminal cancers, asthma, cataract, etc.). They constructed a symptomatic measure of relief based on the incidence of each condition, the average age of those suffering from them, the number of treated patients, and the expected years of survival, into which they factored the years of disability prevented by therapeutic intervention (Bunker, 2001). The overall measure of improved physical or mental function, or prevented pain and suffering, is expressed in "potential years of relief

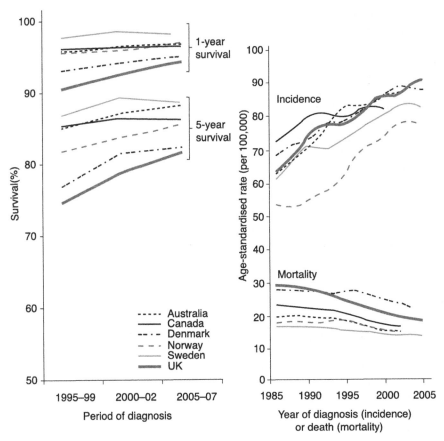

Figure 5.2 Breast cancer survival, incidence and mortality in Australia, Canada, Denmark, Norway, Sweden and the UK

Adapted from: Coleman et al., 2011.

per 100 patients". On average, the interventions achieved relief from approximately five years of poor quality of life per individual (Bunker, 2001). Although providing different and potentially useful results, this technique is based on the inventory approach for mortality described in the next section, and thus is subject to the same methodological problems (Nolte, Bain & McKee, 2009).

The main measures of morbidity are derived from self-reporting of perceived health status in population health surveys. Examples include the *World Health Survey, European Core Health Interview Survey* and various national surveys, such as the *Health Survey for England* and *US National Health Interview Survey*. These typically include a question on self-rated health (usually on a five-point scale, but sometimes on a four-point scale) but the results are not specifically related to health care interventions. They are also subject to potential bias, as those with higher expectations of health often record their health as worse than those with lower expectations, even when they are similar on objective measures. This can, however, be addressed by the use of anchoring vignettes, in which respondents are asked to allocate a health status to an imaginary subject with a specified level of disability (King et al., 2004). While several countries have instituted regular surveys using relevant instruments, data are not necessarily comparable with similar surveys undertaken elsewhere, in particular when the data collection instrument cannot ensure cross-cultural equivalence. Where cross-national comparable instruments have been employed, these frequently tend to cover only a few countries, often building on small samples of uncertain representative power in participating countries. Elsewhere, surveys are not undertaken regularly, or perhaps only once, so data tend to become outdated (Nolte, 2010). Surveys also include a variety of disease-specific measures, some of which may be attributable to health care, such as blood pressure diagnosis and control. Within Europe, the New European Health Survey System (EHSS) promises to be a valuable source, while the *Survey of Health, Ageing and Retirement in Europe* (SHARE), along with the English Longitudinal Survey of Ageing, with which it is compatible, provide valuable data on older people. More detailed discussion of population-based surveys is provided in Chapters 7 and 11.

In some limited cases, the incidence of specific diseases may be useful in comparing health system performance. Thus, the OECD HCQI project includes the incidence of vaccine-preventable diseases (pertussis, measles, hepatitis B) in its set of indicators. The rationale for this is that the incidence of these diseases should be minimal in the presence of appropriate health care intervention (immunization). Variations in notification requirements and prevention practices can affect incidence rates for these conditions.

Routinely collected data on health service utilization, such as inpatient admissions or number of general practitioner (GP) consultations, while often cited as measures of performance, have a limited value. They are often based on unrepresentative samples of activity; may say only a little about those in need of care but not receiving it; and take no account of whether the activity is necessary.

Finally, there are a number of population-based disease registries, although typically established within the framework of research projects. However, not all registries cover entire populations or all population groups (see cancer survival above). In some cases these may be part of international initiatives so that the data are, to some extent, comparable across countries. They may also be quite unrepresentative of the countries in which they are located as they are likely to be based on centres of excellence.

Summary measures

Death rates in industrialized countries have now fallen to historically low levels, giving rise to ageing populations, often with substantial levels of disability. This has led to efforts to combine mortality and disability, with measures such as health-adjusted life expectancy (HALE) and DALYs. The advantage of summary indicators is their ability to combine the key elements of adverse health outcomes – mortality, morbidity and disability. Typically, summary measures of health are divided into two broad categories: health expectancies and health gaps.

Health expectancy is a measure of how long people can expect to live free of certain diseases or limitations to their normal activities (active life expectancy, disability-adjusted life expectancy, health-adjusted life expectancy, etc.). With this measure, less weight is assigned to years lived in less than full health. Healthy life expectancy has been used to establish the relationship between population health and health system inputs in 191 countries (Evans et al., 2001). A recent report of the Commonwealth Fund used healthy life expectancy at age 60 as one of three measures of productive and healthy lives in seven OECD countries (Australia, Canada, Germany, Netherlands, New Zealand, UK and the United States) as one of the measures demonstrating the ability of a health system to ensure long and healthy lives (Davis, Schoen & Stremikis, 2010).

Health gaps quantify the difference between a designated norm for the population (e.g. 75 years in good health) and actual levels of health. These are usually expressed as years of life lost (YLL), which do not include years lived with disability, or DALYs, which do.

The latter involve applying a weighting to years lived with disability so as to reduce their value. This is typically done in one of three ways. The first is the time-trade-off, in which respondents are asked to choose between remaining in a state of ill health for a period of time or being restored to perfect health but with a shorter life expectancy. The second is the standard gamble, where they are asked to choose between remaining in a state of ill health for a period of time or choosing an intervention which may either restore them to perfect health or kill them. The third is the visual analogue scale, in which they are asked to rate a state of ill health on a scale from 0 to 100, with 0 representing death and 100 representing perfect health. Other refinements include placing a higher value on a year of life lived at certain ages (typically between 10 and 55) and a lower value in childhood and old age. The advantage of this approach is "to combine information on mortality and non-fatal health outcomes to represent the health of a particular population as a single numerical index" (Murray & Salomon, 2002).

Key methodological issues facing those using summary measures of health status relate to conceptual differences in the approaches taken and data limitations (Etches et al., 2006). The definitions, measurement and weighting of disability as applied to particular health states are complex and have long been controversial. For example, some commentators have expressed ethical concerns about the way this methodology places a value on life (Gold, Stevenson & Fryback, 2002), exemplified by its use in the Global Burden of Disease project (Lopez et al., 2006).

A further issue, when extended beyond high-income countries, is that mortality data may not be available. In these cases, health outcomes are modelled based on known associations between mortality and other, typically economic, variables. All of these mortality-based measures of population health provide valuable information on the overall progress of nations but say relatively little about the contribution of health care.

At present, comparable health status data are not available for all countries, so existing summary measures of population health are typically based on estimates of the prevalence of various health states (Mathers et al., 2003). This makes it difficult to assess trends over time, as any observed variation may simply reflect changes in data used to generate estimates. Thus, where levels of health are modelled using equations incorporating economic measures, booms or busts can create artificial changes in estimates of life expectancy or disease burden. A New Global Burden of Disease (2010) Study aiming to provide more continuity at corporability to health data across the globe and addressing some of the issues raised in preceding versions were released at the end of 2012.

Most of the indicators mentioned above are available in the public domain, from the WHO (European Health for All database, Global Health Observatory, Global Mortality Database), World Bank (World Development Indicators) or European Commission (Eurostat) websites.

In summary, mortality-based measures of population health are attractive due to their availability and accuracy, particularly for high-income and most of the middle-income countries. The data needed to construct generic mortality indicators are readily accessible in high-income countries and indicators are easy to calculate. Age/disease-specific rates can potentially indicate weaknesses in the health system. Morbidity data are generally less widely available or consistent, often relying on self-reporting and over-representing those who actively seek care. Summary measures of population health combine both mortality and morbidity information; however, the methodology (DALY weightings of health states and age) and validity of measures of health system performance remain controversial. Thus, of the common measures of population health, such as mortality (infant, perinatal, total), life expectancy, morbidity, or summary derivatives, only a select few are able to distinguish the components of the overall burden of disease that are attributable to health systems and those which result from factors arising elsewhere, while disease-specific indicators, such as mortality from IHD or cancer survival rates, can only reflect isolated elements of the overall service. Consequently, assessment of the performance of health care requires identification of the indicators of population health that directly reflect health care (see section 5.6). Differences in data collection and registration practices need to be understood when comparing these indicators across countries or time.

5.5 The contribution of health care to population health

There has been long-standing debate about whether health services make a meaningful contribution to population health (McKee, 1999). In the late 1970s, several authors argued that health care had contributed little to the observed decline in mortality that had occurred in industrialized countries over the preceding century or so. Among them was Thomas McKeown, who showed how much of the decline in mortality from tuberculosis (TB) in England and Wales between 1848–1854 to 1971 predated the introduction of immunization and effective chemotherapy (McKeown, 1979). He explained this decline by factors acting outside the health care sector, such as improvements in living conditions, behavioural change and, most importantly, changes in nutrition (McKinlay & McKinlay, 1977; Cochrane, St Leger & Moore, 1978; McKeown, 1979). Others, such as Illich, argued that developments in health care in the 1950s and 1960s were actually damaging to population health, introducing the term iatrogenesis (physician-produced disease) (Illich, 1976). Illich was especially concerned with the role of medicine as a form of social control.

Recent writers have taken a more nuanced approach. They have noted how there has been a revolution in the therapeutic armamentarium since the 1960s. Thus, Mackenbach showed how the rate of decline in infectious disease mortality doubled in the Netherlands after the introduction of antibiotics in 1946, while mortality rates from common surgical procedures and perinatal conditions improved markedly after the 1930s (Mackenbach, 1996). However, even McKeown's example of TB has been revisited, with more recent work attributing part of the reduction in mortality that predated the introduction of antibiotics to public health interventions, such as the segregation of patients with active disease (Fairchild & Oppenheimer, 1998). Furthermore, a study of changes in age-specific mortality showed how, although the acceleration in the overall death rate was small, the first 10 years after introducing chemotherapy (1945–1955) were marked by striking year-on-year reductions in TB mortality rates among young people in England and Wales (Nolte & McKee, 2004).

At present, therefore, there is a general consensus that, while McKeown and others were broadly correct in pointing to a relatively limited role of curative medical measures in mortality decline prior to the mid-20th century (Colgrove, 2002), the scope of health care and its contribution to population health has progressed dramatically since the mid-20th century. Advances in the pharmaceutical and technology sectors have transformed acute fatal diseases into treatable or manageable conditions (such as infectious diseases and type 1 diabetes). These developments, along with more effective ways of organizing health care (such as introducing multidisciplinary stroke units or integrated screening programmes) and the implementation of evidence-based medicine, have ensured a growing contribution of the health care sector to population health.

This raises the question of how to quantify the contribution of health care to reduced mortality. This is rarely straightforward. In some cases, the impact of health care is self-evident: examples include vaccine-preventable diseases, antibiotic treatment of acute infections and the introduction of insulin for type 1 diabetes. However, more often, the impact of health care is less easily quantifiable. Thus, in the last 30 years, there have been substantial reductions in mortality from many chronic diseases; while health care has contributed to these reductions, there have also been declines in exposure to many common risk factors and, thus, the incidence of disease.

We begin by examining the key approaches that seek to quantify the contribution of health care to population health. These are the inventory approach and the production function approach (Buck, Eastwood & Smith, 1999; Nolte & McKee, 2004). Two others – avoidable mortality and the use of tracers – are described in more detail later in this chapter.

The inventory methodology examines selected health services and their influence on the burden of disease in a target population. McKinlay and McKinlay (1977) noted that much of the decline in mortality in the United States between 1900 and the early 1970s was due to falling deaths from infectious disease, and that at least some of this must have been attributable to medical interventions such as antibiotics and vaccines. They then calculated, for 10 infections, the contribution to the overall mortality decline since 1900 made by reductions in deaths from these infections occurring after the relevant interventions had been introduced. As most of these interventions came about when death rates had already fallen substantially, they estimated that the interventions had contributed only about 3.5% of the total mortality decline. They rejected the idea that there were interventions that might have contributed to falls in any chronic diseases. More recent work by Bunker et al. (1994) sought to quantify the contribution of individual medical interventions to life expectancy and quality of life in the United States between 1950 and 1989, combining published evidence on the effectiveness of specific clinical preventive and curative interventions and data on the prevalence of the corresponding diseases. They estimated that about half of the 7–7.5 year gain in life expectancy observed could be attributed to these activities (Bunker, 2001). A different methodology was adopted by Wright and Weinstein (1998), stratifying the population into those with average or elevated levels of disease risk and those with established disease, and then measuring the impact of preventive and therapeutic interventions on gains in life expectancy. For instance, they estimated that a reduction of cholesterol to 200 mg/dl would result in between 50 to 76 months' gain in life expectancy in a 35-year-old person with elevated cholesterol (>300 mg/dl). In comparison, quitting smoking in a 35-year-old at average risk of cardiovascular disease would yield a 8 to 10 month gain in life expectancy. Cutler and McClellan (2001) looked at the cost of providing improved care, analysing the contribution of technology to five selected conditions and finding that four of them (heart attack, low birth weight, depression, cataracts) had yielded net monetary benefits.

Analyses based on an inventory approach provide essential information about the potential contribution of health care to population health. However, they rest on the assumption that the health gains reported in clinical trials translate directly to the population level (Nolte et al., 2011). This is not necessarily the case (Britton et al., 1999) as trial participants are often highly selected groups, typically excluding elderly people and those with comorbidities, even though these groups often dominate the population that will require treatment. Also, evaluations of individual interventions fail to capture the combined effects of integrated individualized packages of care (Buck, Eastwood & Smith, 1999), or indeed of the entire system, on population health. These findings thus provide only a partial insight into what health systems actually achieve in terms of health gain or how different systems compare (Nolte, Bain & McKee, 2009).

One other method is the production function approach. This typically uses regression analysis to examine how health care inputs (and other explanatory variables) affect a specific health measure (outputs). The findings of such analyses have produced mixed results. Earlier work failed to identify strong and consistent relationships between health care indicators (such as health care expenditure or number of doctors) and health outcomes (such as infant mortality rate or life expectancy), but found socioeconomic factors to be powerful determinants of health outcomes (Martini et al., 1977; Kim & Moody, 1992; Babazono & Hillman, 1994). However, more recent work suggests alternative conclusions. Significant inverse relationships have been established between health care expenditure and infant and premature mortality (Crémieux, Ouellette & Pilon, 1999; Or, 2000; Nixon & Ulmann, 2006), and between the number of doctors per capita and premature and infant mortality, as well as life expectancy at age 65 (Or, 2001).

A related methodology involves comparisons of the ways in which health care systems are organized. A study by Elola, Daponte and Navarro (1995) categorized 17 health systems in Europe into National Health Service (NHS) systems (such as Denmark, Ireland, Italy, Spain and the United Kingdom) and social security systems (such as Germany, Austria and the Netherlands). This analysis concluded that countries with NHS systems achieve lower infant mortality rates than those with social security systems at similar levels of gross domestic product (GDP) and health care expenditure. On the other hand, van der Zee and Kroneman (2007) conducted a longitudinal analysis of trends in Europe from 1970 onwards. Their results suggest that the relative performance of the two types of system changed over time and that social security systems have achieved slightly better outcomes (in terms of total mortality and life expectancy) since 1980, when inter-country differences in infant mortality became negligible. The myriad of other factors involved makes such analyses almost impossible to interpret.

All these approaches have obvious limitations arising from data availability and reliability. However, the production function approach also fails to take account of lagged relationships, as noted by, for example, Gravelle and Blackhouse (1987). An obvious example is cancer mortality, where death rates often reflect treatments undertaken up to five years previously. Their cross-sectional nature is ill-equipped to address causality adequately, and such models often lack any theoretical basis that might indicate what causal pathways may exist (Buck, Eastwood & Smith, 1999). The complex pathway between increased inputs and health outcomes also means that there are likely to be many unrecognized confounders. Analyses undertaken so far tend to lack a sound theoretical basis and, in particular, provide little insight into the mechanisms involved. However, the greatest problem is that the majority of studies of this type employ indicators of population health (for example, life expectancy and total mortality) that are influenced by many factors outside the health care sector. These include policies in sectors such as education, housing and employment, where the production of health is a secondary goal. This raises concern that the observed relationships are due to confounding. An example of the potential pitfalls is provided by the fall in infant mortality in the two formerly divided parts of Germany in the 1990s that, on closer inspection, can be seen to be due to a fall in neonatal mortality in the east (most likely due in large part to improved health care) and in post-neonatal mortality in the west (which has different causes) (Nolte et al., 2000).

5.6 A way forward

The reason why the measures discussed in the previous sections are so often used for performance measurement is because they are available. It is important to ensure that any new performance indicators are driven by what is theoretically meaningful, rather than simply available. As has been noted previously, the fundamental role of performance measurement is to provide the necessary information to support health system improvement (Smith, 2009). Capturing the differences in health system performance in a systematic and comparable way requires other approaches.

The next section of the chapter will discuss two complementary approaches – avoidable mortality and tracers, which have been used in recent years to capture information on different aspects of health systems.

Avoidable mortality

The concept of avoidable mortality was initially developed by Rutstein in the 1970s. It is based on a notion that certain deaths should not occur in the presence of timely and effective medical care (Rutstein et al., 1976). Later, Charlton et al. (1983) proposed a list of specific conditions amenable to health care. In time, this evolved to reflect new epidemiological research and advances in medical care. The concept was adopted by a wide range of researchers in Europe in the 1980s and early 1990s, as it was seen as a potential tool to assess the performance of health systems. The publication of the *European Community Atlas of Avoidable Deaths* and its subsequent editions in 1988, 1991 and 1997 served as a major stimulus for a series of analyses at national level across many of the high-income countries (Nolte & McKee, 2004).

This is, however, an area where there has been some confusion about terminology (Kamarudeen, 2010). Avoidable mortality, in its broadest sense, includes deaths considered to be avoidable by appropriate and timely medical care, as well as those preventable by population-based interventions. 'Amenable mortality' is often considered to be a subset of avoidable mortality, including only those conditions directly amenable to health care, "from which it is reasonable to expect death to be averted even after the condition develops" (Nolte & McKee, 2004). In contrast, 'preventable' deaths are usually taken to include deaths from conditions that can be prevented by population-based interventions but where the contribution of health care may be limited once the condition has developed. Examples include lung cancer, alcoholic liver disease and suicides. These can, however, be used as an indicator of overall government performance, as noted above.

In 2004, Nolte and McKee undertook a systematic review of the work on avoidable mortality then available, revised the list of causes of death considered to be amenable to health care, and applied this to 12 EU countries (Nolte & McKee, 2004). They adopted a definition of a health system that covered primary and hospital care, as well as primary and secondary prevention (including immunization and screening). The objective was to investigate the impact of health care on changing patterns of mortality and life expectancy in the 1980s and 1990s. Since the 1980s, all countries examined had experienced an increase in life expectancy, although the pace of improvement varied. For most of these countries, the greatest reductions in amenable mortality were achieved in the 1980s. During the 1990s, the decline slowed, particularly in the countries where mortality from amenable causes was already low, as in Northern

Europe. However, even there, amenable mortality still continued to fall, albeit at a slower pace.

Newey et al. (2004) demonstrated similar results for the older members of the EU. Notably, most of the countries that had joined the EU in 2004 experienced relatively small reductions in amenable mortality in the 1990s, at a time when their health systems were undergoing major reconfiguration, but the authors (correctly) predicted that several would begin to close the gap in the 2000s, once the major structural and economic reforms had become embedded.

In a subsequent analysis of 19 industrialized countries between 1997–1998 and 2002–2003 (Nolte & McKee, 2008), the largest reductions in amenable mortality were seen in many of the countries with the highest initial levels. However, the United States experienced hardly any reduction from its initial high level, so that it increasingly lagged behind other industrialized countries.

Other research by the same authors has shown how the USSR lagged increasingly far behind western Europe from the mid-1960s onwards, reflecting its failure to modernize its health care system to address the rising tide of chronic diseases (Andreev et al., 2003), while another study showed the acceleration in the rate of improvement of amenable mortality in China, Taiwan following the introduction of national health insurance in the 1990s (Lee et al., 2010). The importance of health care was also apparent from an analysis of trends in amenable mortality in New Zealand (Tobias & Yeh, 2009). This concluded that, over the preceding 25 years, improvements in health care contributed approximately one-third to the overall improvement in life expectancy. Together, these findings support the notion that improvements in access to effective care have a measurable impact in industrialized countries, and that the concept of amenable mortality may provide a valuable indicator of health system performance overall.

The precise composition of lists of causes deemed amenable to health care may not be of great importance. This is the conclusion of a recent report by the OECD (Gay et al., 2011) that compares the impact of two slightly different lists, by Nolte and McKee (2008) and Tobias and Yeh (2009). As Figure 5.3 shows, both produce similar results.

Amenable mortality does, however, suffer from a number of limitations. As an aggregate measure, it summarizes a wide range of causes of death, each reflecting different aspects of the health system. It is therefore necessary to break down the overall figures by cause and age to understand what is driving any change. This may be difficult where there are small numbers in particular groupings, as will be the case in all but the largest countries. Indeed, this is an increasingly important problem as deaths from many causes in those aged under 75 reach very low levels.

Second, aggregate data conceal variations within populations, which can be divided according to geographic, ethnic, socioeconomic and other parameters. Improvements for one group may conceal deteriorations for others (Nolte & McKee, 2008).

There are, however, some more fundamental problems with the concept that must be addressed (Nolte & McKee, 2004). One is the variable lag between

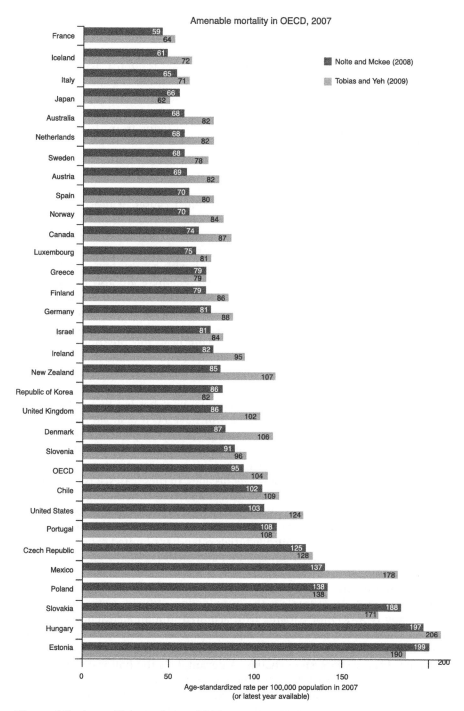

Figure 5.3   Amenable mortality in OECD countries, 2007

Adapted from: Gay et al., 2011.

medical intervention and mortality. In some cases this will be instantaneous, as in the case of resuscitation following cardiac arrest. Here, the outcome can reasonably be attributed to intervention in the same year. However, cancer survival is measured after five years and, while there is often a sharp reduction in survival at the time of treatment, there is a slower decline over several years. Thus, a death may be attributable to treatment decisions up to five years previously. In other cases the lag may be much longer. *Helicobacter* eradication therapy in a young person may save them from dying from stomach cancer several decades later.

Another concern is the changing incidence of disease. Deaths from amenable causes will decline if the incidence is falling regardless of any change in health care, and vice versa.

The original list of amenable causes included causes of death that could be prevented entirely by health care as well as those from which some deaths would be inevitable but this number could be minimized. The former is exemplified by vaccine-preventable diseases such as measles; the latter by IHD, where even in the best performing health care system, there will be some sudden and unobserved deaths. However, there are also many causes of death not considered to be amenable where, in some circumstances, health care can be life-saving. This is true of many cancers for which a small proportion may be identified early making curative treatment possible. An example is cancer of the pancreas. This begs the question what proportion of deaths from a specific cause should be preventable in order for the cause to be considered amenable. This issue has previously been addressed only implicitly.

One approach to doing so is to determine what has led to a reduction in avoidable deaths. In some cases, there will have been a single intervention. The term 'magic bullet' recalls the dramatic benefits of penicillin when it was first given to patients with severe staphylococcal infections in the 1940s. More often, health care will prevent deaths through a combination of interventions introduced incrementally, perhaps over decades. In these cases, it is necessary to look at changes in death rates over considerable time, introducing the problem of attribution as it is necessary to exclude other explanations for observed changes. This is, however, complicated by the limited evidence available. As noted above, randomized controlled trials often have limited external validity, as they frequently exclude both children and older people; those with comorbidities; and, historically, women. Hence, it will often be necessary to draw on natural experiments where it is possible to determine when new treatments were introduced. An example is the introduction of highly active antiretroviral therapy (HAART) for patients with acquired immunodeficiency syndrome (AIDS), where death rates fell very rapidly. In other cases, even where detailed data are unavailable, it may be possible to infer the impact of health care where there has been wider system change. An example is the political transition in Eastern Europe around 1990. The opening of borders to modern pharmaceuticals and ideas of evidence-based medicine made it possible to provide treatment that had been previously denied to sufferers from many chronic diseases. Thus, in countries such as Estonia, there was a rapid decline in mortality from stroke, almost certainly as a result of better treatment of hypertension, at a time when such deaths were increasing in the neighbouring Russian Federation. It may also be necessary to look at historical evidence: conditions such as acute appendicitis became amenable to health care once the introduction of asepsis and anaesthesia made intra-peritoneal surgery possible in the late 19th century. The treatment of hypertension has a shorter history but has still been possible since the late 1950s.

In all previous studies, the definition of amenable deaths has had an upper age limit, reflecting the view that "everyone must die of something". The age limit has increased over time, from 65 to 75, but this creates certain problems. The first is that it is explicitly ageist, as it devalues curative care for those aged over 75. The second is empirical: life expectancy in some countries now exceeds this figure and also there is growing evidence that many types of health care are very effective in older people. If, however, the definition of an amenable cause is one where health care can reduce the death rate by 50% or more, then there is no intrinsic reason to have an upper age limit. However, while conceptually attractive, this also poses problems of obtaining evidence, firstly because older patients are often excluded from trials and, second, because the absence of an observed decline in mortality at older ages at a time when an intervention was being introduced may simply mean that this population was not offered treatment.

Amenable mortality is a dynamic concept. Although most definitions still include infectious diseases such as measles, the numbers of deaths in high-income countries are negligible. In other words, success in tackling causes of death amenable to health care renders these causes obsolete as indicators of future progress. At the same time, new treatments are discovered that render once untreatable conditions treatable, justifying their inclusion in a new categorization. This clearly poses problems for longitudinal analyses.

Finally, the scope for reducing rates of avoidable mortality is greatest in the countries where initial levels are high. As a consequence, the ability to compare health system performance among developed countries is likely to be limited in the future, as the differences will be relatively small. Also, changes in coding of cause of death and in ICD versions may create artefactual discontinuities. It is also necessary to take account of changes in the incidence of underlying disease. For all these reasons, superficial comparisons of amenable mortality may be misleading (Desai et al., 2011). Yet, despite these limitations, the concept of avoidable mortality provides a potentially useful indicator of health system performance. It is, however, important to recognize that high levels should not be taken as definite evidence of ineffective health care, but rather as an indicator of potential weaknesses that require further investigation. These, and some of the earlier problems noted, can be illustrated by reference to renal cancer. In some countries, death rates are increasing and yet, paradoxically, data from cancer registries suggest that five-year survival rates are improving. Several factors must be considered. As this is a smoking-related cancer, the incidence is continuing to increase among women. There have also been advances in treatment, although of uncertain benefit. Finally, reported cancer survival is subject to lead-time bias as the greater use of abdominal imaging techniques in place of barium studies for intestinal problems is identifying many more early tumours.

The tracer concept

Many of the aggregate indicators discussed above say little about what must be done to improve the outcomes of health care so the policy implications are often unclear (Walshe, 2003).The challenge is to develop techniques that can capture performance in a systematic and comparable way. The use of tracer conditions is based on the premise that carefully selected health problems can provide insights into the performance of different elements within the overall health system (Nolte, Bain & McKee, 2006, 2009).

The concept was proposed initially by Kessner, who set out the six criteria for a condition to be used as a tracer (Kessner, Kalk & Singer, 1973):

1. *functional impact*, i.e. requires specific treatment, otherwise resulting in functional impairment;
2. *well defined and easy to diagnose*;
3. *sufficient prevalence* in the population to permit collection of adequate data;
4. *natural history which varies with utilization and effectiveness of health care*;
5. *available techniques of medical management* which are well defined for at least one of the following: prevention, diagnosis, treatment, or rehabilitation;
6. *known epidemiology*.

Over the past 30 years, the application of the tracer methodology has expanded slowly, as it has the potential to identify strengths and limitations of the entire health system. It is important to note that this approach does not assess the quality of care per se, but rather identifies potential strengths and weaknesses of the system's response to tracer conditions.

The process involves the collection of data from a variety of sources, including surveys and interviews with patients, providers and policy-makers. The assessment focuses on the inputs of care (physical, such as facilities and pharmaceuticals; human, such as trained health workers and empowered patients; knowledge, such as evidence-based guidelines; and social, such as social support and communication systems) and their integration.

The selection of health problems suitable for the tracer concept depends on the specific health system features requiring assessment. Thus, public health policies at the system level can be evaluated using vaccine-preventable conditions, while neonatal mortality can be adopted as a possible measure for assessing access to health care (Koupilová, McKee & Holcik, 1998; Nolte et al., 2000).

The increasing burden of chronic diseases, along with their complexity, makes then especially suitable for use as tracers, given that they require the coordinated input of multiple elements of the health system. Various studies have now used diabetes mellitus to evaluate health system performance measurement in high-, middle- and low-income settings (Hopkinson et al., 2004; Beran, Yudkin & de Courten, 2005; Nolte, Bain & McKee, 2006). Diabetes fits the criteria for a tracer condition, as it is well defined, fairly easy to diagnose (WHO, 1999) and common. Diabetes outcomes reflect a range of aspects of health system performance.

Crucially, albeit with some caution, the identification of failings in the provision of care for one chronic disorder can often highlight failings affecting many others. McColl and Gulliford (1993) classify deaths from diabetes among young people as "sentinel health events" that should raise questions about the quality of health care delivery. Effective treatment prevents complications and disability, which is clearly illustrated by the countries with limited access to insulin (Yudkin & Beran, 2003) and by countries where health systems have collapsed (Telishevka et al., 2001).

Despite the availability of effective treatment for diabetes for almost a century, with an extensive evidence base for managing this disorder, there remains substantial variation across health systems in the standards of care people with diabetes receive. Examining a measure based on the ratio of mortality to incidence of diabetes in young people, Nolte, Bain & McKee (2006) found a 10-fold difference among 29 high- and middle-income countries.

A number of instruments are now available for use in tracer studies. The Rapid Assessment Protocol for Insulin Access (RAPIA) has been developed by the International Insulin Foundation as a functional evaluation tool (Yudkin & Beran, 2003). It provides a multilevel assessment of the different elements that influence access to insulin of patients in a given country. Beran, Yudkin and de Courten's 2005 analysis using the RAPIA protocol in Mozambique and Zambia showed that, although insulin supplies were sufficient in these countries, their health systems did not permit appropriate distribution according to need, nor did they ensure adequate provision of additional equipment or the existence of training programmes for health care workers, all factors that increased the risk of misdiagnosis or failure to detect diabetes.

A similar approach was taken in Kyrgyzstan (Hopkinson et al., 2004) and Georgia (Balabanova et al., 2009). These studies identified key failings in integration (ineffective insulin distribution system, lack of necessary equipment, complex pathways) that prevented the delivery of quality care for diabetes patients despite the existing provision of the essential services (insulin supply, training of health professionals, financed care packages).

While these studies have obvious practical implications for the management of diabetes, the use of the tracer approach shows how, even though many inputs may be in place, there can still be critical gaps and a failure to integrate different aspects of the system. Although such studies focus on a single tracer, the problems they identify are often generic. Thus, diabetes can be seen as representative of a much larger group of complex chronic diseases that require long-term treatment by multidisciplinary teams and the active involvement of informed and empowered patients (Nolte et al., 2011).

5.7 Conclusion

Many of the existing measures of population health fail to distinguish the contribution of health care from extraneous factors and those that do suffer from a number of methodological problems. Some of these problems may be insurmountable; however, what is important is to understand them and take them into account when interpreting data, particularly in the context of comparing health systems. Thus, age-standardized mortality from selected causes, coupled with additional information on disease prevalence, incidence and survival, can identify areas that justify in-depth investigation. However, such investigations must respect the many caveats that can affect cross-national comparability.

The concept of amenable mortality is no more than an indicator of potential problems. In international comparisons, it is subject to many methodological limitations and depends on achieving consensus on definitions and the choice of conditions included for analysis. It is a starting point; an accurate diagnosis and conclusions will require much more detailed and iterative examination of the data that contribute to it. The use of the tracer methodology may be part of this further enquiry.

References

Anderson, W.J. and Murtagh, C. (2007) Cancer survival statistics should be viewed with caution, *The Lancet Oncology*, 8(12): 1052–3; author reply 1053–4.

Andreev, E.M. et al. (2003) The evolving pattern of avoidable mortality in Russia, *International Journal of Epidemiology*, 32(3): 437–46.

Anell, A. and Willis, M. (2000) International comparison of health care systems using resource profiles, *Bulletin of the World Health Organization*, 78(6): 770–8.

Arah, O.A. et al. (2006) A conceptual framework for the OECD Health Care Quality Indicators project, *International Journal for Quality in Health Care*, 18(Suppl): 5–13.

Babazono, A. and Hillman, A.L. (1994) A comparison of international health outcomes and health care spending, *International Journal of Technology Assessment in Health Care*, 10(3): 376–81.

Balabanova, D. et al. (2009) Navigating the health system: diabetes care in Georgia, *Health Policy Plan*, 24(1): 46–54.

Beaglehole, R. (1986) Medical management and the decline in mortality from coronary heart disease, *BMJ (Clinical Research Edition)*, 292(6512): 33–5.

Beran, D., Yudkin, J.S. and de Courten, M. (2005) Access to care for patients with insulin-requiring diabetes in developing countries: case studies of Mozambique and Zambia, *Diabetes Care*, 28(9): 2136–40.

Bots, M.L. and Grobbee, D.E. (1996) Decline of coronary heart disease mortality in The Netherlands from 1978 to 1985: contribution of medical care and changes over time in presence of major cardiovascular risk factors, *Journal of Cardiovascular Risk*, 3(3): 271–6.

Brenner, G., Altenhofen, L. and Boqumil, W. (2000) *Gesundheitszustand und ambulante medizinische Versorgung der Bevölkerung in Deutschland im Ost-West-vergleich*. Köln: Zentralinstitut für die kassenärztliche Versorgung.

Britton, A. et al. (1999) Threats to applicability of randomized trials: exclusions and selective participation, *Journal of Health Services Research and Policy*, 4(2): 112–21.

Buck, D., Eastwood, A. and Smith, P.C. (1999) Can we measure the social importance of health care? *International Journal of Technology Assessment in Health Care*, 15(1): 89–107.

Bunker, J.P. (2001) The role of medical care in contributing to health improvements within societies, *International Journal of Epidemiology*, 30(6): 1260–3.

Bunker, J.P., Frazier, H.S. and Mosteller, F. (1994) Improving health: measuring effects of medical care, *The Millbank Quarterly*, 72(2): 225–58.

Charlton, J.R. et al. (1983) Geographical variation in mortality from conditions amenable to medical intervention in England and Wales, *The Lancet*, 1(8326 Pt 1): 691–6.

Cochrane, A.L., St Leger, A.S. and Moore, F. (1978) Health service 'input' and mortality 'output' in developed countries, *Journal of Epidemiology and Community Health*, 32(3): 200–5.

Coleman, M.P. et al. (2008) Cancer survival in five continents: a worldwide population-based study (CONCORD), *The Lancet Oncology*, 9(8): 730–56.

Coleman, M.P. et al. (2011) Cancer survival in Australia, Canada, Denmark, Norway, Sweden, and the UK, 1995–2007 (the International Cancer Benchmarking Partnership): an analysis of population-based cancer registry data, *The Lancet*, 377(9760): 127–38.

Colgrove, J. (2002) The McKeown thesis: a historical controversy and its enduring influence, *American Journal of Public Health*, 92(5): 725–9.

Crawford, S.M. (2010) UK cancer survival statistics. Reflect NHS clinical realities, *BMJ*, 341: c5134.

Crémieux, P.Y., Ouellette, P. and Pilon, C. (1999) Health care spending as determinants of health outcomes, *Health Economics*, 8(7): 627–39.

Cutler, D.M. and McClellan, M. (2001) Is technological change in medicine worth it? *Health Affairs (Millwood)*, 20(5): 11–29.

Davis, K., Schoen, C., Stremikis, K. (2010) *Mirror, Mirror on the Wall: How the performance of the U.S. health care system compares internationally, 2010 update. T.C. Fund.* New York: The Commonwealth Fund (http://www.commonwealthfund.org/Publications/Fund-Reports/2010/Jun/Mirror-Mirror-Update.aspx?page=all, accessed 8 October 2012).

Desai, M. et al. (2010) Two countries divided by a common language: health systems in the UK and USA, *Journal of the Royal Society of Medicine*, 103(7): 283–7.

Desai, M. et al. (2011) Measuring NHS performance 1990–2009 using amenable mortality: interpret with care, *Journal of the Royal Society of Medicine*, 104(9): 370–9.

Dickman, P.W. and Adami, H.O. (2006) Interpreting trends in cancer patient survival, *Journal of Internal Medicine*, 260(2): 103–17.

Elola, J., Daponte, A. and Navarro, V. (1995) Health indicators and the organization of health care systems in western Europe, *American Journal of Public Health*, 85(10): 1397–401.

Etches, V. et al. (2006) Measuring population health: a review of indicators, *Annual Review of Public Health*, 27: 29–55.

Evans, D.B. et al. (2001) Comparative efficiency of national health systems: cross national econometric analysis, *BMJ*, 323(7308): 307–10.

Fairchild, A.L. and Oppenheimer, G.M. (1998) Public health nihilism vs pragmatism: history, politics, and the control of tuberculosis, *American Journal of Public Health*, 88(7): 1105–17.

Fleming, P.J. et al. (1990) Interaction between bedding and sleeping position in the sudden infant death syndrome: a population based case-control study, *BMJ*, 301(6743): 85–9.

Ford, E.S. et al. (2007) Explaining the decrease in U.S. deaths from coronary disease, 1980–2000, *New Engand Journal of Medicine*, 356(23): 2388–98.

FSID (2011) *Factfile 2: Research background to the reduce the risk of cot death advice. Foundation for the Study of Infant Deaths* (fsid.org.uk/document.doc?id=42, accessed 16 October 2012).

Garne, E. et al. (2001) Different policies on prenatal ultrasound screening programmes and induced abortions explain regional variations in infant mortality with congenital malformations, *Fetal Diagnosis and Therapy*, 16(3): 153–7.

Gay, J. et al. (2011) *Mortality amenable to health care in 31 OECD countries: estimates and methodological issues.* Paris: Organisation for Economic Co-operation and Development Publishing (OECD Health Working Papers, no. 55).

Gold, M.R., Stevenson, D. and Fryback, D.G. (2002) HALYs and QALYs and DALYs, Oh My: similarities and differences in summary measures of population health, *Annual Review of Public Health*, 23: 115–34.

Gravelle, H. and Blackhouse, M. (1987) International cross-section analysis of the determination of mortality, *Social Science and Medicine*, 25(5): 427–41.

Hopkinson, B. et al. (2004) The human perspective on health care reform: coping with diabetes in Kyrgyzstan, *International Journal of Health Planning and Management*, 19(1): 43–61.

Illich, I. (1976) *Limits to medicine: Medical nemesis, the expropriation of health*. London: Marion Boyars Publishing.

Jack, R.H. et al. (2003) Geographical inequalities in lung cancer management and survival in South East England: evidence of variation in access to oncology services? *British Journal of Cancer*, 88(7): 1025–31.

Kamarudeen, S. (2010) *Amenable mortality as an indicator of healthcare quality – a literature review*. Newport: Office for National Statistics.

Kelley, E. and Hurst, J. (2006) *Health Care Quality Indicators project: Conceptual framework paper*. Paris: Organisation for Economic Co-operation and Development Publishing (OECD Health Working Paper, no. 23).

Kessner, D.M., Kalk, C.E. and Singer, J. (1973) Assessing health quality – the case for tracers, *New England Journal of Medicine*, 288(4): 189–94.

Kesteloot, H., Sans, S. and Kromhout, D. (2006) Dynamics of cardiovascular and all-cause mortality in Western and Eastern Europe between 1970 and 2000, *European Heart Journal*, 27(1): 107–13.

Kim, K. and Moody, P.M. (1992) More resources better health? A cross-national perspective, *Social Science and Medicine*, 34(8): 837–42.

King, G. et al. (2004) Enhancing the validity and cross-cultural comparability of measurement in survey research, *American Political Science Review*, 98(1): 191–207.

Koupilová, I., McKee, M. and Holcík, J. (1998) Neonatal mortality in the Czech Republic during the transition, *Health Policy*, 46(1): 43–52.

Lalonde, M. (1974) *A new perspective on the health of Canadians; a working document*. Ottawa: Department of National Health and Welfare.

Lee, Y.C. et al. (2010) The impact of universal National Health Insurance on population health: the experience of Taiwan, *BMC Health Services Research*, 10: 225.

Leon, D.A., Vågerö, D. and Olausson, P.O. (1992) Social class differences in infant mortality in Sweden: comparison with England and Wales, *BMJ*, 305(6855): 687–91.

Lopez, A.D. et al. (eds) (2006) *Global burden of disease and risk factors*. New York: Oxford University Press and World Bank.

Mackenbach, J.P. (1996) The contribution of medical care to mortality decline: McKeown revisited, *Journal of Clinical Epidemiology*, 49(11): 1207–13.

Mariotto, A., Capocaccia, R. and Verdecchia, A. (2002) Projecting SEER cancer survival rates to the US: an ecological regression approach, *Cancer Causes and Control*, 13(2): 101–11.

Marques-Vidal, P. et al. (1997) Trends in coronary heart disease morbidity and mortality and acute coronary care and case fatality from 1985–1989 in southern Germany and south-western France, *European Heart Journal*, 18(5): 816–21.

Martini, C.J. et al. (1977) Health indexes sensitive to medical care variation, *International Journal of Health Services*, 7(2): 293–309.

Mathers, C., Salomon, J. and Murray, C. (2003) Infant mortality is not an adequate summary measure of population health, *Journal of Epidemiology and Community Health*, 57: 319.

Mathers, C. et al. (2003) Alternative summary measures of average population health, in C.J.L. Murray and D.B. Evans (eds) *Health Systems Performance Assessment: Debates, methods and empiricism*. Geneva: World Health Organization.

McColl, A. and Gulliford, M. (1993) *Population health outcome indicators for the NHS. A feasibility study*. London: Faculty of Public Health Medicine and the Department of Public Health Medicine, United Medical and Dental Schools of Guy's and St Thomas' Hospitals.

McKee, M. (1999) For debate – Does health care save lives? *Croatian Medical Journal*, 40(2): 123–8.

McKee, M. (2010) The World Health Report 2000: 10 years on, *Health Policy and Planning*, 25(5): 346–8.

McKee, M., Shkolnikov, V. and Leon, D.A. (2001) Alcohol is implicated in the fluctuations in cardiovascular disease in Russia since the 1980s, *Annals of Epidemiology*, 11(1): 1–6.

McKee, M. et al. (1996) Preventing sudden infant deaths – the slow diffusion of an idea, *Health Policy*, 37(2): 117–35.

McKeown, T. (1979) *The role of medicine: dream, mirage or nemesis*. Oxford: Blackwell.

McKinlay, J.B. and McKinlay, S.M. (1977) The questionable contribution of medical measures to the decline of mortality in the United States in the twentieth century, *The Milbank Memorial Fund Quarterly: Health and Society*, 55(3): 405–28.

Murray, C. et al. (eds) (2002) *Summary measures of population health. Concepts, ethics, measurement and applications*. Geneva: World Health Organization.

Newey, C. et al. (2004) *Avoidable mortality in the enlarged European Union*. Paris: Institut des Sciences de la Santé.

Nixon, J. and Ulmann, P. (2006) The relationship between health care expenditure and health outcomes. Evidence and caveats for a causal link, *European Journal of Health Economics*, 7(1): 7–18.

Nolte, E. (2010) *International benchmarking of healthcare quality: A review of literature*. RAND Europe (http://www.rand.org/content/dam/rand/pubs/technical_reports/2010/RAND_TR738.pdf, accessed 8 October 2012).

Nolte, E. and McKee, M. (2004) *Does healthcare save lives? Avoidable mortality revisited*. London: The Nuffield Trust (http://www.nuffieldtrust.org.uk/sites/files/nuffield/publication/does-healthcare-save-lives-mar04.pdf, accessed 8 October 2012).

Nolte, E. and McKee, M. (2008) Measuring the health of nations: updating an earlier analysis, *Health Affairs (Millwood)*, 27(1): 58–71.

Nolte, E., Bain, C. and McKee, M. (2006) Diabetes as a tracer condition in international benchmarking of health systems, *Diabetes Care*, 29(5): 1007–11.

Nolte, E., Bain, C. and McKee, M. (2009) Population health, in P.C. Smith et al. (eds) *Performance measurement for health systems improvement: Experiences, challenges and prospects*. Cambridge: Cambridge University Press.

Nolte, E., et al. (2000) Neonatal and postneonatal mortality in Germany since unification, *Journal of Epidemiology and Community Health*, 54(2): 84–90.

Nolte, E., et al. (2002) The contribution of medical care to changing life expectancy in Germany and Poland, *Social Science and Medicine*, 55(11): 1905–21.

Nolte, E. et al. (2011) Saving lives? The contribution of health care to population health, in J. Figueras, et al.(eds) *Health Systems, Health, Wealth and Societal Well-being: Assessing the case for investing in health systems*. Buckingham: Open University Press (European Observatory on Health Systems and Policies Series).

OECD (2004) *Private health insurance in OECD countries*. The OECD Health Project, OECD Publishing (http://www.oecd-ilibrary.org/social-issues-migration-health/private-health-insurance-in-oecd-countries_9789264007451-en, accessed 8 October 2012).

Or, Z. (2000) Determinants of health outcomes in industrialized countries: a pooled, cross-country, time-series analysis, *OECD Economic Studies*, 30: 53–77.

Or, Z. (2001) *Exploring the effects of health care on mortality across OECD countries*. Paris: Organisation for Economic Co-operation and Development (Labour Market and Social Policy Occasional Paper, no.46).

Richardus, J.H. et al. (1998) The perinatal mortality rate as an indicator of quality of care in international comparisons, *Medical Care*, 36(1): 54–66.

Rutstein, D.D. et al. (1976) Measuring the quality of medical care. A clinical method, *New England Journal of Medicine*, 294(11): 582–8.

Scioscia, M. et al. (2007) A critical analysis on Italian perinatal mortality in a 50-year span, *European Journal of Obstetrics and Gynecology and Reproductive Biology*, 130(1): 60–5.

Scott, A., Campbell, H. and Gorman, D. (1993) Sudden infant death in Scotland, *BMJ*, 306(6871): 211–12.

Smith, P.C. et al. (eds) (2009) *Performance measurement for health system improvement: Experiences, challenges and prospects.* Cambridge: Cambridge University Press.

Telishevka, M., Chenett, L. and McKee, M. (2001) Towards an understanding of the high death rate among young people with diabetes in Ukraine, *Diabetic Medicine*, 18(1): 3–9.

Tobias, M. and Yeh, L.C. (2009) How much does health care contribute to health gain and to health inequality? Trends in amenable mortality in New Zealand 1981–2004, *Australian and New Zealand Journal of Public Health*, 33(1): 70–8.

Tunstall-Pedoe, H. et al. (1999) Contribution of trends in survival and coronary-event rates to changes in coronary heart disease mortality: 10-year results from 37 WHO MONICA project populations. Monitoring trends and determinants in cardiovascular disease, *The Lancet*, 353(9164): 1547–57.

Tunstall-Pedoe, H. et al. (2000) Estimation of contribution of changes in coronary care to improving survival, event rates, and coronary heart disease mortality across the WHO MONICA Project populations, *The Lancet*, 355(9205): 688–700.

Uusküla, M., Lamp, K. and Väli, M. (1998) An age-related difference in the ratio of sudden coronary death over acute myocardial infarction in Estonian males, *Journal of Clinical Epidemiology*, 51(7): 577–80.

van der Pal-de Bruin, K.M. et al. (2002) The influence of prenatal screening and termination of pregnancy on perinatal mortality rates, *Prenatal Diagnosis*, 22(11): 966–72.

Van der Zee, J. and Kroneman, M.W. (2007) Bismark or Beveridge: a beauty contest between dinosaurs, *BMC Health Services Research*, 7: 94.

Verdecchia, A. et al. (2007) Recent cancer survival in Europe: a 2000–02 period analysis of EUROCARE-4 data, *The Lancet Oncology*, 8(9): 784–96.

Walshe, K. (2003) International comparisons of the quality of health care: what do they tell us? *Quality and Safety in Health Care*, 12(1): 4–5.

WHO (1999) *Definition, diagnosis and classification of diabetes mellitus and its complications. Part 1: diagnosis and classification of diabetes mellitus.* Geneva: World Health Organization.

WHO (2000) *The World Health Report 2000 – Health systems: improving performance.* Geneva: World Health Organization.

WHO (2009) *Global health risks: mortality and burden of disease attributable to selected major risks.* Geneva: World Health Organization.

Wiesner, G., Grimm, J. and Bittner, E. (1999) Zum Herzinfarktgeschehen in der Bundesrepublik Deutschland: Prävalenz, Inzidenz, Trend, Ost-West-Vergleich, *Gesundheitswesen*, 61(Suppl 2): 72–8.

Wright, J.C. and Weinstein, M.C. (1998) Gains in life expectancy from medical interventions – standardizing data on outcomes, *New England Journal of Medicine*, 339(6): 380–6.

Yudkin, J.S. and Beran D. (2003) Prognosis of diabetes in the developing world, *The Lancet*, 362(9393): 1420–1.

Zatonski, W.A., McMichael, A.J. and Powles, J.W. (1998) Ecological study of reasons for sharp decline in mortality from ischaemic heart disease in Poland since 1991, *BMJ*, 316(7137): 1047–51.

chapter six

Comparing Health Services Outcomes

Niek Klazinga and Lilian Li

6.1 Introduction

Although the main objective of health services is ultimately to assist individuals in realizing their potential health and thus promote the health of the population, measuring the contribution of health services to health outcomes involves quite distinct challenges. For example, it is essential to ensure that the services being compared are comparable and that proper adjustment is made for differences in the populations being served. Direct indicators of the contribution of health services to health status are available in the form of health service quality measures, such as standardized hospital mortality rates and numerous disease-specific health outcome measures. Routine use of patient-reported outcome measures is also being piloted in England and the Netherlands. For the purposes of international comparison, the OECD HCQI project is an important resource (OECD 2009, 2010a, 2010b, 2011). While such measures offer some indicators of the performance of individual organizations (after suitable adjustment for case-mix and other contextual circumstances), international comparison is complicated by different organizational settings and reporting conventions.

In many performance measurement initiatives, measures of health care process are used in preference to more direct measures of outcome. These have the virtue of administrative convenience, can be measured immediately, and are easier to attribute directly to the efforts of the health services. Furthermore, they reflect compliance with what is considered good practice and, as such, are perceived as a better measure of assessing the quality of health care providers than the more distant outcome parameters that are influenced by so many factors other than the quality of care provision alone. However, they may ignore the ultimate effectiveness or appropriateness of the intervention, and their use pre-judges the nature of response to a health problem, which may not be identical in all settings. Especially in situations where health services are dealing with patients with multi-morbidities, judging health services by standards or guidelines based on single diseases can be misleading.

This chapter focuses on health services outcomes and will discuss: the underlying concepts; different types of health services outcomes; and the present methodological and data challenges. It comprises of the following sections:

- Health services outcomes and health system performance: concepts and constructs
- Measuring the contribution of hospital services to health system performance
- Health outcomes of long-term care services
- Measuring the contribution of primary health care to health system performance
- The contribution of mental health care to health system performance
- Health outcomes in preventive care
- Patient-reported outcome measures (PROMs)
- Summary of data problems
- Conclusions

6.2 Health services outcomes and health system performance: concepts and constructs

Health services are production units that provide health care actions, with the aim of helping users realize their health potential. Health care actions usually involve knowledge and expertise-based professional input, in combination with the application of specific technologies. The organization of production units may vary considerably but the rationale behind it is usually based on ways in which professionals and technologies can be combined to provide services at economies of scale. The hospital is often taken as being the prototype of a health service. However, the health care actions provided in hospitals have changed dramatically over time. In the early decades of the 20th century, hospitals evolved from being nursing homes for the poor and the dying, into the epicentre of modern medicine, becoming the working place for medical specialists and the location for new technologies such as X-ray, anaesthesia and laboratory tests. This resulted in the modern hospital, with its emphasis on clinical admissions and a wide array of diagnostic and therapeutic possibilities. However, with the further advancements of medical technologies and information technology that dissolve the necessity to have various forms of expertise (specialist knowledge) located physically in one place, hospital care is now gradually shifting from relying on inpatient treatment to outpatient and day care services.

This illustrates the fact that health services develop over time, meaning that the possibility of comparing the performance of the same hospital over time, or different hospitals within or between countries with existing differences in capacity to produce health care actions, is naturally difficult.

Also, the aggregate level of production units of health care actions into health services hugely differs. In primary care, physicians (either GPs or specialists) can have solo practices that deliver a concise set of health care actions. However, there is an overlap of health care services with polyclinics and parts of hospital organizations, for example, in the monitoring of patients with a chronic disease (such as diabetes). When Dutch insurers started contracting diabetes care as part of disease management programmes, the units contracted varied from a group of four GPs to organized groups of 80 GPs, or large groups of GPs together with a regional laboratory or academic hospital. Comparing these different organizational units on their performance in delivering high-quality diabetes care poses huge methodological problems.

Linking the performance of individual health services (hospitals, GP practices, community health centres) to health system performance, and thus population health, requires aggregates of various health services that together have the potential of influencing health outcomes (for example, in stroke patients, the combination of GP preventive care, ambulance services, acute interventions, stroke units in the hospital, home care and rehabilitation, i.e. stroke services). Labels such as "organized delivery systems (US)" are often chosen to highlight the necessity to consider a combination of coordinated and/or integrated health services when trying to assess health outcomes on a population level. Thus, health services with respect to health system outcomes alludes to the quality of individual health care actions, nested within production units, nested in organizations, in turn embedded in care delivery organizations, delivering to groups of individuals over a long period of time care that enhances population health.

Health outcomes are also multidimensional. Similar to the concept of health, health outcomes involve not just the absence of death but also the minimization of discomfort and disabilities. As described in Chapter 5, there are many indicators that express the health of populations. Outcome measures that reflect the contribution of health care services to the health of populations can be grouped into outcomes that reflect: the postponement of death (healthy life expectancy, five-year relative survival rates for cancer, case-fatality rates for AMI and stroke); mitigation of disabilities (activities of daily living (ADL), mobility, eyesight, hearing impairment); discomfort (pain, nausea); or other complaints perceived as non-optimal health. When health services are targeted to a specific disease, the measures used to assess the outcome usually try to capture disease-specific outcomes. However, measuring disease-specific outcomes often takes a lot of resources in terms of both time and money, and is not necessarily congruent with the experienced health of an individual. Furthermore, some of the services may only have a long-term outcome, which is not evident in the short term. The outcomes are most obvious when dealing with trauma; If a person breaks their leg and health services (ambulance, hospital, rehabilitation) help the person to regain their walking abilities to a pre-accident state, the outcome measurements would include functionality (walking), lack of disability and the time frame in which the outcome was realized. However, for major categories of disease, such as cancer and cardiovascular diseases, the outcomes are less clear. The ultimate goal is to prolong life (survival rates for cancer, case-fatality rates for AMI and stroke), but this should also be judged against associated disabilities and discomfort. Furthermore, although these outcome parameters may reflect the quality of the therapeutic and rehabilitation services, from a health system perspective they do not necessarily reflect the quality of preventive services (cancer screening, hypertension control), factors outside the health care domain, or the effectiveness of more general health policies (diet, physical exercise, smoking, etc.). Although outcome measures are available, it is paramount first to distinguish clearly the performance of the services being assessed in relation to health system performance before making judgements on the appropriateness of certain outcome measures.

In his recent article, "What is value in health care?" Michael Porter addresses the connection of health services with health system performance (Porter, 2010). In trying to measure value in health care, he considers outcomes as the numerator of the value equation and states that they are inherently condition specific and multidimensional. He proposes a three-tier outcome measures hierarchy where the first tier looks at the health status achieved or retained (measured by survival, or degree of health or recovery); the second tier looks at the process of recovery (measured through time to recovery and return to normal activities, as well as the disutilities of care, e.g. diagnostic errors, ineffective care, treatment-related discomfort, complications, adverse effects); and the third tier addresses the sustainability of health (measured through sustainability of health or recovery, nature of recurrences, and long-term consequences of therapy, i.e. iatrogenic diseases). Although this hierarchy is still open to debate, it is a good attempt at creating a meaningful, conceptual link between the various constructs of health services and health system performance. It also illustrates the huge challenges that remain in the endeavour to transform the present kaleidoscope of health services outcome measures into meaningful information for health system performance improvement.

6.3 Measuring the contribution of hospital services to health system performance

As stated earlier, hospitals are considered by many policy-makers to be the epicentre of health care systems. This notion is largely fuelled by the fact that during the 20th century they became the nucleus of medical technological innovation and remain responsible for a substantial proportion of health care costs. As hospitals differ in their provision of services and are prone to changes in the health care actions they offer due to medical innovation and professionalization, constructing indicators to measure performance between hospitals and over time is difficult. While the majority of indicators have a process or structural nature, four types of outcome indicators that are presently studied and used in many countries are: hospital-standardized mortality rates (HSMRs); case-fatality rates for AMI and stroke; patient safety indicators; and hospital readmission rates.

Hospital-standardized mortality rates

HSMRs were initially developed by Jarman (Jarman et al., 2005; Jarman, 2008). The methodology is based on adjusted hospital mortality rates and used for performance comparison of hospitals. This indicator has been taken up by a number of countries. There have been debates on the validity and usefulness of HSMRs because of inherent methodological and conceptual problems. Experts point out that HSMRs do not account for preventable deaths and observe that a majority of deaths are unavoidable (Black, 2010; Lilford & Pronovost, 2010). Further debates address the challenge of international comparability of data (or lack thereof), given differences across hospital systems and records. One of the key elements of discussion here is the different way in which countries and regions may have organized out-of-hospital palliative care and the resulting chance of persons dying in a hospital. Nonetheless, there remains substantial policy interest in this indicator.

The usability of HSMRs is greatly associated with the quality of coding of secondary diagnoses and administrative databases. Differences in coding practice for causes of death, as well as the varying degree to which mortality statistics are linked to overall death statistics, often frustrate endeavours to use mortality statistics for benchmarking and reporting performance indicators. The development and adoption of the use of unique patient identifiers (UPIs) is therefore essential for future development.

Case-fatality rates for AMI and stroke

Much work is being done in the field of hospital-specific indicators in European countries, such as Belgium, Denmark, France, Germany, Italy, Portugal, Spain, the UK and the Netherlands. Indicators are currently being developed and tested, sourcing mainly from administrative databases and medical records.

Hospital indicators are relevant, as hospitals have become the hub for observing changes in health outcomes because of progress in medical treatment. There are numerous new and improved imaging technologies and laboratory tests that provide rapid and precise diagnosis; powerful drugs that help stabilize patients; and new surgical and interventional approaches that save many lives.

Noteworthy are increased survival rates after acute cardiovascular events, including stroke and AMI, both of which are remarkable illustrations of the impact of medical progress. An AMI occurs when a blood clot occludes a pencil-thin artery supplying blood to the heart so that there is an irreversible loss of cardiac function and, if left untreated, potential heart failure and cardiac arrest. A stroke refers to the same phenomenon occurring in the brain (ischaemic) or the occurrence of bleeding (haemorrhagic stroke). In many industrialized countries, cardiovascular diseases are the leading causes of death but mortality rates have seen a decline since the 1970s (Weisfeldt & Zieman, 2007). This is a remarkable observation, illustrating the impact of hospital services on health outcomes, as the incidence of AMI has not seen a parallel decline (Goldberg, Gurwitz & Gore, 1999).

The reduction in mortality can be attributed to lower acute mortality from AMI due to improved medical treatment in the critical phase (Capewell et al., 1999; McGovern et al., 2001). The introduction of coronary care units in the 1960s (Khush, Rapaport & Waters, 2005) and the advent of treatment aimed at restoring coronary blood flow in the 1990s (Gil, 1999) have dramatically altered care for AMI. Treatment for AMI may now involve thrombolysis (the administration of intravenous drugs that dissolve the blood clot) and then percutaneous coronary intervention (a catheter is advanced into the patient's coronary artery and the clot pushed away with an inflatable balloon). Alternatively, cardiologists use coronary stents, whereby tiny wire tubes are inserted to keep the artery from closing up again. Because research shows that the time lapse between an AMI and the re-opening of the artery is critical to prognosis, other care processes have also changed. Various drugs, such as aspirin and heparin, are now administered by emergency medical personnel as patients are being transported to hospital. Emergency departments have instituted procedures to ensure that patients also receive these medical treatments within minutes of arrival.

The evidence base supporting these treatments is impressive, thanks to many rigorously designed clinical trials. These care processes, which have been codified into practice guidelines as standard practices of care, provide a foundation for the construction of outcome indicators, reflecting the final result of care. Over the years, numerous indicators, particularly for AMI care, have been developed and have gained wide acceptance. One such example is the 30-day case-fatality rate for AMI, which was one of the first HCQI indicators selected by the OECD subcommittee for cardiac care.

Despite the strong conceptual and scientific basis for measuring quality of care for acute cardiovascular conditions, the collection of data for such indicators remains challenging, particular at the international level, where issues of comparability are prevalent. Indicators often require information from individual patient medical records (for example, the time between the patient's arrival at the hospital and start of thrombolysis and whether medication is prescribed once patients are released from the hospital) and this is only available at the local level because few countries have national data collections.

However, there are sufficient data available for 30-day case-fatality rates for AMI, ischaemic stroke and haemorrhagic stroke (Figure 6.1).

Figure 6.1 shows age- and sex-standardized in-hospital case-fatality rates within 30 days of admission for AMI. There is a nearly tenfold difference between the highest fatality rate (Mexico 21.5%) and the lowest rate (Denmark 2.3%), while the average rate is 5.3%. Well below the average is the cluster of Nordic countries (Norway, Denmark, Sweden and Iceland). It should be noted that the reported rates may be influenced by differences in hospital transfers, average lengths of stay and emergency retrieval times. Certain countries have a special system of emergency care, whereby emergency medical technicians are accompanied by specialist physicians trained in advanced life support when retrieving critically ill patients. In these cases, a higher number of patients may reach the hospital alive but die shortly after admission because of failed stabilizing. Along similar lines, other countries often transfer unstable cardiac patients to tertiary care centres, which could cause a downward bias in case-fatality rates, assuming the transfers are recorded as live discharges.

Several methodological challenges remain because of data limitations. The indicator requires tracking every patient for 30 days after initial hospital admission in order to define survival status. This obliges the use of UPIs, which most countries still do not have. Consequently, the indicator uses implied data;

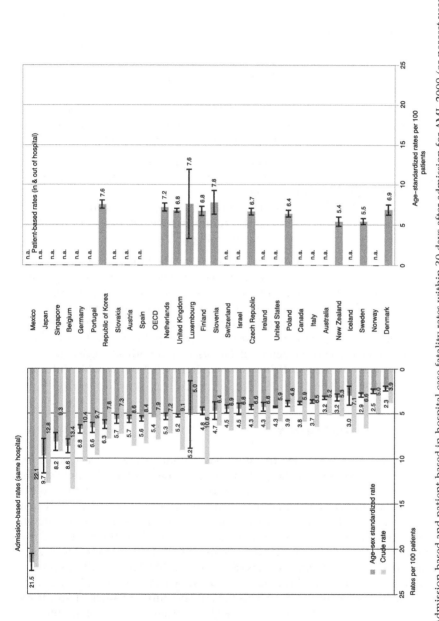

Figure 6.1 Admission-based and patient-based in-hospital case-fatality rates within 30 days after admission for AMI, 2009 (or nearest year)

Note: Rates age–sex standardized to 2005 OECD population (45+). 95% confidence intervals represented by H.

Source: OECD, 2011.

it assumes that patients who have been discharged before 30 days have survived, which is far from ideal, although various inter-country analyses have suggested that the errors introduced by this implication are small. It is also important to adjust for differential patient risk profiles in international comparisons, but there is a lack of information to do so thoroughly.

Figure 6.2 shows reductions in the case-fatality rates for AMI between 2001 and 2009 in the labelled countries. These reductions reflect improvements in care and, particularly for Canada, in the rapid reopening of occluded arteries (Fox et al., 2007; Tu et al., 2009).

Comparative work by WHO and the OECD on administrative databases has identified the following generic problems in assessing outcome measures from health services, such as case-fatality rates on AMI from hospitals:

- quality of coding practices for administrative databases (ICD9 or ICD10);
- lack of nationally and internationally standardized procedure codes;
- lack of coding for secondary diagnoses;
- lack of coding for whether a certain condition was present at admission; and
- lack of opportunities for linking the administrative databases of individual hospitals with other databases (e.g. by using a UPI).

In fact, retrieving the appropriate data from medical records also poses problems. Methodological flaws are still reported, even though techniques for performing audits on medical and nursing records are improving. Most countries still lack sufficient usage of electronic health records (EHR), which act as the primary source of data for calculating performance indicators. The optimization of EHRs for population statistics is hindered by political rather than technical problems. Further deterrent factors include privacy legislation and insufficient focus on standardizing data requirements from a public information perspective.

Patient safety indicators

Within hospital services, patient safety has become a major focal point for performance assessment in the past 10 years. Subsequent to the publication of *To err is human* in the US (Kohn, Corrigan & Donaldson, 1999), the EU introduced a number of activities to organize policy development and research in this area. In 2007, a meeting was held in Porto (Portugal) to provide an overview of ongoing research efforts (WHO, 2007) and, in the next year, the EU funded EUNetPaS (European Network for Patient Safety), a project seeking to coordinate various national efforts (EUNetPaS, 2008). Since 2012 this project has been continued as a Joint Action on Patient Safety (European Network on Patient Safety and Quality of Care; PAsQ). WHO has further launched inventory programmes of ongoing research on a global scale. To date, a number of European countries have carried out studies to assess the magnitude of adverse events using data from medical records. To this end, several countries have also implemented adverse event reporting programmes, set up and administered by national patient safety agencies. There is a growing body of knowledge on topics such as safety culture, medication errors, reducing hospital infections,

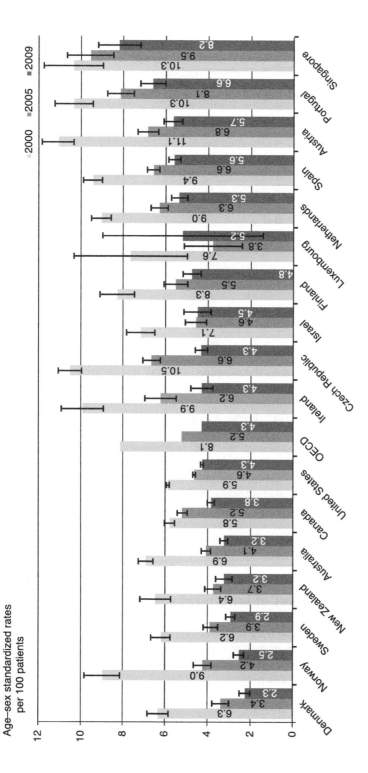

Figure 6.2 Reduction in in-hospital case-fatality rates within 30 days after admission for AMI, 2000–09 (or nearest year)

Note: Rates age–sex standardized to 2005 OECD population (45+). 95% confidence intervals represented by H.
Source: OECD, 2011.

and the implementation of safety systems. OECD's HCQI project has been working on internationally comparative patient safety indicators (PSIs), such as foreign bodies left after surgery, obstetric trauma, accidental punctures and postoperative deep venous thromboses (Drösler et al., 2009, 2012).

With respect to data collection, the challenges relating to patient safety indicators are similar to those found in data collection for other quality indicators on hospital services. Noteworthy are the following:

- many studies depend on the quality of medical records;
- EHRs are often an inadequate source for necessary data;
- many administrative systems have a dearth of secondary diagnosis coding, interfering with the calculation of PSIs;
- these administrative databases often do not record other medical conditions present at admission; and
- linking databases within the hospital (laboratory or pharmacy), or outside the hospital (primary care databases), is either not possible or not allowed.

Readmission rates

Readmission rates have gained popularity as an outcome measure of health care despite being a proxy outcome measure for hospital services, as unplanned hospital readmission cannot always be attributed to the quality of care delivered by professionals working in the hospital and may instead be a function of the performance of other health care services (such as home care or GP services). Since the United States initially employed readmission rates, a growing number of European countries also consider it as an outcome measure of health services and, as such, measure readmission rates systematically. The extent to which readmission rates are regarded as valid and proper is reported in a recent literature study (Fischer, Anema & Klazinga, 2012).

The study points out two main challenges in the use of readmission rates. First, there are conceptual challenges to the definition of "% of readmission to hospital" with regards to time frame, the type of readmissions included (avoidable, emergency, planned) and the applicable case-mix adjustment. Moreover, the actual relationship between this indicator and the quality of care is in need of more supporting evidence.

6.4 Health outcomes of long-term care services

Measuring the quality of long-term care services is of high importance given the global ageing population trend and the present morbidity and disability patterns associated with chronic diseases. Unfortunately, the complexity of chronic care, with services provided in different levels and settings, has very much hampered the identification of possible quality indicators. Types of services may range from home care services, nursing homes, homes for the elderly, assisted living arrangements to many other organization types that offer a combination of nursing, medical, social and domestic services. The majority of existing quality indicators focus on process elements, and client experiences are an important outcome element. Although medical outcomes are only a part of the overall performance of long-term care services, some quality indicators have a specific focus on chronic diseases, for example, diabetes or dementia. In many countries, often as part of disease management programmes, attempts are made to assess the health care outcomes of a specific disease like diabetes by looking at the rates of undesirable outcomes such as foot amputations, renal failure and blindness (diabetic retinopathy). However, the related medical care (such as appropriate use of insulin and medication to control blood-sugar levels) is as much a performance measure of the functioning of the general medical services provided by GPs or medical specialists as a measure of the performance of the nursing services. Overall, it is hard to pinpoint medical outcome measures to the performance of long-term care institutions, so nursing-related indicators, such as bed sores and patient falls, tend to be the only ones used. Future development in this area could assess care services according to their micro, meso and macro levels, so as to circumvent the challenges associated with the multidimensional characteristic of chronic care (McKee & Nolte, 2009). Overall, medical outcomes might be less appropriate to measure the performance of long-term care services than nursing outcomes, more generic health outcomes and measures of patient experiences.

Quality indicators for long-term care for the elderly are also limited by a plethora of technical and conceptual problems. The fact that long-term care is provided in both home and institutional settings creates difficulties in standardizing data collection and reporting conventions (Mor et al., 2009). Recent years have seen some countries, such as the United States, Canada, Finland and Switzerland, beginning to use InterRAI, a standardized data collection system containing a minimum data set and 18 resident assessment protocols as a data validation endeavour (InterRAI, 2006). The current dearth of uniform data on long-term care for the elderly is a primary hindrance to performance assessment, so the adoption of new methods, for example InterRAI, is imperative. The OECD has also recognized the need to identify indicators for long-term care for the elderly and has ongoing efforts to this end. However, quality measurement of chronic diseases is at present considered to be part of the work on performance of primary care systems.

6.5 Measuring the contribution of primary health care to health system performance

The significance of primary care lies in its effectiveness in preventing illness and death, and in its association with a more equitable distribution of health in populations. Thus, as the *World Health Report 2008* states, the primacy of monitoring quality improvements in primary care is now more crucial than ever, because primary care systems are an essential element for an efficient and effective health system (Starfield, Shi & Macinko, 2005; Kringos et al., 2010). Furthermore, the European Commission identified in its recent health strategic approach (2008–2013), the objective to "foster good health in ageing, recognising the global population ageing trend and the subsequent demands on health". The simultaneous increase in the demand for health care and the reduction in the working population suggest that health care expenditure will see a significant increase as a proportion of GDP. However, EU Commission projections estimate that rises in health care expenditure due to an ageing population could be greatly reduced (by up to 50%), suggesting that the usefulness of primary care in mitigating and managing the impact of chronic diseases cannot be underestimated. Consequently, there is increased interest in primary care quality.

Thus, the OECD HCQI project also gives priority to identifying, selecting and implementing quality in primary care. The project further addressed the quality of chronic care, specifically in relation to diabetes and cardiac disease, two of the most common chronic diseases in industrialized countries. In 2004, an OECD Health Technical paper publication, *Selecting indicators for the quality of health promotion, prevention and primary care at the systems level in OECD countries* (Marshall et al., 2006), laid out a selection of indicators for health prevention and primary care that were considered by an expert panel to be sufficiently relevant to policy, as well as scientifically sound, for potential use in international data collection. The panel concluded that "avoidable events" could be useful for capturing problems in the delivery of primary care, especially preventable hospital admissions for conditions that would benefit more from ambulatory care.

Conceptual challenges

Given that primary care systems involve complex and fluid practices in varying community, social and acute care backdrops, designing indicators for assessing quality in primary care is far from simple. The wide variation in payment and contractual organization for primary care services across countries inevitably translates into differences in the scope of data collection possible, consequently affecting the ability to measure one aspect consistently across health systems. Nonetheless, there has been progress in the development of a small collection of comparable quality indicators. Indicators have been developed based on evidence, but significant challenges in ensuring construct consistency across OECD countries remain. Potentially preventable admissions are currently being used in a number of countries.

Operational and methodological challenges

International differences in both data coverage and comprehensiveness further frustrate efforts in making measures of quality of primary care systems available. Despite progress in the international collection of data, the most robust source for deriving indicators in primary care remains hospital administrative data. Indicators such as readmission rates are, after all, proxy indicators of primary care that provide indirect measures of primary care quality. As such, they do not provide a complete assessment of a primary care system's quality of care. Recently the OECD has started to expand its work on quality indicators in primary care by exploring the potential of using national medication prescription data for making international comparisons.

In the future, full understanding of the underlying mechanisms that produce inter-country performance variations, and the extent to which the observed variation is a function of differences in quality of care or an artificial deduction from data, will be fundamental to the development of quality indicators.

Figure 6.3 presents normalized hospital admission rates for asthma, chronic obstructive pulmonary disease (COPD), diabetic acute complications and

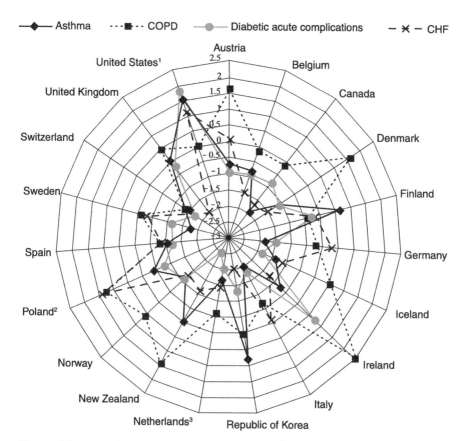

Figure 6.3   Avoidable hospital admission rates, 2007

Notes: The number of hospital admissions for people aged 15 years and over per 100 000 population; age- and sex-standardized rates in relation to the OECD average. Values have been normalized for ease of interpretation. Data from Austria, Belgium, Italy, Poland, Switzerland and the United States refer to 2006. Data from the Netherlands refer to 2005.
1. Data do not fully exclude day cases.
2. Data include transfers from other hospitals and/or other units within the same hospitals, which marginally elevates the rates.
3. Data for CHF include admissions for additional diagnosis codes, which marginally elevates the rates.
CHF: congestive heart failure; COPD: chronic obstructive pulmonary disease.

Source: OECD, 2010b.

congestive heart failure (CHF) for 2007. It illustrates the variation of admissions rates and quality between countries. Quality is visually displayed by distance, where the closer a line is to the centre the lower the volume of potentially preventable admissions. The significant variations in this graph suggest that, if these indicators do indeed measure quality, then countries perform better in certain areas but not others.

6.6 The contribution of mental health care to health system performance

Mental health problems are common, affecting all sections of society and every age group (WHO, 2001; Eaton, 2008; Fajutrao et al., 2009). Mental health care services are provided in a number of settings: within the community, through primary health care, in general and psychiatric hospitals, and in specialized mental health institutions. In recent decades, policy-makers and service-planners in most OECD countries have changed their approach to mental health services, moving away from large psychiatric hospitals and long-stay institutions to an increasing reliance on home and community care.

Because systems of care vary markedly across countries, assessing the quality of mental health care services for evidence-based policy is no easy task (Hermann et al., 2006). Two indicators considered suitable for international comparison are unplanned schizophrenia and bipolar disorder readmission rates (Figures 6.4 and 6.5). In theory, a reduction in average length of stay in many high-income countries is more likely if appropriate levels of community-based care and support are in place. Conversely, any increase in readmission rates could be perceived as a potential indicator of poor-quality initial treatment or community services.

There remain certain challenges for cross-country comparison of readmission rates, because of the freedom service users have to move between different public and private hospitals in addition to the number of cross-referrals. In reality, the availability of national indicator data suitable for international comparison is extremely limited (Garcia-Armesto, Medeiros & Wei, 2008) due to the complex nature of mental health disorders; the differences in diagnostic and therapeutic practices; institutional government barriers; as well as differences in the coding and reporting of mental health care within and between countries. For example, suicide or average life expectancy could be considered as outcome indicators, because the majority of suicides (and therefore a reduction in life expectancy) are often linked to mental health problems (Wilkinson, 1982). However, there are major confounders because of differences in the reporting of death (Renvoize & Clayden, 1990; Kelleher et al., 1998) and differences in the actual care settings and patterns of diagnosis. For example, strict anonymization protocols would be required to make full use of this tool while preserving confidentiality.

In order to measure the outcome of mental health care, for example by using average life expectancy of people once diagnosed with schizophrenia or bipolar disorder, data on treatment and procedures, together with mental morbidity, individual data and specific mortality data would be required. It is essential that mental health-related information systems are further improved so that

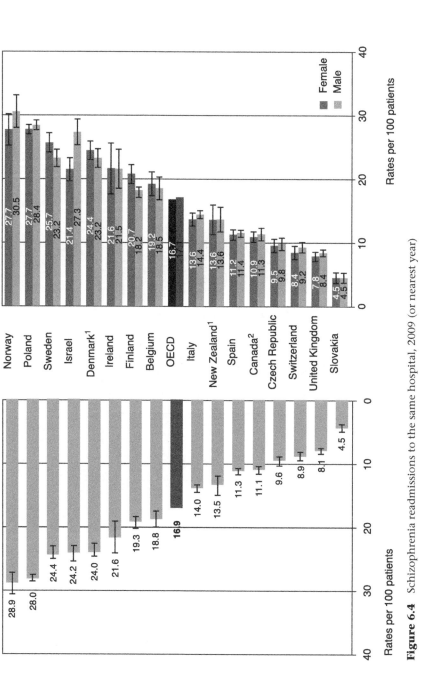

Figure 6.4 Schizophrenia readmissions to the same hospital, 2009 (or nearest year)

Note: Rates age–sex standardized to 2005 OECD population. 95% confidence intervals represented by H.
1. Data do not include patients with secondary diagnosis of schizophrenia and bipolar disorder.
2. Only readmissions within 30 days of the intial hospitalization were counted as readmissions.
Source: OECD, 2011.

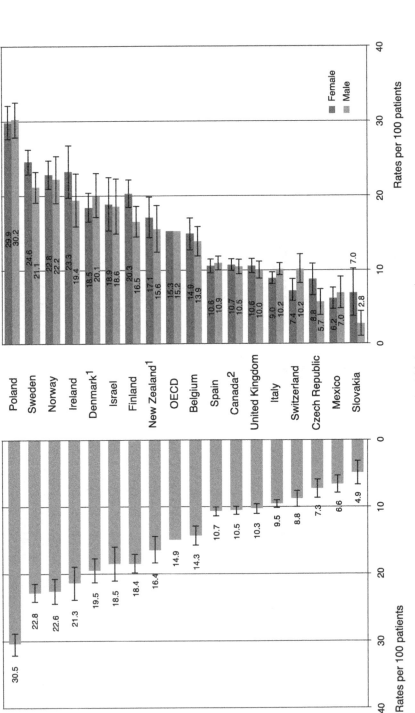

Figure 6.5 Bipolar disorder readmissions to the same hospital, 2009 (or nearest year)

Note: Rates age–sex standardized to 2005 OECD population. 95% confidence intervals represented by H.
1. Data do not include patients with secondary diagnosis of schizophrenia and bipolar disorder.
2. Only readmissions within 30 days of the intial hospitalization were counted as readmissions.

information for comparisons is readily available. While confidentiality is a serious challenge (mental health conditions are more prone to raise privacy and data protection issues than most other areas of care), an expansion of the availability of UPIs is of huge importance. It would signify a significant step forward in terms of the ability to track patients across different settings, facilities and levels of care. Several countries are already undertaking reform along these lines and so an improvement in the availability of data can be expected soon.

6.7 Health outcomes in preventive care

Screening

While screening can be conducted for a variety of infectious diseases as well as non-communicable diseases like hypercholesterolaemia, here the screening rates cited refer to cancer. Screening is of great interest to policy-makers because of the significant bearing it may have on survival prospect. Although, from a health system perspective, screening rates are process measures rather than outcome measures, in many performance reports, they are presented as 'intermediate' outcomes and a signal of compliance with national screening programmes. With reference to breast cancer, countries adopt cancer screening to varying extents; some have endorsed national screening (Finland, Ireland and the Netherlands), while others have local and opportunistic screening (Czech Republic and United States) (Figure 6.6).

Several methodological issues persist in data collection for and comparability of cancer screening indicators in combination with other cancer outcome information, such as five-year survival rates and cancer mortality rates. These include: data sourcing (e.g. surveys versus registries); heterogeneity in cancer survival and screening reporting periods; age standardization; the extent to which country data are nationally representative; and, perhaps most importantly, a lack of cancer staging data. The current mix of nationally and non-nationally representative data renders cross-national comparisons confusing and even invalid. It is difficult to adjust screening and survival rates for different demographic and social profiles between countries. As screening rates are only an intermediate outcome, staging data is crucial for completing an assessment of whether increases in measured survival are due to the earlier detection of cancer. Staging data would facilitate finding a conclusion as to whether screening and survival rates are explicitly correlated. As risk factors for cancer become better understood, the future advancement of screening will not only involve genetics but will also be more explicitly targeted to certain population groups.

6.8 Patient-reported outcome measures (PROMS)

Although initially used in clinical trials to measure outcomes, there is growing interest in using PROMS for more generic outcome measurement. PROMS are

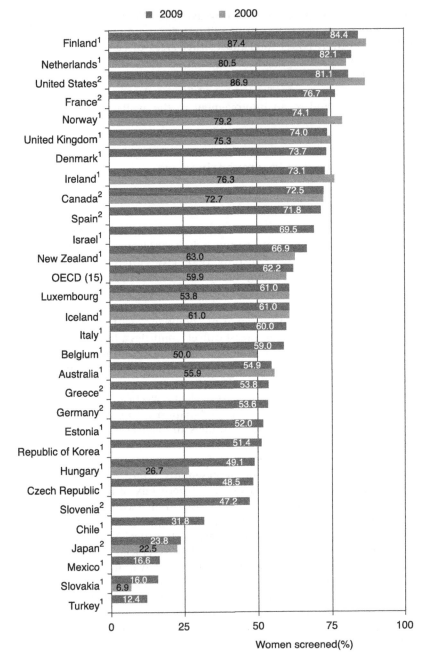

Figure 6.6 Mammography screening, percentage of women aged 50–69 screened, 2000–09 (or nearest year)

Note: 1. Programme. 2. Survey.
Source: OECD, 2011.

not only able to capture and regularly assess aspects of health that are of most concern to patients, but are also argued to be essential for the assessment of patient need and communication between patient and provider in routine care (Fitzpatrick, 2009; Greenhalg, 2012; Hildon, 2012; Worth et al., 2012).

PROM instruments belong to two distinct categories: generic, which are developed to be relevant to the widest possible range of health problems; and specific, which are disease- or condition-specific instruments intended to be relative to a specific disease, or specific aspect or dimension of illness. The argument for specific measures is that they are more sensitive to change in the health-related quality of life produced by an intervention because they contain a higher proportion of supposedly relevant items for the illness and intervention being studied.

By far the most commonly used generic measure, also translated into at least 50 languages, is the Short Form 36 (SF36), a questionnaire with 36 standard questions enquiring about the respondent's health during the past month (Ware and Sherbourne, 1992). Disease-specific PROMs, such as the Arthritis Impact Measurement Scales and Parkinson's Disease Questionnaire (PDQ-39), are used in the belief that they are necessary to identify the small but important benefits and harms associated with novel interventions and clinical trials. In contrast to traditional questionnaires with fixed items, individualized instruments elicit an individual's personal goals and concerns by requiring respondents to state, for example, the five most important areas of their lives affected by a disease or health problem. Unfortunately, individualized instruments are very time-consuming and often involve complex interviews.

To date, there is little evidence of PROMs being used extensively or on an ongoing basis in a health care system for performance assessment. In the UK, PROMs are used at the national level to measure health gain in four clinical procedures: hip and knee replacements; groin hernias; and varicose veins, as shown in Table 6.1 (NHS, The Information Centre 2010). In the Netherlands PROMs have been systematically introduced in mental health care since 2010.

The uptake of PROMs is hindered largely by comparability issues, especially in content validity and the relative importance of different criteria. Indeed, these questionnaires are not only considered to be costly and time-consuming, but also to be potentially intrusive and burdensome to patients, therefore running

Table 6.1 Health status measures used in the PROMs questionnaires (UK)

Procedure	Condition-specific	Generic
Unilateral hip replacement	Oxford Hip Score	EQ-5D
Unilateral knee replacement	Oxford Knee Score	EQ-5D
Groin hernia surgery	None	EQ-5D
Varicose vein surgery	Aberdeen Varicose Vein Questionnaire	EQ-5D

Source: UK Department of Health, 2009.

the risk of jeopardizing the professional client relationship. The future will tell whether PROMs become an integral part of health services delivery.

6.9 Summary of data problems

The current construction of measures of health outcomes related to health services performance, as described in the previous paragraphs, depends on five sources of information:

- administrative databases;
- birth and death statistics (mortality data);
- electronic health records;
- population- and patient-based surveys (i.e. responsiveness); and
- specific registries (for specific diseases and specialities, such as hip replacement or surgical complication).

Birth and death statistics

Birth and death statistics, which are widely available in most countries, are the oldest data source for international comparative studies. Administrative systems that register births and deaths are complete and robust, where causes of death are coded in an internationally comparable manner. However, one main limitation with death data is the lack of secondary diagnosis, which is useful for assessing quality of care in certain areas of health services. For example, given that people diagnosed with schizophrenia or bipolar disorder are associated with excess mortality rates, then average life expectancy, as a proxy measure for the quality of mental health, is dependent entirely on secondary diagnosis data. Data on secondary diagnosis are essential for presenting accurate estimates of the number of people dying who have previously experienced a specific disease in their life. The use of UPIs can help resolve such problems by creating a link between death registries and other potentially relevant administrative databases, like hospital information databases. The sharing of information that UPIs create between primary sources (death registries) and secondary sources (other health information systems) can help to supplement information deficits.

National registries

Efforts within the OECD on HCQI rely heavily on national registries for data on communicable diseases and cancer. A growing number of countries are implementing disease-, procedure- or speciality-specific registries, such as diabetes and surgery registries, providing useful information on quality of care. However, limitations in data coverage, as well as data-coding differences, weaken the international comparability of data. In the future, more complete and standardized codification of staging information for cancer care would facilitate better comparisons in this area.

Administrative databases

Data derived from administrative databases, such as claims, billing, vital records and service utilization, are being increasingly used for quality monitoring purposes. However, these databases often lack important patient care information, including physical examination and laboratory results. Nonetheless, there are numerous advantages to drawing on administrative data for quality monitoring purposes. Not only are data typically accessible and inexpensive, they are also available for a wide range of patient services, both inpatient and outpatient. In addition, these data are likely to be up-to-date, a distinct advantage when seeking to measure quality of care.

Electronic health records

Many countries are adopting health ICT to improve the organization and accessibility of health care information feeds and processes. Such developments are crucial, especially in the face of an increasingly complex range of information feeds associated with similarly multidimensional care processes. EHR systems have become an essential component of health systems that are in pursuit of high-quality, efficient and safe health care processes.

Assuming that ongoing problems with the development of EHRs, such as the lack of standardization and unstructured text, are adequately addressed, their contribution to monitoring and assessing quality could be enormous. For example, consider the recent automated web-based risk assessment tool used in New Zealand for cardiovascular disease among adults aged 45 and over. While this data collection is primarily for clinical management purposes, the data may potentially also be used for monitoring population health and measuring health care performance.

Population surveys

Population surveys are common and cover a range of topics, such as health status, living standards, drug use and prevalence of specific diseases. These surveys provide valuable information on health and health trends because the nature of the surveys is longitudinal and has been collected over multiple years. Surveys can be conducted at both national and subnational levels and data are collected via post, telephone or personal interviews. However, some main drawbacks are the associated monetary expense, the high methodological demands, and the questionable reliability for certain types of condition.

Summary of methodological problems

While various methodological problems have been identified in this chapter, the underlying challenge seems to be the validity of outcome measures of health services. The concern for validity stems in part from the problems in the availability, quality and, consequently, reliability of data. In addition, when outcome measures are taken from one country and used directly in another (e.g. readmission rates), or are linked to financial incentives, validity becomes a prime concern. Within the literature, validity is referred to in four categories: face validity, content validity, construct validity and criteria validity.

- *Face* validity suggests that the outcome measure is supported by experts.
- *Content* validity suggests that underlying research supports the indicator.
- *Construct* validity suggests that observed differences in the outcome measure are related to variations in other measures that are supposed to measure the same underlying phenomenon, for example, do hospitals with a higher HSMR also have higher complication rates?
- *Criteria* validity suggests that any reporting of outcome measures is associated with levels of compliance with evidence-based process measures. Criteria-based studies with a focus on patient safety indicators may be rare but provide the best evidence.

The past 10 years have seen a steep increase in studies on the validity of health outcomes measures related to health services performance. The next 10 years will demonstrate whether outcome measures will be introduced into the practice of policy-makers and health services managers with the necessary accompanying research and development work on the testing of validity and reliability, and whether (national) information infrastructures will strike a balance between privacy and data protection concerns on the one hand and the generation of data for quality and safety governance on the other.

6.10 Conclusions

Assessment of health services and health system performance by means of outcome measures is increasing in popularity. Imperative to an appropriate assessment of outcome-based performance measures are well-defined boundaries of 'health services' and 'health systems'. In particular, the underlying construct of health care actions, which are performed in production units, nested in separate health services as part of the larger organized delivery system of health services, should be made explicit. The three-tier hierarchical model of outcome measures proposed by Porter (2010) should be studied further, especially for understanding and improving the relationships between measurements on the micro, meso and macro levels of the health system.

Thus far, outcome measures can only capture a limited set of dimensions of the broad 'health concept' and seem to focus on mortality (case-fatality rates and HSMRs); adverse events and complications (patient safety indicators); and re- and avoidable admissions (hospital care, mental health care, primary care). Far less prevalent are broader outcome measures in areas such as disabilities and discomfort. In fact, preventive services rely on 'screening rates', in essence, intermediate process measures interpreted alongside outcome measures (survival rates). This application of intermediate outcomes, in addition to the recent adoption of PROMs in the UK as outcome indicators for disease-specific care, exemplify that future development in outcome indicators may well diverge from the existing forms.

As one of the main methodological issues in the development of outcome indicators is data quality and availability, any further development in measuring health outcomes is conditional to the enhancement and expansion of current data sources. This will entail: the further use of UPIs to link various data sources; the use of secondary diagnosis codes and present-at-admission codes; the standardization of procedure codes to increase the potential for case-mix adjustments for outcome measures; and the further development and testing of new measures such as RAI, PROMs and other measures that can use EHRs and patient surveys as their main data source Contingent on privacy and data protection regulation, and supported by the necessary R&D to test reliability and validity, health outcome measures, capturing health services outcomes, will become an increasingly important part of health system performance assessment.

References

Black, N. (2010) Assessing the quality of hospitals, *BMJ*, 340: c2066.

Capewell, S. et al. (1999) Increasing the impact of cardiological treatments. How best to reduce deaths, *European Heart Journal*, 20(19): 1386–92.

Drösler, S.E. et al. (2009) Application of patient safety indicators internationally: a pilot study among seven countries, *International Journal for Quality in Health Care*, 21(4): 272–8.

Drösler, S.E. et al. (2012) International comparability of patient safety indicators in 15 OECD member countries: a methodological approach of adjustment by secondary diagnoses, *Health Services Research*, 47(1 Pt 1): 275–92.

Eaton, W. et al. (2008) The burden of mental disorders, *Epidemiologic Reviews*, 30: 1–14.

EUNetPaS (2008) *European Network for Patient Safety (EUNetPaS)* (http://ns208606.ovh. net/~extranet, accessed 8 October 2012).

Fajutrao, L. et al. (2009) A systematic review of the evidence of the burden of bipolar disorder in Europe, *Clinical Practice and Epidemiology in Mental Health*, 5: 3.

Fischer, C., Anema, H.A. and Klazinga, N.S. (2012) The validity of indicators for assessing quality of care: a review of the European literature on hospital readmission rate, *European Journal of Public Health*, 22(4): 484–91.

Fitzpatrick, R. (2009) Patient-reported outcome measures and performance measurement, in P.C. Smith et al. (eds) *Performance measurement for health system improvement: Experiences, challenges and prospects.* Cambridge: Cambridge University Press.

Fox, M. et al. (2007) The clinical effectiveness and cost-effectiveness of cardiac resynchronisation (biventricular pacing) for heart failure: systematic review and economic model, *Health Technology Assessment*, 11(47): iii–iv, ix–248.

Garcia-Armesto, S., Medeiros, H. and Wei, L. (2008) *Information availability for measuring and comparing quality of mental health care across OECD countries.* Paris: Organisation for Economic Co-operation and Development Publishing (OECD Health Technical Paper, no. 20).

Gil, V. (1999) Right ventricular dysfunction in left dysfunction caused by ischemia: conditioning factors and implications, *Revista Portuguesa de Cardiologia*, 18(12): 1163–72.

Goldberg, R., Gurwitz, J. and Gore, J. (1999) Duration of, and temporal trends (1994–1997) in, prehospital delay in patients with acute myocardial infarction: the Second

National Registry of Myocardial Infarction, *Archives of Internal Medicine*, 159(18): 2141–7.

Greenhalgh J, et al. (2012) How do doctors refer to patient-reported outcome measures (PROMS) in oncology consultations? *Quality of Life Research*, Jun 16 [Epub ahead of print].

Hermann, R. et al. (2006) Quality indicators for international benchmarking of mental health care, *International Journal for Quality in Health Care*, 1(Suppl): 31–8.

Hildon, Z. et al. (2012) Clinicians' and patients' views of metrics of change derived from patient reported outcome measures (PROMs) for comparing providers' performance of surgery, *BMC Health Services Research*, 12: 171.

Institute for Healthcare Improvement (2003) *Move your dot: Measuring, evaluating, and reducing hospital mortality rates*. Cambridge, MA: Institute for Healthcare Improvement.

InterRAI (2006) *Long Term Care Facilities (LTCF)* (http://www.interrai.org/index.php?id=97, accessed 8 October 2012).

Jarman, B. (2008) In defence of the hospital standardized mortality ratio, *Healthcare Papers*, 8(4): 37–42.

Jarman, B. et al. (2005) Monitoring changes in hospital standardised mortality ratios, *BMJ*, 330(7487): 329.

Kelleher, M.J. et al. (1998) Religious sanctions and rates of suicide worldwide, *Crisis*, 19(2): 78–86.

Khush, K., Rapaport, E. and Waters, D. (2005) The history of the coronary care unit, *Canadian Journal of Cardiology*, 21(12): 1041–5.

Kohn, L.T., Corrigan, J.M. and Donaldson, M.S. (eds) (1999) *To err is human: building a safer health system*. Washington, DC: National Academy Press.

Kringos, D.S. et al. (2010) The breadth of primary care: a systematic literature review of its core dimensions, *BMC Health Services Research*, 10: 65.

Lilford, R. and Pronovost, P. (2010) Using hospital mortality rates to judge hospital performance: a bad idea that just won't go away, *BMJ*, 340: c2016.

Marshall, M. et al. (2006) OECD Health Care Quality Indicator Project. The expert panel on primary care prevention and health promotion, *International Journal for Quality in Health Care*, 18(Suppl 1): 21–5.

McGovern, P.G. et al. (2001) Trends in acute coronary heart disease mortality, morbidity, and medical care from 1985 through 1997: the Minnesota heart survey, *Circulation*, 104(1): 19–24.

McKee, M. and Nolte, E. (2009) Chronic care, in P.C. Smith et al. (eds) *Performance measurement for health system improvement: Experiences, challenges and prospects*. Cambridge: Cambridge University Press.

Mor, V. et al. (2009) Long-term care quality monitoring using the interRAI common clinical assessment language, in P.C. Smith et al. (eds) *Performance measurement for health system improvement: Experiences, challenges and prospects*. Cambridge: Cambridge University Press.

NHS, The Information Centre (2010) s (http://www.ic.nhs.uk/statistics-and-data-collections/hospital-care/patient-reported-outcome-measures-proms, accessed on 12 July 2012).

OECD (2009) *Health at a Glance 2009*. Paris: Organisation for Economic Co-operation and Development.

OECD (2010a) *Health at a Glance Europe 2010*. Paris: Organisation for Economic Co-operation and Development.

OECD (2010b) *Improving value in health care: measuring quality*. Paris: Organisation for Economic Co-operation and Development.

OECD (2011) *Health at a Glance 2011*. Paris: Organization for Economic Co-operation and Development.

Porter, M.E. (2010) What is value in health care? *New England Journal of Medicine*, 363(26): 2477–81.

Renvoize, E. and Clayden, D. (1990) Can the suicide rate be used as a performance indicator in mental illness? *Health Trends*, 22(1): 16–20.

Starfield, B., Shi, L. and Macinko, J. (2005) Contribution of primary care to health systems and health, *Milbank Quarterly*, 83(3): 457–502.

Tu, J.V. et al. (2009) National trends in rates of death and hospital admissions related to acute myocardial infarction, heart failure and stroke, 1994–2004, *Canadian Medical Association Journal*, 180(13): E118–25.

UK Department of Health (2009) *Guidance on the routine collection of Patient Reported Outcome Measures (PROMs).* London: Department of Health (http://www.dh.gov. uk/en/Publicationsandstatistics/Publications/PublicationsPolicyAndGuidance/ DH_092647, 6 June 2012).

Ware, J.E. Jr and Sherbourne, C.D. (1992) The MOS 36-item short-form health survey (SF-36). I. Conceptual framework and item selection, *Medical Care*, 30(6): 473–83.

Weisfeldt, M. and Zieman, S. (2007) Advances in the prevention and treatment of cardiovascular disease, *Health Affairs (Millwood)*, 26(1): 25–37.

WHO (2001) *The World Health Report 2001 – Mental Health: new understanding, new hope.* Geneva: World Health Organization.

WHO (2007) *Patient safety research – shaping the European agenda.* Geneva: World Health Organization (http://www.who.int/patientsafety/events/07/26_09_2007/en/index. html, accessed 8 June 2012).

Wilkinson, D.G. (1982) The suicide rate in schizophrenia, *British Journal of Psychiatry*, 140: 138–41.

Worth, A. et al. (2012) Systematic literature review and evaluation of patient reported outcome measures (PROMs) for asthma and related allergic diseases, *Primary Care Respiratory Journal*, Sep 21 (doi: 10.4104/pcrj.2012.00084 [Epub ahead of print].

chapter seven

Conceptualizing and Comparing Equity Across Nations

Cristina Hernández-Quevedo and Irene Papanicolas

7.1 Introduction

Spending on health systems worldwide has reached an all-time high, and yet there is still a wide level of heterogeneity in health status across populations. Within countries there exist differences in health status between populations from different geographical regions, ethnic groups and socioeconomic strata, which can be explained by differences in living conditions, including absolute and relative income, education, employment, housing and transport. Lifestyle choices, such as diet, housing, job control, physical exercise, smoking and alcohol consumption, clearly have an effect on health and are also influenced by social factors (Marmot & Wilkinson, 1999). The health system also plays a role in explaining these health inequalities (Holland, 1986; Mackenbach, Bouvier-Colle & Jougla, 1990; Nolte & McKee, 2004).

Despite general agreement that equity is an important objective of health systems, there is little consensus as to what is meant by equity, how it relates to other concepts, such as equality and fairness, and how it conforms to competing paradigms of justice. While the terms equity and equality both derive from the Latin *aequus* meaning 'equal, fair and just', in their application they have come to represent different notions. Equality is used to convey a notion of equal division of some entity, while equity implies notions of fairness or justice. It is often implied that notions of equality are equitable, although there is frequently a lack of clarity as to what 'entity' should be equal, such as income, wealth, opportunity, capability, or – in the health services literature – well-being, health and/or health care.

In many areas of the health system, such as access to care, we do find notions of equality to be associated with equity. This is referred to as 'horizontal equity', where there is equal treatment of individuals who are equal in a relevant respect, such as 'equal access for equal need'. However, this principle does not hold in all areas of the health system and, in some areas such as health finance, the same distribution of resources is not always perceived to be fair. In such cases, what is equal is not necessarily equitable and what is equitable is not always equal. For this reason, tax systems or health financing systems are often constructed according to principles of 'vertical equity', where groups with unequal needs are treated according to their inequality.

The distinction between equality and equity becomes even more pronounced when considering the achievement of equal health outcomes (for example, equal mortality and morbidity). This task implies eliminating incidental inequalities between individuals, including differences in income, education, housing, but also lifestyle and even genetics. As Oliver and Mossialos (2004) note, this is potentially undesirable because it requires too many restrictions on the ways people may choose to live their lives. However, equity in health outcomes (or attaining less unequal health outcomes) may be a more practical and desirable objective as it focuses efforts on mitigating those circumstances where policy can influence the factors associated with varying outcomes while allowing certain 'acceptable' differences. This echoes Le Grand's argument that inequality in health care use is not inequitable if it is the result of different choices or preferences (Le Grand, 1987,1991).

While equity and equality are not always synonymous, it is also not always clear when this is the case, or what alternative distribution would be more equitable. The assessment of when a distribution should be altered, and how it should be redistributed, requires some form of ethical judgement to be made. While many different paradigms of justice exist, and can be used by policy-makers, different perspectives may produce conflicting assessments of equity (Table 7.1). Thus, the first difficulty in conceptualizing equity in the health system is deciding upon an ethical paradigm with which to assess equity.

The second factor that creates difficulties in conceptualization relates to the selection of a paradigm. While policy-makers may adopt different paradigms as a basis to inform their judgements, there is no ground upon which to select one paradigm universally above all others. Indeed, we live in a pluralistic society in which there exists a diversity of views across policy-makers and societies, and where people are entitled to their own views and personal values. Yet, the diversity in normative perspectives surrounding equity often makes it difficult to agree upon a common starting point from which to assess it. This is a problem encountered in all areas of the public sphere where, in order to form policies, a method of agreement needs to be reached to determine who decides what paradigm to adopt and how they make a decision.

Finally, the third factor relates to another area where differences of judgement occur: the assessment of how narrow or broad the boundaries of the health system are, i.e. what is deemed to be within the context of the health system? Policy-makers must make trade-offs between policy objectives when deciding how to allocate the public budget. Determining the boundaries of the health

Table 7.1 Selected ethical paradigms applied to equity

Ethical paradigm	Main principles	Health policy focus
Libertarian	Preserving personal liberty and ensuring minimum health care standards are achieved. Health care is a privilege not a right.	Free market
Utilitarian	Use resources efficiently to produce the most 'good'.	Cost–benefit analysis
Contractarian	Social and economic institutions should be arranged to maximally benefit the least well-off.	Social exclusion
Community	The well-being of the community as a whole must be protected and ensured.	Public health
Egalitarian	Access to health care is a fundamental human right therefore should not be influenced by income or wealth. Care should be financed according to ability to pay and delivery organized so that everyone has the same access to care.	Health and health care disparities

Adapted from: Aday et al., 2004; Roberts et al., 2008; Allin, Hernández-Quevedo & Masseria, 2009.

system will identify to what extent the health system is accountable for differences in health status between groups. At the national level, clarity of boundaries is important for policy-makers in order to best inform discussions and in carrying out health reforms. At the international level, agreement upon boundaries is necessary to ensure that comparisons are meaningful and methodologically sound.

Recognizing that ethical perspectives and the assignment of boundaries can differ across countries, this chapter does not intend to prescribe which view of equity should be adopted by policy-makers. As disparities in health status are identified, it is up to nations to decide how important it is for these to be corrected. Our views about health equity are not what matters, and so this chapter will not discuss what countries *should* do; instead we are concerned with ensuring that stakeholders are aware of the tools available to them to use in order to measure their performance with regards to the policies they have chosen to advocate. More broadly, the discussion in this chapter will be set in the wider context of equity and socioeconomic determinants of health.

In practice, research on health equity is concerned with one or more of four main variables: health outcomes; health care utilization/access; health care financing; and responsiveness (O'Donnell et al., 2008b). This chapter will focus on these four areas, considering for each: why equity is an important consideration; the supply and demand side factors that contribute to inequities; and the tools and data resources available for measurement. The chapter concludes by reviewing the current limitations in methods and data, before making recommendations for future research and policy.

7.2 Inequalities in health outcomes

While the concept of 'equity' in health is understood and defined in different ways, the study of equity lies in the motivation to understand, and address, the systematic health disparities that exist among different population groups. Discussions of equity and fairness often take a central role in policy debates, whether the focus is on equity in the delivery of health care or on the distribution of health status across different groups in society. At the international level, discussions surrounding equity have focused on identifying and targeting the disparities between richer and poorer countries, but also on investigating the differences in the health disparities between groups within countries.

Van Doorslaer and Van Ourti (2011) note that the measurement and assessment of total inequalities in health and health care have received relatively little attention, with few empirical contributions (Le Grand, 1978, 1987; Wagstaff & van Doorslaer, 2004). The majority of empirical measurement and research has focused on social determinants of health outcomes and numerous studies have demonstrated that the health of populations is related to socioeconomic factors and the organization of society (Marmot & Wilkinson, 1999, 2003). Not only are there large disparities in health status between countries with different levels of wealth, but there are also large differences in the mortality and morbidity of people belonging to different socioeconomic groups within the same country. Even within some of the most affluent countries in the world, evidence shows that people with a lower income, poorer education or low social status have significantly lower life expectancy and suffer from more illnesses than their richer, more educated counterparts. Table 7.2 presents evidence of different socioeconomic sources of inequality from cross-country studies within the EU.

Even where countries have been outlining equity objectives for a long time, there is evidence that inequalities between the poor and the better-off persist. Poor individuals are consistently more likely to suffer higher rates of mortality and morbidity than the richest individuals, and they are less likely to have access to health care. Information on inequities in health outcomes can provide useful knowledge about the demand and supply of health care, which can be helpful in directing policy. On the demand side, the size of health inequality will inform the inequalities in the *need* for health care, across different groups of the population (Olsen, 2011); while on the supply side, information on the size and cause of health inequalities is useful to inform how public monies should be allocated across sectors, as well as within the health system, to maximize health gain in the population.

Key variables

Health status

In order to conduct any national or international analysis of health inequality, some measure of health outcome across the population groups of interest is necessary. In practice, empirical analyses have used measures of health outcome at both the aggregate and individual levels. At the aggregate level, examples

Table 7.2 Some evidence on social determinants of health in Europe

Source of inequality	Evidence	Reference(s)
Education-related inequalities in SAH	Austria, Denmark, Italy, the Netherlands, Norway, Spain, UK, West Germany	Kunst et al. (2005)
Education-related inequalities in chronic diseases	Belgium, Denmark, Finland, France, Italy, the Netherlands, Spain, UK	Dalstra et al. (2005)
Income-related inequalities in health	Belgium, Denmark, Finland, France, the Netherlands, Norway, UK	Mackenbach et al. (2005)
Income-related inequalities in health limitations	Austria, Belgium, Denmark, England, Finland, France, Germany, Greece, Ireland, Italy, Luxembourg, the Netherlands, Portugal, Spain, UK	Hernández-Quevedo et al. (2006)
Education and material deprivation as important determinants of SAH	Czech Republic, Estonia, Hungary, Latvia, Lithuania, Russia	Bobak et al. (2000)
Education-related inequalities in health generally stable over time (1994–2004)	Estonia, Latvia, Lithuania, Finland	Helasoja et al. (2006)

SAH: self-assessed health.

of population health variables used are: life expectancy (Regidor et al., 2003); disability-free life expectancy (DFLE) (Matthews, Jagger & Hancock, 2006); health-adjusted life expectancy (HALE); quality-adjusted life years (QALYs) (Gerdtham & Johannesson, 2000; Burström, Johannesson & Diderichsen, 2005); and disability-adjusted life years (DALYs). However, given the data requirements for the analysis of socioeconomic inequalities, most of the empirical studies in this area use individual health outcome indicators (see Chapter 5 for more information on these types of indicators).

The first challenge to measuring inequalities in health outcomes is finding a robust and widely available indicator with which to measure them. There are a number of different individual health outcome measures that have been used in this area (Box 7.1), ranging from subjective measures such as self-assessed health (Nummela et al., 2007) to more objective measures of health like biological markers (Johnston, Propper & Shields, 2009). In the middle of this spectrum are the quasi-objective indicators, such as: the SF36 physical functioning score (Marmot, 2005); indicators of specific illnesses or disease areas, such as coronary heart disease (Hemmingsson and Lundberg, 2005) or mental health (García-Álvarez et al., 2007); measures of limiting long-standing illness (Eikemo et al., 2008); and body mass index (BMI) (Kopp & Rethelyi, 2004).

Self-assessed health (SAH) is the most common subjective measure of individual health, providing an ordinal ranking of perceived health status, which is generally available in socioeconomic surveys at both national and

Box 7.1 Measures of health outcomes

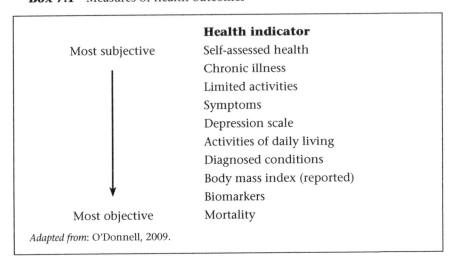

	Health indicator
Most subjective	Self-assessed health
	Chronic illness
	Limited activities
	Symptoms
	Depression scale
	Activities of daily living
	Diagnosed conditions
	Body mass index (reported)
	Biomarkers
Most objective	Mortality

Adapted from: O'Donnell, 2009.

international levels. The health question usually asks the respondent to rate their general health, sometimes including a time reference (they are asked to rate their health over the last twelve months), or an age benchmark (they are asked to assess their current health compared to individuals of their own age). Respondents are often given five categories to choose from, ranging from very good or excellent to poor or very poor; this also varies in practice.

In the literature, SAH has been used in numerous studies which have investigated: the relationship between health and socioeconomic status (Ettner, 1996; Deaton & Paxson, 1998; Smith, 1999; Benzeval, Taylor & Judge, 2000; Salas, 2002; Adams et al., 2003; Frijters, Haisken-DeNew & Shields, 2005); the relationship between health and lifestyles (Kenkel, 1995; Contoyannis, Jones & Rice, 2004); and the analysis of socioeconomic inequalities in SAH (van Doorslaer et al., 1997). SAH has been found to be a powerful predictor of subsequent mortality (Idler & Kasl, 1995; Idler & Benyamini, 1997) and this predictive power does not vary across socioeconomic groups (Burström & Fredlund, 2001). Moreover, it is a good predictor of subsequent use of medical care (van Doorslaer et al., 2000) and of inequalities in mortality (van Doorslaer & Gerdtham, 2003).

However, there are debates surrounding the validity of SAH as a measure of health status. Some researchers have suggested that perceived health does not correspond with actual health (Bound, 1991). The main concerns are that, as a subjective measure of health, SAH may be prone to measurement errors. Indeed, numerous studies have identified the existence of differential reporting of health across individuals or groups of individuals with the same health status. In particular, the association between self-assessed health and mortality is often mediated by geographic location, psychosocial factors (e.g. social integration, stress), gender, age, and socioeconomic position (Idler & Benyamini, 1997; Berkman & Kawachi, 2000; Cattell, 2001; Sen, 2002; Lindeboom & van Doorslaer, 2004; Kievit et al., 2005) Thus, self-reported health is not only a function of actual health status, but also of individuals' or population groups' perceptions of health.

This systematic use of different threshold levels by different population groups reflects the existence of reporting bias and this source of measurement error has been termed: "state-dependent reporting bias" (Kerkhofs & Lindeboom, 1995); "scale of reference bias" (Groot, 2000); and "response category cut-point shift" (Sadana et al., 2000; Murray et al., 2001). This occurs if subgroups of the population use systematically different cut-point levels when reporting their SAH, despite having the same level of 'true health'. Essentially, different groups appear to interpret the question within their own specific context and therefore use different reference points when they are responding to the same question. It has been shown by Bago d'Uva et al. (2008) that correcting for reporting differences generally increases income-related inequalities in health. This is specifically a concern in cross-country studies, given that respondents from different cultural and national settings may have different reference levels of health, as response categories may not mean the same thing. In a cross-country study, Jurges (2007) found that there are considerable differences in cross-country reporting styles, and that failing to account for these may yield misleading results when comparing health across countries.

Various approaches to correcting for reporting bias have been developed in the literature. The first approach is to condition on a set of objective indicators of health and argue that any remaining variation in SAH reflects reporting bias. For example, Lindeboom and van Doorslaer (2004) used Canadian data and the McMaster Health Utility Index as their quasi-objective measure of health, finding some evidence of reporting bias by age and gender, but not by income. However, this approach relies on having a sufficiently comprehensive set of objective indicators to capture all the variation in true health. The second is to use health vignettes, such as those currently included in the *World Health Survey* (Murray et al., 2001; Kapteyn, Smith & van Soest, 2004; Bago d'Uva et al., 2008). The third is the examination of biological markers of disease risk in the countries considered for comparison. Studies such as Banks et al. (2006) combine self-reported data with biological data, which might result in less ambiguous results. Also, Johnston and colleagues report that the income gradient appears significant when using an objective measure of hypertension measured by a nurse rather than the self-reported measure of hypertension included in the *Household Survey of England* (Johnston, Propper & Shields, 2009).

As individuals tend to evaluate their own health relative to that of their peers, objective measures of health status such as physicians' assessments or hospital stays are thought to be the best for comparative purposes. However, the availability of objective measures of health, such as biomarkers, is restricted to very specific national surveys. At the European level, neither the *European Community Household Panel Survey* (ECHP) nor the *European Union Survey of Income and Living Conditions* (EU-SILC) include objective measures. Only the *Survey of Health, Ageing and Retirement in Europe* (SHARE) and the forthcoming *European Health Interview Survey* include objective (for example, walking speed, grip strength) and quasi-objective (for example, ADL, symptoms) measures of health.

Together with their limited availability, biomarkers may also be subject to bias and are not included in longitudinal data. The main methodological challenge lies with the standardization of data collection, as variations may arise from different methods of collection, for example, a person's blood pressure may vary according to the time of day it is taken. In fact, information on the details of objective health collection is often not provided. These measurement errors are particularly problematic if correlated with sociodemographic characteristics, hence, biasing estimates of social inequalities. Collecting biological data also tends to reduce survey response rates, which limits the sample size and representativeness (Masseria et al., 2007). The limitation of biological markers to cross-sectional data is an important disadvantage as using longitudinal data allows the exploration of the dynamic relationship between health, socioeconomic status and access to health care (Hernández-Quevedo, Jones & Rice, 2008).

One way of identifying individual reporting behaviour regarding health is to examine variations in the evaluation of given health states represented by hypothetical vignettes (Tandon et al., 2003; Kapteyn, Smith & van Soest, 2004; King et al., 2004; Salomon, Tandon & Murray, 2004). The vignettes represent fixed levels of latent health, and hence, all the remaining variation in their rating can be attributed to reporting behaviour (Box 7.2). This could be analysed in relation to observed characteristics. On the assumption that individuals rate the vignettes in the same way as they rate their own health, it is possible to identify a measure of health that is purged of reporting heterogeneity.

Other surveys that include vignettes are SHARE and the WHO *World Health Surveys*, 2002–2003 (Üstün et al., 2003). Murray et al. (2003) evaluate the vignette approach to the measurement of health, in the domain of mobility, using data from 55 countries covered by the *WHO Multi-Country Survey Study on Health and Responsiveness* (WHO-MCS, 2000–2001). The principal objective of their analysis is to obtain comparable measures of population health that are purged of cross-country differences in the reporting of health. Reporting of health is allowed to vary with age, sex and education, but there is no

---

Box 7.2   Example of a vignette

The following is an example of an instrument containing three vignettes for the domain of mobility. For each vignette, the respondent is asked to determine how much difficulty [*name in example*] had in moving around. Response categories range from: extreme difficulty/severe difficulty/ moderate difficulty/no difficulty.

- Paul is an active athlete who runs long distance races of 20km twice a week and plays soccer with no problems.
- Vincent has a lot of swelling in his legs due to his health condition. He has to make an effort to walk around his home as his legs feel heavy.
- George has a brain condition that makes him unable to move. He cannot even move his mouth to speak or smile. He can only blink his eyelids.

Source: Masseria et al., 2007.

detailed examination of these dimensions of reporting heterogeneity, or of the impact on measured health disparities. Bago d'Uva et al. (2006) use differences in reporting of health based on six domains (sex, age, urban/rural location, education and income) and assess to what extent estimated disparities in health change when reporting differences are purged from the health measures. They find that, although homogeneous reporting by sociodemographic groups is significantly rejected, the size of the reporting bias in health disparities is not large.

Measure of variation

Very few empirical studies in the area of equity have focused on total health inequalities (van Doorslaer & van Ourti, 2011). Most assessments focus on socioeconomic inequalities as a result of social class (Kelleher et al., 2003), self-reported education (Silventoinen et al., 2005), and disposable household income (Nummela et al., 2007). Box 7.3 outlines the potential sources of a socioeconomic gradient, which might well differ across the individual's life-cycle. In order to associate differences in health outcomes with any of these factors, it is necessary to be able to group the outcome measures by any of the socioeconomic variables being examined.

Box 7.3   Potential sources of socioeconomic gradient

- Current Income ($Y = Y_p + Y_e$)
  - o Permanent income (Y_p)
  - o Random income (Y_e)
- Wealth ($W = S+H+F+I$)
  - o Savings wealth (S)
  - o Housing wealth (H)
  - o Financial wealth (F)
  - o Inherited wealth (I)
- Knowledge (K)
  - o Education
  - o Ability
  - o Informal knowledge
  - o Health knowledge
- Environmental effects (E)
  - o Personal environment (individual effects)
    - Marriage
  - o Neighbourhood effects (contextual effects)
  - o Peer effects (endogenous effects)
    - Social interactions

Source: Costa-Font & Hernández-Quevedo, 2012.

Most high-income countries have databases that include information on income and education. These can take the form of household-based surveys, which are conducted regularly and occasionally contain information on subjective health status, or can be collected through other administrative databases. In some countries, data linkage allows these indicators across different databases to be grouped together; however, this requires a method to identify individuals across data. Often, these identifiers do not exist for reasons of privacy and protection. Studies on international comparisons mostly make use of cross-country surveys, which collect information on income, health and, possibly, education.

Information on wealth, knowledge and environmental effects is often limited. Thus, many empirical assessments fail to account for these parameters. These omissions limit our understanding of inequalities. For example, most available income data are based on current income and do not include information on wealth; hence, only a few studies have managed to disentangle the effect of permanent income (e.g. Eberth and Gerdtham, 2008). Other important factors associated with income, such as knowledge and social environment, are also not usually controlled for, which can bias results and leave many possible explanations uncovered.

Measurement techniques

With adequate comparable data on health outcomes and social, economic or demographic variables, there are a few different measurement techniques that can be used to determine the extent of inequity in health within or across countries, either in absolute or relative terms. Several methodologies exist to measure inequalities in health and these are often grouped differently in the literature (Mackenbach & Kunst, 1997; Regidor, 2004a, 2004b; Harper & Lynch, 2006). The different methodologies also differ in their degree of complexity, ranging from the construction and comparison of simple ratios across groups, to more complex regression models. Following the classification provided by Mackenbach and Kunst (1997), we will review the following methods: gap measures (e.g. rates of difference); correlation and regression measures (e.g. relative index of inequality and slope index of inequality); and Gini-like coefficients (e.g. concentration index).

Gap measures

Gap measures, such as rate differences and rate ratio measures are simple measures of the difference in health between two population groups. For example, we could measure the level of health of the lowest income group of a society (measured by the first quintile of income) and the richest income group (fifth quintile) (de Looper & Lafortune, 2009). While gap measures are easy to construct and interpret, using easily accessible data, they have several drawbacks. Gap measures provide a range or a measure of the gap between two groups, but no information on intermediate categories. Moreover, they do not take into consideration the size of the groups, which does not facilitate cross-country analysis. Hence, these measures are limited in that they don't take into account the whole distribution and nor can other confounding factors be easily controlled for.

Correlation and regression measures

Regression analysis allows researchers to take into account the whole range of health outcomes and to control for confounding factors. This method can be used to create measures such as the slope index of inequality (SII) and the relative index of inequality (RII), which are better able to capture the socioeconomic dimension of health distribution. The SII is defined as the slope of the regression line showing the relationship between the level of health in each socioeconomic group and the hierarchical ranking of each group on the social scale. By construction, the SII is sensitive to the average health status of the population. The RII, obtained by dividing the SII by the average level of health of the population (Regidor, 2004b), corrects for this, and thus is a better choice of indicator for cross-country comparisons. An application of these methods can be found in Sassi (2009).

Gini-like coefficients

Increasingly, new methods based upon the analysis of income distribution, have dominated the empirical literature on measurement of inequalities in health outcomes (Wagstaff & van Doorslaer, 2000). These techniques based on regression analysis allow for a more sophisticated analysis that enables researchers to take into account the whole population. In this chapter we will review the Lorenz curve as applied to health, the concentration curve and the various indices of health inequality that can be constructed using these curves.

Lorenz curve and Gini coefficient

The Lorenz curve and Gini coefficients in health are based upon the tools, of the same name, used to measure income distributions within a population. When applied to health, these tools allow the measurement of the distribution of 'pure' inequalities in health variables across a population, or overall inequalities.[1] The Lorenz curve is constructed by plotting the cumulative proportions of the population on the horizontal axis. Individuals are ranked by their level of health, from the sickest to the healthiest individual, and plotted against the cumulative proportions of health on the vertical axis. If the distribution of health across a population were equal, the Lorenz curve would represent a 45-degree line, such as the perfect equality line in Figure 7.1. In most cases, there is an unequal distribution of health in the population and so the Lorenz curve is convex, as illustrated in Figure 7.1. The further away the curve lies from the line of equality, the larger the level of inequalities in health.

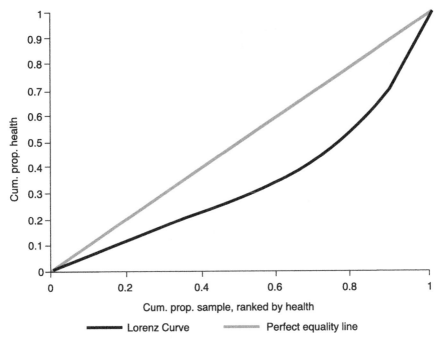

Figure 7.1 Lorenz curve for health status

This inequality can also be captured in numeric form by the Gini index, which is defined as twice the area between the 45-degree line and the Lorenz curve, or calculated using the following formula:

$$G = 2/\mu \text{cov}(\gamma_i, R_i) \tag{7.1}$$

where μ is the average health of the population, y_i is the health variable considered, and R_i the ranking of individuals in the health distribution.[2]

Concentration curve and index

While the Lorenz curve and Gini index provide information on the overall inequality of a population, they do not provide information on the social gradient in health. The Lorenz curve is univariate, in that it investigates the variation of health across the population. An analysis of the variation of health by social groups requires a multivariate analysis, where the distribution of health is plotted against the distribution of social status (measured by income, level of education, etc.). An extension of the Lorenz curve allows for this multivariate analysis. The concentration curve (CC), and its corresponding index, the concentration index (CI), indicate the level of income-related health inequality within a population, in relative terms (Wagstaff, van Doorslaer & Paci, 1989).

Figure 7.2 illustrates the CC for a measure of health limitations; in this figure, the sample/population of interest is ranked by socioeconomic status, rather than level of health. Assuming income is used as the relevant ranking variable, the horizontal axis indicates the cumulative proportion of individuals ranked from the poorest and progressing through the income distribution up to the richest. This relative income rank is then plotted against the cumulative proportion of health limitations on the vertical axis in order to construct the CC. Thus, the CC represents the cumulative percentage of health limitations relative to the cumulative percentage of the population ranked from the poorest to the richest (if income is the socioeconomic variable of interest). In Figure 7.2 this corresponds to the concave curve.

If there was perfect equality in health across the different population groups, the CC would be equal to a 45-degree line. This line would indicate perfect equality, such that the poorest 20% of individuals experience 20% of the illness in the population. In Figure 7.2, the concave CC lies above the line of equality, indicating a pro-poor distribution of health limitations, with poor individuals concentrating a disproportionate level of health limitations, e.g. 20% of health limitations in this society. The size of inequality can be summarized by the health CI, which is given by twice the area between the CC and the 45-degree line.

The CI is a measure of the degree of association between an individual's level of health and his relative position in the income distribution, derived from the location of the CC relative to the line of equality. There are various ways of expressing the CI algebraically (Wagstaff & van Doorslaer, 2000; O'Donnell et al., 2008b). The one that is most frequently used in the literature is:

$$C = \frac{2}{\mu} \sum_{i=1}^{N} (y_i - \mu)(R_i - \tfrac{1}{2}) = \frac{2}{\mu} \operatorname{cov}(y_i, R_i) \tag{7.2}$$

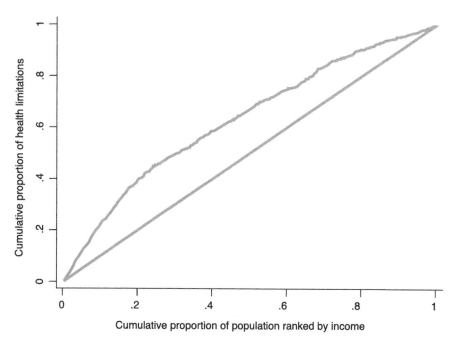

Figure 7.2 Concentration curve for an indicator of health limitations

known as the 'convenient covariance' method as it provides a more convenient formula or device for computation (Kakwani, 1980; Jenkins, 1988). Expression (7.2) shows that the value of the CI is a measure of the association between individual health (y_i) and the individual's relative rank (R_i), scaled by the mean of health in the population (μ). The whole expression is multiplied by 2, to ensure that the CI ranges between –1 and +1. A positive (negative) value of the CI implies that the health outcome is concentrated among the rich (poor). It is important to highlight that, if the CI equals zero, this does not mean an absence of inequality but an absence of the socioeconomic gradient in the distribution, i.e. an absence of inequality associated to socioeconomic characteristics.

In their review of measures of health inequalities, Wagstaff, Paci and van Doorslaer (1991) point out the advantages of the CC and CI over other indicators: they are able to capture the socioeconomic dimension of health inequalities; they use information from the whole income distribution rather than just the extremes; they offer the possibility of visual representation through the CC; and finally, they allow checks of dominance relationships.

Standardization of the concentration index

A demographic standardization of the health distribution aims to describe the distribution of health by socioeconomic status, conditional on other factors such as age and sex (O'Donnell, 2008b). Assuming the researcher is interested in measuring the magnitude of avoidable inequalities in health, in cross-country analyses, the CI must account for the role that demographic factors play in generating such inequality in each of the countries considered. Thus, the index is standardized by age and gender, variables that may be considered policy-irrelevant.

For this purpose, the literature proposes two alternative methods: a direct standardization and an indirect standardization method, which are explained in detail elsewhere (see O'Donnell et al., 2008b). The direct standardization requires the use of grouped data but the number of groups considered will influence the magnitude of the CI (Kakwani, Wagstaff & van Doorslaer, 1997). An example of direct standardization is provided by van Doorslaer and colleagues (1997). The indirect standardization method can be applied to individual-level data, which consider those variables we would like to standardize for. However, it has been argued that the indirect standardization method underestimates the level of inequalities in health when the standardizing variables are correlated with income (Gravelle, 2003). Some applications can be found in Wagstaff and van Doorslaer (2000) and, more recently, Costa-Font, Hernández-Quevedo & McGuire (2011).

Decomposition analysis

Further information as to the source of the inequalities in health can be identified using a decomposition analysis. The CI approach allows the decomposition of overall inequalities in health by the contribution of 'need' and 'non-need' variables (Wagstaff, van Doorslaer & Watanabe, 2003; O'Donnell et al., 2008b). Using the results from the regressions used to construct the CC, we can also measure the contribution of different variables to the total inequality being measured. The variables being considered will vary by the data available for inclusion in the analysis.

The decomposition analysis assumes that the contribution of each variable to total inequality is the product of three factors (divided by the mean value of the dependent variable): firstly, the relative weight of that variable (measured by its mean); second, its income distribution (Gini coefficient for income itself and the CI for all other variables); and finally, the marginal effect on the health model (linear regression coefficient). Together with these deterministic components, there is also a residual component that reflects the income-related inequality in health that is not explained by systematic variations in the regressors with respect to income. This value should approach zero for a well-specified model.

Equity and efficiency trade-off

A discussion that is common in the area of equity in health outcomes concerns the so-called 'equity–efficiency' trade-off. This trade-off refers to the conflicting attainment of two goals in the presence of scarce resources: improving the health status of the population as well as the equity of health outcomes. Wagstaff (2002) has described this as a normative trade-off in the literature, where policy-makers may be willing to sacrifice some aggregate health for more equality of health. While more aggregate or average health is considered a good thing, inequality of health around the average is negatively valued. This trade-off between the achievement in terms of average health and the level of inequality will depend on the level of aversion to inequality of the policy-maker, with a level of aversion to inequalities that could range from zero (only focusing on 'efficiency', defined as improving the average health of the population or higher) to infinity. The higher the level of aversion to inequalities in health, the more weight is given to the worse-off in that society.

The standard CI does not capture the equity–efficiency trade-off. However, Wagstaff (2002) has established an index of health achievement, which summarizes the equity–efficiency trade-off for different degrees of inequality aversion, given by the following expression:

$$IHAv = \mu 1 - C(v) = 1ni = 1 \, nyiv \, (1 - R_i)(v - 1), \tag{7.3}$$

where y_i is the measure of health for individual i and R_i is their relative rank in the socioeconomic distribution. The different degrees of inequality aversion are represented by v.

This index has been applied to comparative cross-country analysis by Hernández-Quevedo et al. (2006), showing how different weights provided to poorer individuals can alter the achievement of the different countries according to health in the EU15. Meheus and van Doorslaer (2008) and Xu

(2006) also apply this index, using the *Demographic and Health Surveys* and the *US Current Population Survey*, respectively. Some recent OECD work that has attempted to understand and quantify the equity and efficiency trade-off, using panel data regressions and data envelopment analysis (see Chapter 10), found that countries with the lowest inequalities in health status also tend to enjoy the highest average health status (Joumard, André & Nicq, 2010).

The equity–efficiency trade-off also applies to the delivery of health care (Gulliford, 2003). While an efficient health service may provide the greatest aggregated amount of access for a given level of resources, being efficient does not imply that access is distributed fairly between groups (Williams, 1997). Hence, inequities may be reduced but with an associated cost which may not always be socially acceptable.

Long-term inequalities in health

One of the main limitations of existing approaches to measuring inequalities in health is a failure to consider the longitudinal perspective. When studying a series of cross-sectional samples of the population across time, it is not possible to understand how changes in an individual's income are related to changes in their health; cross-sectional data cannot detect the effect of change in income ranks over time (for example, downwardly income mobile individuals have poorer than average health). Hence, a long-run perspective, where income is averaged over a series of periods for each individual, may be considered when longitudinal data are available.

Jones and López-Nicolás (2004) show that income-related health inequality can be either greater or smaller in the long run as compared to the short run. This difference can be measured through an index of health-related income mobility, based on the CI, called the mobility index (MI) (Box 7.4). The MI measures the covariance between levels of health and fluctuations in income

Box 7.4 Construction and application of the mobility index

The MI measures the covariance between levels of health and fluctuations in income rank over time and is given by the following expression:

$$M^T = 1 - \frac{CI^T}{\sum_t w_t CI^t} = \frac{2}{N \sum_t \bar{y}^t CI^t} * \left(\sum_i \sum_t (y_{it} - \bar{y}_t)(R_i^t - R_i^T) \right),$$

$$w_t = \frac{\bar{y}^t}{T \bar{\bar{y}}^T},$$

and

(i) $\bar{y}^t = \dfrac{\sum_i y_{it}}{N} \; i = 1, \ldots, N; \; t = 1, \ldots, T,$

(ii) $\bar{\bar{y}}^T = \dfrac{\sum_t \sum_i y_{it}}{NT} = \dfrac{\sum_t \bar{y}^t}{T},$

where y_{it} is a cardinal measure of illness for individual i (i = 1, . . ., N) at time t (t = 1, ..., T); $y_i^T = (1/T) \sum_t y_{it}$ is the average for individual i after T periods; R_i^t is the relative rank of individual i in the income distribution in period t; R_i^T is the relative rank of individual i in the distribution of average income after T periods. For a more detailed explanation on how to calculate long-run inequalities and the mobility index, see, for example, Jones and López-Nicolás (2004) and Hernández-Quevedo et al. (2006).

Hernández-Quevedo et al. (2006) constructed long-term concentration indices and mobility indices for various European countries (see Table 7.3). The long-term concentration indices (CI^T) are negative for all the countries; hence, there are long-term income-related inequalities in health, with health limitations more concentrated among those with lower incomes. The largest long-term socioeconomic inequalities in health limitations can be seen in Cyprus, while the smallest correspond to Poland (in absolute terms). The long-term concentration index for Poland has a value of –0.04, which implies that in the long term health limitations are more concentrated among individuals in the bottom of the income distribution. The MI has a value of 0.32, thus a failure to take into account the mobility of individuals in the income distribution over time when calculating long-term inequalities in health would result in a 32% overestimation of inequalities in health limitations.

The majority of the mobility indices are positive, indicating there is lower long-run income-related inequality in health limitations than would be inferred by the average of the short-run indices. However, for some countries such as Austria, Czech Republic, France, Latvia, Slovakia, mobility indices are negative. This suggests that in these countries, downwardly income mobile individuals are more likely to suffer health limitations than upwardly mobile individuals. Comparing the absolute size of the overall mobility index across the countries, we can see that the greatest value corresponds to Belgium and the lowest to the United Kingdom.

Source: Hernández-Quevedo, Masseria & Mossialos, 2010b.

---

rank over time. If income rankings remain constant over time, long-term inequalities equal the (weighted) average of the short-run CIs. If people switch ranks over the T periods, and these changes are systematically related to health, MI differs from zero. If MI is positive, then upwardly income mobile individuals – in the sense that their rank in the long-run distribution of income is greater than their rank when income is measured over a short period – enjoy a smaller than average level of illness. Of course, this means that downwardly mobile individuals would tend to have a greater than average level of illness. In these circumstances, long-run income-related health inequality would be greater than the average of the short-run measures.

Table 7.3 Long-term concentration indices and mobility indices, 2005–2007

	CI^T	MI
BE	–0.20	0.17
CZ	–0.19	–0.21
EE	–0.16	0.21
ES	–0.12	0.15
FR	–0.13	0.00
IT	–0.11	0.08
CY	–0.26	0.01
LV	–0.20	–0.12
LT	–0.17	0.04
LU	–0.09	0.14
HU	–0.10	0.08
NL	–0.17	0.01
AT	–0.13	–0.02
PL	–0.04	0.32
PT	–0.11	0.08
SI	–0.17	0.07
SK	–0.12	–0.07
FI	–0.10	0.14
SE	–0.12	0.01
UK	–0.21	–0.01

[T]The 'adjusted' concentration index.

Source: Hernández-Quevedo, Masseria & Mossialos, 2010b.

Although the CI is widely used to measure inequalities in health, there are several known methodological issues, highlighted in the literature, which make it difficult to use for comparative purposes. The first main issue is that the bounds of the CI depend on the mean of the health variable, making comparisons across populations with different mean health levels problematic (Wagstaff, 2005). Another issue is that different rankings are obtained when comparing inequalities in health with inequalities in ill health (Clarke et al., 2002). Finally, it has been argued that if the health variable has a qualitative nature, then the index becomes arbitrary. Given these three issues, Erreygers (2009) suggested a new corrected CI that can be used to compare groups of individuals that could present different levels of average health.

Taking into account the usual CI given by expression (7.2), the corrected CI can be calculated as follows:

$$E(h) = \frac{4\bar{y}}{y^{max} - y^{min}} * C(y) \tag{7.5}$$

where $\bar{y}$ is the mean of the health variable, y^{max} and y^{min} are the extremes of the health variable and C(y), the 'old' CI. Without this correction, the CI will depend on average health and it may result in incorrect comparisons of inequalities in health among the countries analysed. Hernández-Quevedo, Masseria and Mossialos (2010a, b) calculate the CI and adjusted CI using the same data. When comparing these results, one can observe differences in the magnitude and trends of inequalities in health limitations in several countries.

Data limitations

Although comparative indicators on inequality of health and equity in access to health care are available at the European and non-European levels, current equity indicators derived from past and ongoing projects and datasets may be misleading for policy-makers. There are still various factors that contribute to a lack of good comparable information, which makes it difficult to make adequate cross-country comparisons. The first of these factors is the lack of datasets providing a longitudinal perspective. This makes it difficult to determine how policies related to inequalities in health are performing.

Another factor is the limited understanding of the variables explaining health production processes and sources of inequalities, including the role of mental conditions along with cognitive biases in measuring self-reported health. Without a proper framework to consider all the processes that can influence health and the reporting of health, measurement may be misleading. However, even in areas where we do have an idea that there is an effect on health production, limited data make it difficult to measure. One such area is environmental effects, where there is little recorded information that can be linked to existing health variables; thus, it is very difficult to measure how sensitive inequalities in health are to this factor. Similarly, there is inadequate identification of what stands behind measures of socioeconomic position, namely, different income sources and measures of wealth and social environmental controls. The effects of the latter differ across the life-cycle.

Finally, most measures make wide use of self-reported measures of health status given their availability in harmonized datasets. While the availability of these datasets allows international comparisons to be made, there are several limitations to this indicator, which are aggravated by the lack of measures of calibration available in some datasets but not in others. One of the main concerns behind the use of self-assessed health measures is its reliability as a good predictor of objective health status as a whole.

7.3 Inequities related to the health system

The methodologies and concepts reviewed thus far have been focused on measuring the distribution in health across different groups of society. However, a large body of equity research is concerned more specifically with the assessment of the fairness in the distribution of health care. It is important to note, however, that most inequalities in health do not arise from inequalities in access to and delivery of medical care. Indeed, while empirical assessments differ, it is acknowledged that medical care plays a limited role in improving the health of the population relative to other inputs (from other sectors) (see Chapter 5). Nevertheless, a large body of work exists to assess equity within the health system. Aday et al. (2004) refer to this research as 'procedural equity' in contrast to the wider study of disparities in health across groups, which they refer to as 'substantive equity'.

Many international and national HSPA programmes do evaluate health systems based on their ability to ensure that individuals in need of health care receive effective treatment, and even financial protection (see Chapter 2). These egalitarian principles are also echoed in various policy documents and declarations (Allin, Hernández-Quevedo & Masseria, 2009). For this reason, research has been carried out to assess the extent to which procedural equity is achieved within and across health systems. Many health system frameworks identify equity as an intermediate goal, contributing to the final goals of health improvement, responsiveness and efficiency. Thus, the main focus of procedural equity tends to be on the extent to which equity allows these goals to be achieved for the population.

With regard to health improvement, there is a focus on understanding the extent to which there are barriers to the delivery of medical care, or inequitable access to health care. A key area relating to access, often referred to in its own right, is the study of the financial barriers to medical care. Finally, there is also concern about how equitable the system is with regard to other major goals, such as responsiveness and quality. This section will review the terminology, variables and methods associated with equity measurement in these areas.

Equity of access

The equitable distribution of health care is a principle subscribed to in many countries, often explicitly in legislation or official policy documents. Egalitarian equity goals distinguish between horizontal equity (the equal treatment of equals) and vertical equity (appropriate unequal treatment of unequals). In health care, most attention, both in policy and research, has been given to the horizontal equity principle, defined as "equal treatment for equal medical need, irrespective of other characteristics such as income, race, place of residence, etc." (Wagstaff, van Doorslaer and Paci, 1991; van Doorslaer et al., 2000; Wagstaff & van Doorslaer, 2000; O'Donnell et al., 2008b). To define inequity of access, it is usual to distinguish between need variables that 'ought to' affect the use of health care and non-need variables that 'ought not' (Gravelle, Morris & Sutton, 2006). Many studies of horizontal inequity focus on the relationship between use of need and non-need variables after controlling or standardizing for need.

Key variables

Access

In many empirical research papers concerned with equity of access, the terms *access* and *utilization* are used indistinctively, implying that an individual's use of health services is proof that he/she can access these services (Allin, Hernández-Quevedo & Masseria, 2009). However, utilization is not equivalent to access (Le Grand, 1982; Mooney, 1983). Access refers to opportunities, whereas utilization is the manifestation of those opportunities. Differences in utilization could be either due to acceptable reasons (e.g. personal preference) or unacceptable reasons, e.g. information about service availability, direct costs (e.g. user charges), or indirect costs (e.g. transport, lost wages) (Masseria et al., 2007). Le Grand (1982) suggests that access may be best understood in terms of the time and money costs that individuals incur in using health care facilities.

A comprehensive definition of access is that put forward by Whitehead and colleagues, who state that: access refers to the ability to secure a range of health services of a certain degree of quality, while in possession of a certain amount of information, and subject to a specified maximum level of personal inconvenience and cost (Whitehead et al., 1997). Therefore, a distinction must be made between 'having access' (the possibility of using a service if required) and 'gaining access' (actually using a service) (Masseria et al., 2007). A precondition for access is service availability, or the supply of services. Once users have the potential to access care, there are other supply and demand side facts that may limit their possibility of using those health services. On the supply side, there might be financial barriers, such as prohibitive payments; or organizational barriers, such as geographical distance or waiting times that prohibit timely treatment. On the demand side, there might be social or cultural barriers, or even individual preferences, that prohibit individuals from seeking access. Measures of access must encompass these different factors, while equity of access needs to be considered for all groups in society, which may differ in terms of need, socioeconomic status, culture, language or religion.

While some indicators of access capture certain dimensions of it, such as waiting times, service availability and out-of-pocket payments, access can rarely be observed or measured directly; utilization, however, can be. Indeed, many cross-country analyses use data collected on utilization through standardized multi-country surveys, such as the ECHP survey, its replacement EU-SILC and the SHARE database for older individuals. In all these surveys, information about individual use of health services is captured by asking the individual whether and how many times he/she visited a GP/specialist/dentist/emergency care. While these surveys provide valuable information on the use of health care across Europe, they do not capture the groups that seek care but cannot access it.

In an effort to better measure this group of individuals, a new variable, 'self-reported unmet need', was introduced when EU-SILC was launched. This variable identifies the individuals who were unable to receive the health care they felt they needed over a predefined period of time, and why (financial barriers, preferences, lack of time etc.).

Unmet need has been studied at the European level, identifying a strong association with both income and health, with those reporting unmet need being more likely to report worse health and have a lower level of income (Koolman, 2007). Studies based on SHARE data also show an association between foregone care and income. Mielck et al. (2007) found a higher likelihood of foregone care among individuals with a lower income in all countries studied. Increasingly, unmet need type variables have also been introduced by other surveys, such as the *Commonwealth Fund International Health Policy Survey* and the *European Social Survey* (ESS), which cover a different group of countries. Each survey focuses on different aspects of unmet need; the Commonwealth Fund puts an emphasis on financial barriers and service availability, while the ESS measures perceptions of unmet need in the future (Box 7.5).

Need

Another variable that must be defined in order to measure 'equal access for equal need' is need. There has been considerable debate surrounding the definition of 'need' (Wagstaff & van Doorslaer, 2000; Williams & Cookson, 2000). Culyer and Wagstaff (1993) have provided four definitions for need. These are:

- current level of ill health;
- capacity to benefit from health care;
- expenditure a person ought to have to restore health; and
- the minimum amount of resources required to exhaust an individual's capacity to benefit.

In practice, need is usually captured by the first definition, that is, variables that report the level of health and morbidity for the individual (such as self-reported health status, incidence of chronic illness or health limitations in daily activity, etc.), together with demographic factors such as age and gender. While these measure the burden of illness, they fail to capture important areas of health services, such as preventive care or public health, which can have large effects on health status. The second definition of need, the capacity to benefit from health care, addresses this shortcoming. This definition encompasses not just the existence of a health problem but the possibility of intervening so as to improve health status.

The third and fourth definitions put forward by Culyer and Wagstaff (1993) reflect 'need' with respect to the resource constraints that are present in all health systems. The first considers a value judgement, that is, some absolute maximum amount that should be spent on an individual to restore health, while the other reflects cost–effectiveness, that is, the minimum amount required to exhaust an individual's capacity to benefit.

Measurement techniques

The main methodological techniques available for measuring inequity in access are: a simple comparison of rates of access for different groups of the

Box 7.5 Examples of unmet need questions in multi-country health surveys

---

1. EU Statistics on Income and Living Conditions (EU-SILC)

- Was there any time during the last 12 months when you personally really needed a medical examination or treatment for a health problem but you did not receive it?
- (Yes, No)
- If respondent answered 'Yes', what was the main reason for not consulting a medical specialist?
- Could not afford to (too expensive)
- Waiting list
- Could not take time off work (or could not take time off from caring for children or others)
- Too far to travel or no means of transport
- Fear of doctor/hospitals/examinations/treatment
- Wanted to wait and see if problem got better on its own
- Didn't know any good doctor or specialist; other reason)

2. Commonwealth Fund International Health Policy Survey

Was there a time when you (fill in blank with 1–3) because of cost in the past year?

1. Did not fill a prescription for medicine or skipped doses.
2. Had a specific medical problem but did not visit a doctor.
3. Skipped or did not get a medical test, treatment, or follow-up that was recommended by a doctor.

(Yes, No, Not sure, Decline to answer)

- Last time when you needed medical care in the evening, on a weekend or on a holiday, how easy or difficult was it to get care without going to the emergency department?
- (Very easy, Easy, Somewhat difficult, Very difficult, Never needed care in the evenings, weekends or holidays, Decline to answer)

3. European Social Survey (ESS)

- During the next 12 months how likely is it that you will not receive the health care you really need if you become ill?
- (Not at all likely, Not very likely, Likely, Very likely, Don't know)

---

population; the use of regression methods such as adjusted odds ratios, which are a measure of association; and the Gini-like coefficients such as the horizontal inequity index. A comprehensive review of the methods summarized in this section can be found in Allin, Hernández-Quevedo and Masseria (2009). An earlier reference for the theoretical and methodological framework of the analysis of equity in access to health care can be found in Wagstaff and van Doorslaer (2000).

Rates of access

Rates of access are summary measures that allow comparisons to be made between different population groups. This approach is useful when a particular measure of access or utilization is needed for a specific population group. Rates of access are calculated by splitting the population into different groups, defined according to socioeconomic status, income, race or any other variable of interest. Absolute and relative access rates can be calculated to compare the differential access between the groups; the absolute measure considers the difference in rates of access between the selected group and the reference group, while the relative measure reports the ratio of the rates between the selected and reference groups. In order to avoid bias, it is important to consider the size of the population groups.

Regression methods

Using a regression model, it is possible to quantify how much a change in one socioeconomic or demographic factor will influence access to care, keeping all other factors constant. Regression methods allow the analysis of individual-level data for access by socioeconomic variables and need. The predictive ability of the model will be determined in part by the data available to measure access and the explanatory variables the researcher wants to examine. Common explanatory variables used in regression methods include measures of need (usually proxied by age, gender and health variables) and socioeconomic status (such as income, education or employment) for each individual.

Inequity indices

The main index used to measure horizontal equity of access is the horizontal inequity index (Kakwani, Wagstaff & van Doorslaer, 1997). The horizontal inequity index is based on the CI explained in detail above. Both these measures derive from the Gini coefficient and Lorenz curve, which were first developed to graphically represent income distributions and measure income inequalities. Figure 7.3 illustrates the concentration curves used to measure inequity in utilization, following the indirect method of standardization of use of health care.[3] Like the CC in Figure 7.2, the horizontal axis shows the cumulative proportion of the population ranked by income, in percentages. The vertical axis shows the cumulative proportion of use of medical care of that population, also shown in percentages. Two curves are mapped onto these axes using information about individuals' utilization of care and their needs (proxied by demographics plus health status and morbidity variables). The first curve measures the actual distribution of medical care (LM(R)), and the second, (LN(R)), the distribution of needs-predicted medical care. The diagonal represents the 45-degree line, which is the line of equality. This would show an equal distribution, where

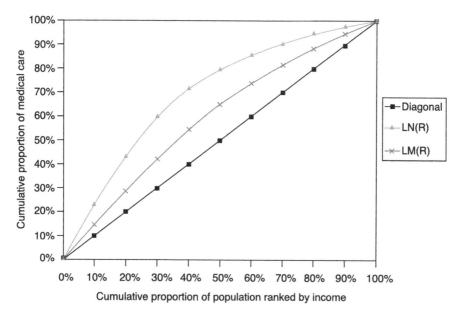

Figure 7.3 Concentration curves to measure inequity in utilization

10% of the population consumes 10% of care available and 20% of the population consumes 20% of care available. Deviations from this line can denote the degree of inequality of what we are investigating, with C corresponding to the CI associated to the actual use of medical care and C*, the CI for needs-predicted use of health care.

Thus, the amount of horizontal equity, measured by the horizontal index, can be calculated as the difference between the two curves (LM(R) – LN(R)) or, similarly, the difference between the concentration indices (C – C*). When the horizontal index is greater than zero, it indicates pro-rich inequity in health care (health care more concentrated among the rich, for equal need). If the horizontal index equals zero, there is no inequity and, if it is less than zero, it indicates pro-poor inequity in health care. This index has been used extensively in the literature on measuring equity in health care access (van Doorslaer et al., 2006). It can be calculated for different types of care and are able to provide useful information on the degree of inequity in access within and across countries. The horizontal indices calculated in van Doorslaer et al. (2006) for primary and secondary care illustrate how this metric can be used for cross-country comparison.

The figure indicates horizontal inequities in the use of GP services and specialists, controlling for the health care needs of individuals. For specialist services, in particular, it appears that in all countries the richest individuals are using more specialists' services than is proportionate to their income level. This level of inequity is lower for GP visits, with some countries such as Spain and Greece exhibiting a negative horizontal index, with a disproportionate concentration of GP visits among the poorest individuals.

7.4 Equity in financing

There has been long-standing interest in equity of financing among international organizations and various countries. Concern over financial barriers to access to health care has been reflected in the growing attention this issue has received in policy discussions and performance assessments in this area. In 2000, the *World Health Report* (*WHR2000*) highlighted 'fairness in financing' as one of the intrinsic objectives of the health system. More recently, the *WHR2010* called for all countries to move towards universal health coverage for their populations. In parallel, a growing number of indicators and measurement techniques in this area have become available. These are discussed in detail in Chapter 8.

In the measurement of equity in finance, the focal point is the extent to which health care payments are related to ability to pay. There are three main classifications of the financing systems found in industrialized countries: progressive (payments are an increasing proportion of ability to pay, such as income taxes); proportional (payments represent a constant proportion of ability to pay, such as payroll taxes); and regressive (payments are a decreasing proportion of ability to pay, such as out-of-pocket payments). In this context, vertical equity is assessed in order to understand the extent to which those with unequal ability to pay incur differential payments towards health care. From an egalitarian perspective, an equitable health care financing system is one in which payments for health care are positively related to ability to pay; in other words, those who are able to pay more towards health care should do so.

Methodological techniques

There are various measurement tools that seek to quantify the extent to which health care payments burden different members of society, and most of these are reviewed extensively in Chapter 8. These variables tend to focus on the size of payments incurred by health care users, and to what extent these payments are impoverishing. While these indicators will demonstrate the extent to which citizens are not protected against poverty by illness, they do not directly measure the disparity in financing between groups. One simple extension that allows for the measurement of equity in financing is to tabulate the average incomes and health care payments by income groups (Hurst, 1985).

While this methodology provides more information as to the different payments by income, it does not allow for cross-country comparison of how progressive different systems are. Yet, the tools discussed previously, such as the Lorenz curve, Gini coefficient and CC, are able to indicate the progressivity of a health system and allow for cross-country comparisons. One important extension of the Lorenz curve is the Kakwani index, which measures the extent to which a tax system departs from proportionality and allows for cross-country comparisons of the progressivity of health care financing systems.

The Kakwani progressivity index

The Kakwani index of progressivity is often used to measure how progressive or regressive the financing of a health system is. It is based on the Lorenz curve outlined above. The Kakwani index is calculated using the Lorenz curve for pre-tax income and the tax CC, which plots the cumulative proportions of the population, ranked according to pre-tax income against the proportions of total tax payments. The area between these curves represents the index of progressivity. If the index is negative, the system is regressive and –2 is the lowest value it can take, while the highest value it can take is 1.

The sign of the index will be determined by the curves; if the CC lies below the Lorenz curve (as indicated in Figure 7.4), then the distribution of premiums is progressive, as it indicates that at any cumulative level of pre-tax income, the cumulative fraction of tax paid is lower than the cumulative fraction of pre-tax income. Thus, if the curves were reversed, such that the CC was above the Lorenz curve, the system would we regressive. If the two curves were to coincide, the distribution of premiums would be equal to the distribution of pre-premium income. Thus, another way to understand the Kakwani index is as the difference between the Gini coefficient of the post-tax curve and the pre-tax curve, or the difference between the CI and the Gini coefficient (Wagstaff & van Doorslaer, 2000).

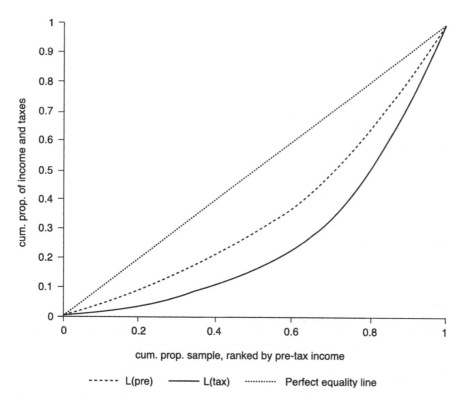

Figure 7.4 Kakwani index: pre-tax income and taxes

Data sources to measure equity in finance are listed in Wagstaff et al. (1999), who provide a cross-country analysis of the redistributive effect of health care financing arrangements in 12 OECD countries.[4] For Asian countries, Rannan-Eliya and Somanathan (2006) show the difficulties of empirical measurement of the progressivity of the health care financing, given the existence of multiple financing mechanisms and lack of accurate data on the share of financing of the different mechanisms, amongst others. Comparative analysis for 13 Asian countries has been provided within the Equitap[5] project by O'Donnell et al. (2004). Their results are consistent with earlier evidence from Europe, where general revenue financing is associated with greater progressivity relative to social insurance.

7.5 Equity in other health system goals

In principle, equity can be measured in relation to any of the other health system goals, such as responsiveness or quality, to understand if there is an equitable distribution in attainment of these goals across the population or between different demographic or socioeconomic groups. At an international level, it may be of interest to compare not only the average attainment of these goals but also their distribution across the population. This was reflected in *WHR2000*, where measuring both the absolute attainment and distribution of not only health improvement but also health system responsiveness, were established as goals of a health system.

While equity in these areas is a concern, especially in the measurement of procedural equity, there has been very little work to assess how much it is achieved within and across health systems. With regards to responsiveness, the main equity concern is to establish whether there are systematic differences in satisfaction, client orientation or patient autonomy across different population groups or countries. The analysis of inequality in responsiveness, and quality, is mostly studied in the context of procedural equity through their association to access or financing of health services (Jones et al., 2010). These measurements usually consist of some assessment of the variation in different goals across population groups, treatment facilities or nations.

7.6 Conclusions

The literature in Europe has documented that inequalities favouring the better-off exist in all European countries, both with respect to the use of health care and with respect to the distribution of health itself, and that the degree of inequality is particularly associated with education, income and job status (Hernández-Quevedo et al., 2006; Hernández-Quevedo, Jones & Rice, 2008). However, there is some debate around how this information should be interpreted, particularly with regard to the direction of causality and the policy implications this holds. This section will outline some of the key debates in this area before concluding with policy recommendations for international comparisons.

Key issues for international comparisons

International comparisons in the area of equity are important to further our understanding of substantive and procedural equity. In the study of substantive equity, benchmarking and comparisons can allow policy-makers to better understand not only if average health status is comparable to other countries, but also if there is a greater or lesser degree of variation amongst the population and across different groups of the population. Comparisons can also be informative for the study of procedural equity, in so much as they allow policy-makers to better understand how well their health system contributes to providing health improvement for all groups, as well as financial protection, responsiveness, access and high-quality services relative to others. Despite the various policy uses international comparisons may hold, there are also challenges in carrying out and interpreting international comparisons in the area of equity. These can broadly be classified into issues of data availability, data limitations, issues of measurement and issues of interpretation.

Table 7.4 illustrates the main equity considerations in the areas of substantive and procedural equity. While various methodological techniques for measuring attainment in these areas exist, there is difficulty in finding the necessary data. In order to conduct any analysis of substantive equity, it is necessary to have data on the health status of the population; international comparisons require this data to be collected across populations in a comparable way. Chapter 5 and section 7.2 in this chapter review the many difficulties this presents, in terms of both data availability and data validity. Measures are limited to outcome measures, and there are few or no data on morbidity. Moreover, longitudinal data are lacking, making it difficult to compare and understand changes in time. While objective measures of health status are the most reliable for comparative purposes, there is limited availability of such indicators for international comparisons. Most of the international measures of health status used are based on subjective measures, which can vary according to demographic and socioeconomic factors within countries, and also due to national and cultural differences across countries. If not adjusted for, these biases may lead to misleading results. On a positive note, the past decade has seen great advances in the methodologies available to standardize outcome measures, and these have been increasingly applied to international surveys.

As Table 7.4 indicates, more data are necessary to compare the social gradient in health within and across different countries. In addition to the data on health status, comparable information on demographic and socioeconomic information needs to be provided. There are only a few surveys providing this type of information across various nations that can be used to study this dimension. However, data on socioeconomic information are available nationally through other social surveys and administrative databases. In future, great progress could be made in research in this area, both nationally and internationally, through the move to EHR and data linkage.

In the study of procedural equity, the information requirements become more severe. To compare equity in access or utilization within or across countries, measures of 'access' and 'need' are necessary. However, the indicators used to measure these concepts are often not ideal; utilization is commonly used as

Table 7.4 Main areas of equity measurement

Equity consideration	What it measures	Selected measurement techniques	Data requirements
Substantive equity	The distribution of health across the population	Gap measures Correlation and regression measures Lorenz curve	Data on health status for a population
Equity in health	The distribution of health across different socioeconomic groups	Gap measures Correlation and regression measures Concentration curve	Data on health status and socioeconomic characteristic of interest (i.e. income, social status, education, etc.) for a population
Equity in health across different socioeconomic groups	The distribution of health care by medical need across the different socioeconomic groups	Rates of access Regression methods Horizontal index	Data on health status, socioeconomic characteristics, and access
Procedural equity	The distribution of health care payments across the population and/or different socioeconomic groups	Index of fair financing Kakwani progressivity index	Data on income, health payments, possibly health status
Equity of access	The distribution of responsiveness across the population and/or different socioeconomic groups The distribution of quality across the population and/or different socioeconomic groups	Variations in goal achievement across different groups	Data on goal and socioeconomic group
Equity in financing			
Equity in other health system goals (i.e. responsiveness, quality)			

a proxy for access, even though this may not capture some of the key groups having difficulties in access to health care. Some work has been done in this area to develop indicators of 'unmet need' or 'opportunity', which are able to provide more accurate assessments of 'access'. Need is often measured by the level of ill health, together with demographic characteristics of the individual; however, this fails to capture the capacity of patients to benefit from other areas of health care, such as public health, prevention or health promotion. At the international level, surveys are the main source of cross-national information; however, these are subject to reporting bias and comparability issues. Comparable information on inequities in responsiveness is very limited. The *World Health Survey* has collected information across a wide number of countries; this is homogenous across countries and benefits from the inclusion of vignettes, however, the information is only provided for one year and, hence, there is no possibility of capturing the longitudinal dimension of this domain across countries. Chapter 9 discusses this issue in more detail. Overall, the main data availability constraints for analysing procedural equity across countries are:

1. the limited outcome indicators available, resulting in a reliance on subjective measures;
2. the limited potential for linkage across national and international data; and
3. the lack of longitudinal data that account for the life-cycle of the individual.

Finally, the issues of interpretation were touched upon briefly in the opening section of this chapter, and have to do with the different ethical frameworks stakeholders use to evaluate equity. Citizens and government, patients and doctors, and national and international policy-makers may all hold different beliefs about what constitutes an equitable distribution of health and/or health care. Moreover, individuals within these groups will also have differing opinions about what is fair or equitable. In the national arena, these differences manifest themselves in policy debates, often about the size of the welfare state or redistributive mechanisms. The difficulty in conducting international comparisons then, is to choose which ethical framework to adopt. This is most obvious when deciding how to compare procedural equity across systems, when not all subscribe to policies such as universal coverage. However, it is also relevant when comparing substantive equity among countries with different welfare states. In these contexts, should equity be interpreted according to the eyes of the interpreter or relative to national objectives?

Conclusions, policy recommendations and the way forward

It is evident that considerable data challenges exist if policy-makers want to be able better to assess and understand the causes of inequities in health and health care, both at national and international levels. Good-quality evidence to guide policy is in short supply and there is a need for new and more consistent data for comparative national-level analyses. Moreover, an additional challenge for policy-makers is to assess the impact their policies have on health inequalities. This requires the implementation of well-designed evaluative studies, particularly those that are able to take advantage of natural experiments to produce a case and control group (changes in employment opportunities, housing provision or cigarette pricing).

There are promising new developments which have the potential to make international comparisons in equity easier, such as the move towards EHR and linkage with other data sources. However, there are some specific areas of policy interest, where information remains limited for cross-country analyses (Table 7.5). Comparative information in these areas could be of use to policymakers by indicating potential areas on which to focus, that might lead to a reduction of health inequalities and access to health care but that have not been exploited. In some of these areas national data are collected but there is no data available that can be used to draw international comparisons.

Finally, the data limitations faced by low- to middle-income countries are more pronounced than those in high-income countries, which have been largely the focus of this chapter. Most empirical analysis of equity of access has been conducted in the context of developed countries, although some research projects have also extended these techniques to developing countries (such as

Table 7.5 Areas of equity research with limited data for international comparisons

Area of interest	Equity implication and potential lessons from comparisons
Substantive equity	
Inequity in health-related behaviours (i.e. smoking, alcohol consumption, diet)	Inequities in these behaviours can lead to inequities in health status. International comparisons can provide information on: • the differences of risky behaviours across nations; • how these differences are linked to different health status; • potential policies that can be successful at minimizing these risky behaviours.
Inequalities in psychosocial stressors	Anxiety and stress may be more prevalent among lower-income groups due to more severe lifestyle restrictions and, in turn, negatively influence mental and physical health. International comparisons can provide information on: • the differences in prevalence of psychosocial stressors across nations and regions; • how these differences are linked to mental and physical health status; • potential factors that can be successful at minimizing these stressors (cultural, environmental, social, etc.).
Inequalities in environmental determinants, such as social support and social integration	Such environmental determinants may be influential to individuals' understanding of health and opportunities to access health. International comparisons can provide information on: • the differences in the level of environmental determinants across nations; • the link between these differences and access to, use of and satisfaction with the health system.

Intergenerational inequalities	Inequities can be sustained across time through genetics, culture, environment and lifestyle, which are passed from one generation to the next.
	International comparisons can provide information on:
	• the differences in the level of intergenerational inequalities in each nation;
	• the persistence of these inequalities across nations over time.
Inequities of health for minorities	Often minorities within a national population will also have differential health status due to a combination of socioeconomic, cultural and even genetic factors.
	International comparisons can provide information on:
	• the differences in the level of inequity in health status for minorities within each country.

Procedural equity

Inequity in quality of care	Inequalities of quality of care are studied in so much as they relate to access, but not as a result of other factors. In practice, quality of care can also vary across patients due to a variety of socioeconomic and even cultural factors.
	International comparisons can provide information on:
	• the differences in the distribution of quality across countries;
	• the different factors associated to the distribution of quality.
Inequity of access to social care	Many patients are discharged from the health care system to the social system (such as those seeking long-term care). Access and coverage requirements to the social care system are likely to influence the health status of these patients.
	International comparisons can provide information on:
	• the differences in access to social care across countries;
	• the differences in health status associated with the different structures of social care available.
Inequities of access for minorities	Often minorities within a national population will also have differential access to the health care system.
	International comparisons can provide information on:
	• The differences in the level of inequity in access to health care for minorities within each country.

the Equitap project). Yet, given the additional data constraints present in these countries, different methodological issues may arise, particularly linked to the availability of limited income data. Given that information on living standards may not be available or reliable, household wealth is used as an indicator of socioeconomic status rather than income. This is derived from information on household ownership of durable goods and housing characteristics, by using principal components analysis to derive the weights. Literature on the calculation of a wealth index has been developed in this context (Kanbur, 2006) and an application can be found in Filmer and Pritchett (2001). Moreover, the more pressing concern for low- and middle-income countries lies in assessing the extent of financial protection that individuals receive from the government.

In order to facilitate international comparisons of equity in health and health care, there must be an important effort from national and international institutions to create good-quality available and comparable data. This requires:

1. harmonization across countries in the definitions of key variables and collection instruments;
2. the collection of individual level information on health and key determinants of health and health care access;
3. greater use of data linkages at the national level to allow for disaggregation by key determinants.

Notes

1 'Pure' inequalities or overall inequalities refer to overall health inequalities in the population (i.e. without taking into account the socioeconomic dimension of these inequalities).
2 For an application of these, see Wagstaff & van Doorslaer (2004).
3 See O'Donnell et al. (2008b) for more details on direct versus indirect methods of standardization.
4 In this study, progressivity is measured using a Kakwani index, which equals the difference between the CI for payments (e.g. taxes, social insurance, private insurance, direct payments) and the Gini coefficient for household gross (that is, pre-payment) income, with heterogeneous results across countries.
5 Equitap (Equity in Asia-Pacific Health Systems) is a project that includes more than 15 research teams in Asia and Europe, with the objective of examining equity in national health systems in the Asia-Pacific region. It is funded by several European and Asian institutions, including the European Commission and the World Bank.

References

Adams, P. et al. (2003) Healthy, wealthy and wise? Tests for direct causal paths between health and socioeconomic status, *Journal of Econometrics*, 112: 3–56.

Aday, L.A. et al. (2004) *Evaluating the Healthcare System: Effectiveness, efficiency, and equity*, 3rd edn. Chicago: Health Administration Press.

Allin, S., Hernández-Quevedo, C. and Masseria, C. (2009) Measuring equity of access to health care, in P.C. Smith et al. (eds) *Performance measurement for health system improvement: Experiences, challenges and prospects*. Cambridge: Cambridge University Press.

Bago d'Uva, T. et al. (2006) *Does reporting heterogeneity bias the measurement of health disparities?* York: University of York (HEDG Working Paper, 06/03).

Bago d'Uva, T. et al. (2008) Does reporting heterogeneity bias the measurement of health disparities? *Health Economics*, 17(3): 351–75.

Banks, J. et al. (2006) Disease and disadvantage in the United States and England, *JAMA*, 295(17): 2037–45.

Benzeval, M., Taylor, J. and Judge, K. (2000) Evidence on the relationship between low income and poor health: is the government doing enough? *Fiscal Studies*, 21: 375–99.

Berkman, L.F. and Kawachi, I. (eds) (2000) *Social Epidemiology*. New York: Oxford University Press.

Bobak, M. et al. (2000) Socioeconomic factors, material inequalities, and perceived control in self-rated health: cross-sectional data from seven post-communist countries, *Social Science and Medicine*, 51(9): 1343–50.

Bound, J. (1991) Self-reported versus objective measures of health in retirement models, *Journal of Human Resources*, 26: 106–38.

Burström, B. and Fredlund, P. (2001) Self-rated health: is it as good a predictor of subsequent mortality among adults in lower as well as in higher social classes? *Journal of Epidemiology and Community Health*, 55: 836–40.

Burström, K., Johannesson, M. and Diderichsen, F. (2005) Increasing socioeconomic inequalities in life expectancy and QALYs in Sweden 1980–1997, *Health Economics*, 14(8): 831–50.

Cattell, V. (2001) Poor people, poor places, and poor health: the mediating role of social networks and social capital, *Social Science and Medicine*, 52(10): 1501–16.

Clarke, P.M. et al. (2002) On the measurement of relative and absolute income-related health inequality, *Social Science and Medicine*, 55(11): 1923–8.

Contoyannis, P., Jones, A. and Rice, N. (2004) The dynamics of health in the British Household Panel Survey, *Journal of Applied Econometrics*, 19(4): 473–503.

Costa-Font, J. and Hernández-Quevedo, C. (2012) Measuring inequalities in health: What do we know? What do we need to know? *Health Policy*, 106(2): 195–206.

Costa-Font, J., Hernández-Quevedo, C. and McGuire, A. (2011) Persistence despite action? Measuring the patterns of health inequality in England (1997–2007), *Health Policy*, 103: 149–59.

Culyer, A.J. and Wagstaff, A. (1993) Equity and equality in health care, *Journal of Health Economics*, 12: 431–57.

Dalstra, J.A. et al. (2005). Socioeconomic differences in the prevalence of common chronic diseases: an overview of eight European countries, *International Journal of Epidemiology*, 34(2): 316–26.

Deaton, A.S. and Paxson, C.H. (1998) Aging and inequality in income and health, *American Economic Review*, 88, 248–53.

de Looper, M. and Lafortune, G. (2009) *Measuring disparities in health status and in access and use of health care in OECD countries*. Paris: Organisation for Economic Co-operation and Development Publishing (OECD Health Working Papers, no. 43).

Eberth, B. and Gerdtham, U-G. (2008) *Why is inequality in obesity more pro-rich in Scotland than in England? The role of permanent income in decomposition analysis*. Aberdeen: Working Paper Health Economics Research Unit, University of Aberdeen.

Eikemo, T.A. et al. (2008) Health inequalities according to educational level in different welfare regimes: a comparison of 23 European countries, *Sociology of Health and Illness*, 30(4): 565–82.

Erreygers, G. (2009) Correcting the concentration index, *Journal of Health Economics*, 28(2): 504–15.

Ettner, S.L. (1996) New evidence on the relationship between income and health, *Journal of Health Economics*, 15(1): 67–85.

Filmer, D. and Pritchett, L.T. (2001) Estimating wealth effects without expenditure data – or tears: an application to educational enrollments in states of India, *Demography*, 38(1): 115–32.

Frijters, P., Haisken-DeNew, J.P. and Shields, M.A. (2005) The causal effect of income on health: evidence from German reunification, *Journal of Health Economics*, 24: 997–1017.

García-Álvarez, A. et al. (2007) Obesity and overweight trends in Catalonia, Spain (1992–2003): gender and socioeconomic determinants, *Public Health Nutrition*, 10(11A): 1368–78.

Gerdtham, U-G. and Johannesson, M. (2000) Income-related inequality in life-years and quality-adjusted life-years, *Journal of Health Economics*, 19(6): 1007–26.

Gravelle, H. (2003) Measuring income related inequality in health: standardization and the partial concentration index, *Health Economics*, 12(10): 803–19.

Gravelle, H., Morris, S. and Sutton, M. (2006) Economic studies of equity in the consumption of health care, in A.M. Jones (ed.) *The Elgar Companion to Health Economics*. Cheltenham: Edward Elgar Publishing Ltd.

Groot, W. (2000) Adaptation and scale of reference bias in self-assessments of quality of life, *Journal of Health Economics*, 19(3): 403–20.

Gulliford, M. (2003) Equity and access to health care, in M. Gulliford and M. Morgan (eds) *Access to Health Care*. London: Routledge.

Harper, S. and Lynch, J. (2006) *Methods for measuring cancer disparities: using data relevant to Healthy People 2010 cancer-related objectives*. Washington, DC: National Cancer Institute (http://seer.cancer.gov/publications/disparities, accessed 6 June 2012).

Helasoja, V. et al. (2006) Trends in the magnitude of educational inequalities in health in Estonia, Latvia, Lithuania and Finland during 1994–2004, *Public Health*, 120(9): 841–53.

Hemmingsson, T. and Lundberg, I. (2005) How far are socioeconomic differences in coronary heart disease hospitalization, all-cause mortality and cardiovascular mortality among Swedish males aged 40–50 attributable to negative childhood circumstances and behaviour in adolescence? *Int J Epidemiol*, 34(2): 260–7.

Hernández-Quevedo, C. and Costa-Font, J. (2012) Inequalities in health: Why do we care? How do we care? What can we do about them? in *Elsevier Handbook of Health Policy* (forthcoming).

Hernández-Quevedo, C., Jones, A.M. and Rice, N. (2008) Persistence in health limitations: a European comparative analysis, *Journal of Health Economics*, 27(6): 1472–88.

Hernández-Quevedo, C., Masseria, C. and Mossialos, E.A. (2010a) Analysing the socioeconomic determinants of health in Europe: new evidence from EU-SILC. *Eurostat: Methodologies and Working Papers*, 2010 edn. Luxembourg: Eurostat, European Commission.

Hernández-Quevedo, C., Masseria, C. and Mossialos, E.A. (2010b) Methodological issues in the analysis of the socioeconomic determinants of health using EU-SILC data. *Eurostat: Methodologies and Working Papers*, 2010 edn. Luxembourg: Eurostat, European Commission.

Hernández-Quevedo, C. et al. (2006) Socioeconomic inequalities in health: a comparative longitudinal analysis using the European Community Household Panel, *Social Science and Medicine*, 63(5): 1246–61.

Holland, W.W. (1986) The 'avoidable death' guide to Europe, *Health Policy*, 6(2): 115–17.

Hurst, J. (1985) *Financing health care in the US, Canada and Britain*. London: Kings Fund.

Idler, E.L. and Benyamini, Y. (1997) Self-rated health and mortality: a review of twenty-seven community studies, *Journal of Health and Social Behavior*, 38(1): 21–37.

Idler, E.L. and Kasl, S.V. (1995) Self-ratings of health: do they also predict change in functional ability? *Journal of Gerontology*, 50B: S344–53.

Jenkins, S. (1988) Calculating income distribution indices from micro-data, *National Tax Journal*, 41(1): 139–42.

Johnston, D., Propper, C. and Shields, M. (2009) Comparing subjective and objective health measures: implications from hypertension for the estimated income/health gradient, *Journal of Health Economics*, 28: 540–52.

Jones, A.M. and López-Nicolás, A. (2004) Measurement and explanation of socio-economic inequality in health with longitudinal data, *Health Economics*, 13(10): 1015–30.

Jones, A.M. et al. (2010) *Inequality and polarisation in health systems' responsiveness: a cross-country analysis.* York: Health Econometrics and Data Group, University of York (HEDG Working Paper 10/27).

Joumard, I., André, C. and Nicq, C. (2010) *Health care systems: efficiency and institutions.* Paris: Organisation for Economic Co-operation and Development (OECD Economics Department Working Paper, no. 769).

Jurges, H. (2007) True health vs response styles: exploring cross-country differences in self-reported health, *Health Economics*, 16: 163–78.

Kakwani, N.C. (1980) *Income inequality and poverty: methods of estimation and policy application.* New York: Oxford University Press.

Kakwani, N., Wagstaff, A. and van Doorslaer, E. (1997) Socioeconomic inequalities in health: measurement, computation and statistical inference, *Journal of Econometrics*, 77: 87–103.

Kanbur, R. (2006) The policy significance of inequality decompositions. *Journal of Economic Inequality*, 4(3): 367–74. (http://www.springerlink.com/content/648g28j08222j5n3/, accessed 30 September 2012).

Kapteyn, A., Smith, J.P. and van Soest, A. (2004) *Self-reported work disability in the US and the Netherlands.* RAND Labour and Population Working Paper (http://www.rand.org/pubs/working_papers/WR206.html, accessed 6 June 2012).

Kelleher, C.C. et al. (2003) Socio-demographic predictors of self-rated health in the Republic of Ireland: findings from the National Survey on Lifestyle, Attitudes and Nutrition (SLAN), *Social Science and Medicine*, 57(3): 477–86.

Kenkel, D. (1995) Should you eat breakfast? Estimates from health production functions, *Health Economics*, 4(1): 15–29.

Kerkhofs, M. and Lindeboom, M. (1995) Subjective health measures and state dependent reporting errors, *Health Economics*, 4(3): 221–35.

Kievit, W. et al. (2005) *The longitudinal association between objective clinical measures and patient self-reporting information in rheumatoid arthritis.* The 27th Annual Meeting of the Society for Medical Decision Making, 21–24 October 2005.

King, G. et al. (2004) Enhancing the validity and cross-cultural comparability of measurement in survey research, *American Political Science Review*, 98(1): 191–207.

Koolman, X. (2007) *Unmet need for health care in Europe. Comparative EU statistics on income and living conditions: issues and challenges.* Proceedings of the EU-SILC conference. Helsinki: Eurostat.

Kopp, M.S. and Rethelyi, J. (2004) Where psychology meets physiology: chronic stress and premature mortality – the Central-Eastern European health paradox, *Brain Research Bulletin*, 62(5): 351–67.

Kunst, A.E. et al. (2005) Trends in socioeconomic inequalities in self-assessed health in ten European countries, *International Journal of Epidemiology*, 34(2): 295–305.

Le Grand, J. (1978) The distribution of public expenditure: the case of health care, *Economica*, 45(178): 125–42.

Le Grand, J. (1982) *The Strategy of Equality.* London: Allen & Unwin.

Le Grand, J. (1987) Inequalities in health: some international comparisons, *European Economic Review*, 31: 182–91.

Le Grand, J. (1991) *Equity and choice: An essay in economics and applied philosophy.* London: HarperCollins Academic.

Lindeboom, M. and van Doorslaer, E. (2004) Cut-point shift and index shift in self-reported health, *Journal of Health Economics*, 23(6): 1083–99.

Mackenbach, J.P., Bouvier-Colle, M.H. and Jougla, E. (1990) "Avoidable" mortality and health services: a review of aggregate data studies, *Journal of Epidemiology and Community Health*, 44(2): 106–11.

Mackenbach, J.P. and Kunst, A.E. (1997) Measuring the magnitude of socioeconomic inequalities in health: an overview of available measures illustrated with two examples from Europe, *Social Science and Medicine*, 44(6): 757–71.

Mackenbach, J.P., et al. (2005) The shape of the relationship between income and self-assessed health: an international study, *International Journal of Epidemiology*, 34(2): 286–93.

Marmot, M. (2005) Social determinants of health inequalities, *The Lancet*, 365(9464): 1099–104.

Marmot, M. and Wilkinson, R.G. (eds) (1999) *Social determinants of health*. Oxford: Oxford University Press.

Marmot, M. and Wilkinson, R.G. (eds) (2003) *Social determinants of health*, 2nd edn. Oxford: Oxford University Press.

Masseria, C. et al. (2007) *What are the methodological issues related to measuring health and drawing comparisons across countries? A research note.* Brussels: DG Employment and Social Affairs, European Observatory on the Social Situation and Demography.

Matthews, R.J., Jagger, C. and Hancock, R.M. (2006) Does socioeconomic advantage lead to a longer, healthier old age? *Social Science and Medicine*, 62: 2489–99.

Meheus, F. and van Doorslaer, E. (2008) Achieving better measles immunization in developing countries: does higher coverage imply lower inequality? *Social Science and Medicine*, 66(8): 1709–18.

Mielck, A. et al. (2007) *Association between access to health care and household income among the elderly in 10 western European countries. Tackling health inequalities in Europe: An integrated approach.* Rotterdam: Erasmus MC Department of Public Health.

Mooney, G. (1983) Equity in health care: confronting the confusion, *Effective Health Care*, 1: 179–85.

Murray, C.J.L. et al. (2001) *Enhancing cross-population comparability of survey results.* Geneva: WHO/EIP (GPE Discussion Paper, no. 35).

Murray, C.J.L. et al. (2003) Empirical evaluation of the anchoring vignettes approach in health surveys, in C.J.L. Murray and D.B. Evans (eds) *Health Systems Performance Assessment: Debates, methods and empiricism.* Geneva: World Health Organization.

Nolte, E. and McKee, M. (2004) *Does healthcare save lives? Avoidable mortality revisited.* London: Nuffield Trust.

Nummela, O.P. et al. (2007) Self-rated health and indicators of SES among the ageing in three types of communities, *Scandinavian Journal of Public Health*, 35(1): 961–71.

O'Donnell, O. (2009) Measuring health inequalities in Europe. Methodological issues in the analysis of survey data, *Eurohealth*, 15(3): 10–14.

O'Donnell, O. et al. (2004) *Who pays for health care in Asia?*, Colombo, Sri Lanka: Equitap Project (Equitap Working Paper Number 1).

O'Donnell, O. et al. (2008a) Who pays for health care in Asia? *Journal of Health Economics*, 27(2): 460–75.

O'Donnell, O. et al. (2008b) *Analyzing health equity using household survey data.* Washington, DC: World Bank Institute.

Oliver, A. and Mossialos, E. (2004) Equity of access to health care: outlining the foundation for action, *Journal of Epidemiology and Community Health*, 58(8): 655–8.

Olsen, J.A. (2011) Concepts of equity and fairness in health and health care, in S. Glied and P.C. Smith (eds) *The Oxford Handbook of Health Economics*. Oxford: Oxford University Press.

Rannan-Eliya, R. and Somanathan, A. (2006) Equity in health and health care systems in Asia, in A.M. Jones (ed.) *The Elgar Companion to Health Economics*. Cheltenham: Edward Elgar Publishing Ltd.

Regidor, E. (2004a) Measures of health inequalities: Part 1, *Journal of Epidemiology and Community Health*, 58: 858–61.

Regidor, E. (2004b) Measures of health inequalities: Part 2, *Journal of Epidemiology and Community Health*, 58: 900–3.

Regidor, E. et al. (2003) Trends in the association between average income, poverty and income inequality and life expectancy in Spain, *Social Science and Medicine*, 56(5): 961–71.

Roberts, M.J. et al. (2008) *Getting health reform right: A guide to improving performance and equity*. Oxford: Oxford University Press.

Sadana, R. et al. (2000) *Comparative analysis of more than 50 household surveys on health status*. Geneva: World Health Organization (GPE Discussion Paper, no. 15).

Salas, C. (2002) On the empirical association between poor health and low socioeconomic status at old age, *Health Economics*, 11: 207–20.

Salomon, J., Tandon, A. and Murray, C.J.L. (2004) Comparability of self-rated health: cross-sectional multi-country survey using anchoring vignettes, *BMJ*, 328(7434): 258.

Sassi, F. (2009) Health inequalities: a persistent problem, in J. Hills, T. Sefton and K. Stewart (eds) *Towards a more equal society?* Bristol: The Policy Press.

Sen, A. (2002) Why health equity? *Health Economics*, 11(8): 659–66.

Silventoinen, K. et al. (2005) Educational inequalities in the metabolic syndrome and coronary heart disease among middle-aged men and women, *International Journal of Epidemiology*, 34(2): 327–34.

Smith, J.P. (1999) Healthy bodies and thick wallets, *Journal of Economic Perspectives*, 13(2): 145–66.

Tandon, A. et al. (2003) Statistical models for enhancing cross-population comparability, in C.J.L. Murray and D.B. Evans (eds) *Health Systems Performance Assessment: Debates, methods and empiricism*. Geneva: World Health Organization.

Üstün, T.B. et al. (2003) The World Health Surveys, in C.J.L. Murray and D.B. Evans (eds) *Health Systems Performance Assessment: Debates, methods and empiricism*. Geneva: World Health Organization.

van Doorslaer, E. and Gerdtham, U-G. (2003) Does inequality in self-assessed health predict inequality in survival by income? Evidence from Swedish data, *Social Science and Medicine*, 57(9): 1621–9.

van Doorslaer, E. and van Ourti, T. (2011) Measuring inequality and inequity in health and health care, in S. Glied and P.C. Smith (eds) *The Oxford Handbook of Health Economics*. Oxford: Oxford University Press.

van Doorslaer, E. et al. (1997) Income-related inequalities in health: some international comparisons, *Journal of Health Economics*, 16(1): 93–112.

van Doorslaer, E. et al. (2000) Equity in the delivery of health care in Europe and the US, *Journal of Health Economics*, 19(5): 553–83.

van Doorslaer, E. et al. (2006) Inequalities in access to medical care by income in developed countries, *Canadian Medical Association Journal*, 174(2): 177–83.

Wagstaff, A. (2002) Inequality aversion, health inequalities and health achievement, *Journal of Health Economics*, 21: 627–41.

Wagstaff, A. (2005) The bounds of the Concentration Index when the variable of interest is binary, with an application to immunization inequality, *Health Economics*, 14(4): 429–32.

Wagstaff, A. and van Doorslaer, E. (2000) Equity in health care finance and delivery, in A.J. Culyer and J.P. Newhouse (eds) *Handbook of Health Economics*. Amsterdam: North-Holland.

Wagstaff, A. and van Doorslaer, E. (2004) Overall versus socioeconomic health inequality: a measurement framework and two empirical illustrations, *Health Economics*, 13(3): 297–301.

Wagstaff, A., Paci, P. and van Doorslaer, E. (1991) On the measurement of inequalities in health, *Social Science and Medicine*, 33(5): 545–57.

Wagstaff, A., van Doorslaer, E. and Paci, P. (1989) Equity in the finance and delivery of health care: some tentative cross-country comparisons, *Oxford Review of Economic Policy*, 5(1): 89–112.

Wagstaff, A., van Doorslaer, E. and Watanabe, N. (2003) On decomposing the causes of health sector inequalities with an application to malnutrition inequalities in Vietnam, *Journal of Econometrics*, 112: 207–23.

Wagstaff, A. et al. (1999) Equity in the finance of health care: some further international comparisons, *Journal of Health Economics*, 18(3): 263–90.

Whitehead, M. et al. (1997) As the health divide widens in Sweden and Britain, what's happening to access to care? *BMJ*, 315(7114): 1006–9.

Williams, A. (1997) Intergenerational equity: an exploration of the 'fair innings' argument, *Health Economics*, 6(2): 117–32.

Williams, A. and Cookson, R. (2000) Equity in health, in A.J. Culyer and J.P. Newhouse (eds) *Handbook of Health Economics*. Amsterdam: North-Holland.

Xu, K.T. (2006) State-level variations in income-related inequality in health and health achievement in the US, *Social Science and Medicine*, 63(2): 457–64.

chapter eight

Measuring and Comparing Financial Protection

Rodrigo Moreno-Serra,
Sarah Thomson and Ke Xu

8.1 Financial protection and health system performance

A key dimension of universal health coverage, which aims to ensure that everyone can access needed and effective health services, is that access to treatment for illness or injury should not lead to financial hardship (WHO, 2010a). WHO's seminal report on health systems performance, published in 2000, drew global attention to the issue of financial protection under the broad rubric of 'fair financing', a concept it identified as a major health system goal[1] in recognition of the wider social value of promoting fairness through the health system (WHO, 2000; McIntyre, 2010). As a result, efforts to secure financial protection in health are often regarded as primarily intended to enhance equity. Although this is a valid point of view, it underplays the vital role financial protection plays in enhancing efficiency.

In this chapter we define financial protection as the extent to which people are protected from the financial consequences of ill health (WHO, 2000; WHO, 2010a). We begin by highlighting the policy importance of financial protection and its relationship to health system performance, then engage in a detailed analysis of the strengths and limitations of different methods of measuring financial protection within and across countries, and their usefulness to policy-makers.

Why do people need financial protection?

The need for financial protection is closely linked to three factors. First, there is uncertainty about the timing and severity of an episode of illness or injury. Unanticipated health care needs[2] have an opportunity cost because financial resources that could have purchased things like food and clothing must instead be spent on health services. Second, health care can be very expensive, both in absolute and relative terms: even low-cost health services may create financial hardship for poorer households. In response, people may forego needed health services or pay for them and risk being impoverished. Third, ill health or injury may be associated with loss of earnings, which also heightens the risk of poverty.

How can financial protection be secured?

International research demonstrates that financial protection in health is secured by sharing the risk of financial loss across groups of people (pooling) and by spreading this risk over time (pre-payment) (Xu et al., 2007). Pooling and pre-payment help to: alleviate the financial consequences of uncertainty regarding health care need; remove financial barriers to accessing health services; and decrease the incidence of financial hardship associated with ill health (WHO, 2010a). In most countries, health financing policy therefore aims to facilitate some form of pooling and pre-payment arrangement. This 'insurance function' can be achieved in a range of ways, for example, through the pooling of tax revenues, or compulsory or voluntary contributions from individuals and employers.

The extent of pooling and pre-payment in a health system influences the degree of coverage people enjoy, in terms of coverage breadth (the universality of health benefits), scope (the range of benefits covered) and depth (the proportion of benefit cost covered by pooled resources). In turn, the quality of coverage determines whether people are adequately protected against the financial consequences of ill health. Policy-makers therefore have a variety of tools with which to promote both coverage and financial protection within the health system.

Much of the literature on financial protection in health focuses on the negative effects of uncertainty regarding health care need and the high cost of health services. There is less emphasis on loss of earnings, probably reflecting the fact that many countries provide protection from lost earnings through other forms of social security, such as entitlement to sickness leave or disability benefits. Historically, however, the risk of lost earnings due to ill health (and, for employers, the risk of a reduced or less productive labour force) has been a major stimulus for the development of pooling and pre-payment arrangements. As the range, effectiveness and cost of health services available has grown, so the need for financial protection specifically from health care payments has expanded.

Why is financial protection a policy concern?

Financial protection can make a significant contribution to two policy goals: efficiency and equity. With regard to efficiency, the welfare gains generated by financial protection accrue to individuals, to the health system and to the wider economy. The efficiency-enhancing effects of health insurance (including insurance for long-term care) are well established (see, for example, Knight (1921) or Barr (2004)). Risk-averse individuals gain from the security of knowing they will not face financial hardship if they become ill and do not therefore have to set aside large amounts of money or other assets in order to be able to cover the maximum financial loss possible; instead, they make regular payments reflecting the average risk of the pool in question. This brings benefits beyond the individuals concerned. At a societal level, there will be scope for efficiency gains if the benefits of extended financial protection outweigh the costs required to achieve it. At the level of the health system, pooled pre-paid resources can be more effectively matched to health need than health care financed directly out-of-pocket, allowing health gain to be maximized.[3] At a macroeconomic level, removal of the need for individuals to hoard wealth to pay for health care may increase national consumption and investment, boosting economic growth.

Without financial protection, inability to pay for health care may lead people to forego or postpone the use of health services. At the health system level, this can generate inefficiencies through reduced health outcomes and through greater use of resources at a later stage if deteriorating health requires more expensive treatment (for example, emergency care as opposed to a visit to a primary care provider). The negative macroeconomic consequences of inadequate financial protection are also well documented (Commission on Macroeconomics and Health, 2001). Paying for urgent health care often forces families to sell their productive assets, undermining national efforts to reduce poverty. Those who lack the required capital to generate income and pay off their debts in the future may be caught in a 'poverty trap', which can affect the educational attainment and earning potential of younger generations if children are forced to leave school prematurely and enter the labour force to help make ends meet. By lowering work productivity, poorer health can also translate into lower wages, higher turnover of labour force and lower profitability for enterprises, making the country less attractive to foreign direct investment and impairing economic growth.

Adequate financial protection tends to have a positive impact on both equity of access to health care and equity in financing health care.[4] Access to the highest attainable standard of health for every citizen, encompassing among other factors access to medical care and medicines, without associated risk of financial hardship or impoverishment, has been recognized as a fundamental human right and a central component in reversing health system inequities (Backman et al., 2008; WHO, 2010a). While all except the extremely wealthy stand to benefit from financial protection, poorer and less healthy people are more likely to face financial hardship due to ill health, since they are usually less able to cope with uncertainty about health care need than the rich (for instance, through access to insurance and credit mechanisms). The removal of financial barriers to accessing health care for previously under-served groups of people will, in turn, help improve health outcomes within these groups –promoting equity in health – and across the whole population. Enhancing financial protection improves equity in financing to the extent that financial protection is secured through pre-payment and therefore lowers reliance on direct or out-of-pocket payments made at the point of use (usually the most regressive form of health care financing) (Wagstaff & van Doorslaer, 2000a).

How can we measure financial protection?

Measuring the incidence and magnitude of direct payments for health care, using data from household surveys, forms the basis for assessing and comparing financial protection within and across countries. Research to date has focused on the extent to which these direct payments are 'catastrophic', relative to some threshold of household income, or 'impoverishing', relative to some pre-defined poverty line. However, a major weakness of current metrics is their failure to recognize that inability to pay may deter access to necessary care, resulting in very low or no reported household expenditure on health. In addition, conventional measures of financial protection cannot say much about the specific drivers of financial risk in a health system. This has led some to suggest that coverage indicators for key health services should be used to complement information about catastrophic and impoverishing health spending (see, for instance, WHO, 2010a).

The rest of the chapter is structured as follows. Section 8.2 describes the main instruments used to measure financial protection, highlighting their strengths and limitations. Section 8.3 discusses important methodological and data issues, as well as research priorities for developing more accurate and informative indicators. Section 8.4 outlines what currently used metrics can and cannot say about health system performance. Section 8.5 concludes with a summary of the chapter's key points.

8.2 Current measurement instruments: strengths, limitations and debates

The multidimensional nature of financial protection makes it extremely difficult to develop a single indicator capturing the full extent to which people are protected from health shocks. It is therefore of little surprise that a single measure of financial protection has yet to emerge as universally accepted in the literature for the purposes of health system performance assessment. This does not mean that there has been no progress in the field. The more recent literature has focused on the incidence and magnitude of household health spending, mainly (and often exclusively) in the form of out-of-pocket payments.

Out-of-pocket spending on health care

A simple strategy to gain insight into how far people are protected from the financial consequences of illness is to look at the contribution of direct or out-of-pocket payments to the financing of the health system.[5] The substantial literature on this finds that a high share of out-of-pocket payments is usually associated with a high risk of financial hardship when health care is needed for those who can afford to access health services, and partial or total lack of access to care for the poorest households (Preker, Langenbrunner & Jakab, 2002; Baeza & Packard, 2006). This association occurs in countries at all stages of economic development, and is particularly strong in low-income countries, where out-of-pocket spending levels are often extremely high (see Figure 8.1). In countries like Guinea, Tajikistan, Nigeria, Georgia and Cameroon, for example, out-of-pocket expenditures accounted for more than 70% of total health spending in 2007, indicating a much higher relative risk of financial hardship due to health care payment.

There is also a good deal of literature on the positive effect of policies to lower out-of-pocket spending levels as a way of enhancing financial protection, both in low- and high-income country settings. For example, using data from the *Vietnam Living Standards Surveys* for 1993 and 1998, Sepehri et al. (2006) found that the Vietnamese social health insurance scheme reduced out-of-pocket spending by between 28% and 35% at the mean income level over that period, with larger effects for individuals with lower incomes. Research shows similar results for the introduction and expansion of Medicare[6] in the United States (Finkelstein & McKnight, 2008; Millett et al., 2010).

Cross-country analysis of the relative importance of out-of-pocket spending in financing health care is useful for comparative assessment of financial risk. However, out-of-pocket expenses represent only one side of the coin. To examine whether people are protected from the financial consequences of illness requires comparison of living standards with and without having to pay for health care. This allows researchers to determine the number or fraction of individuals spending a large proportion of their disposable income on health care payment, where 'large' means that payments exceed some threshold in terms of the chosen living standard measure. In the following sub-sections we examine the two main ways of doing this.

Catastrophic spending on health care

Recent empirical literature often equates financial protection (or the lack thereof) with the incidence of health care spending deemed 'catastrophic' (e.g. Xu et al., 2003a, 2007; van Doorslaer et al., 2007). The latter is usually defined as occurring if a household's share of health care spending lies above a predefined income threshold (a household income aggregate which serves as a measure of living standards). A household's actual health care spending, normally obtained from household expenditure or multipurpose surveys, should ideally be contrasted with its ability or capacity to pay for health care in the absence of illness. Such capacity to pay is not directly observed from surveys, representing a counterfactual that must be constructed from the household's reported expenditures.

Defining household capacity to pay, health care payments and the catastrophic threshold

Most studies compute a measure of household income based on total spending without any health care payments (often labelled pre-payment income) to reflect living standards in the absence of a health shock. In order to better

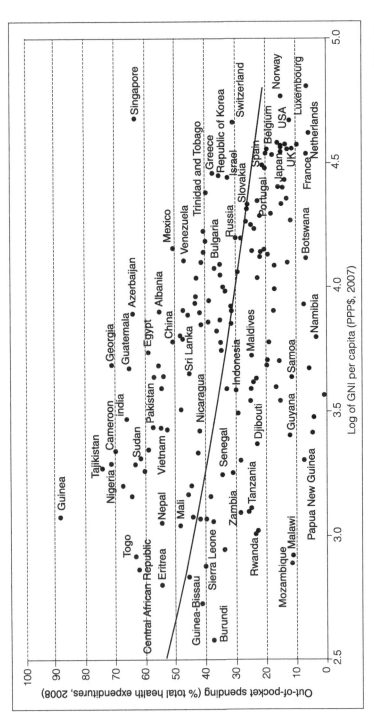

Figure 8.1 Per capita gross national income and out-of-pocket payments as a share of total health expenditures, 164 countries (2007–08)

Source: WHO, 2010b.

reflect a household's capacity to pay for health care, some studies (for example, Xu et al., 2007) use a spending aggregate that excludes subsistence expenditures (spending on things like food and shelter). Health care payments are then compared to the non-subsistence pre-payment spending levels. Health care payments are normally calculated as the sum of the household's out-of-pocket expenditures made directly to providers, excluding any pre-payment such as contributions to health insurance schemes or medical savings accounts. The choice of threshold above which health care payments are defined as catastrophic is unavoidably arbitrary and ultimately a normative choice. The usual practice has been to specify a threshold of between 10% and 40% of pre-payment income (see, among others, Pradhan & Prescott, 2002; Wagstaff & van Doorslaer, 2003; van Doorslaer et al., 2007; Xu et al., 2007). Sensitivity analysis seems warranted after a threshold has been chosen and, to address distributional issues (see below), the analyst may also set different thresholds for richer and poorer households.

Measuring the extent of catastrophic spending in a health system

The incidence of catastrophic spending in a health system can be assessed in various ways depending on the analyst's objectives.[7] The dominant approach has been to compute count measures (number or fraction) of individuals or households whose health care payments exceed the predefined catastrophic threshold. For instance, in the broadest international study of catastrophic health care spending, Xu et al. (2007) examined 116 household surveys (spanning the period 1990–2003) for 89 countries at all levels of economic development. Using a threshold of 40% of a household's pre-payment income, the authors find large differences across countries. The incidence of catastrophic health care spending ranges from virtually zero in the Czech Republic and Luxembourg to 9–11% of households in Nicaragua, Brazil and Viet Nam. The data imply that the incidence of financial catastrophe generally falls below 1% only when out-of-pocket payments represent less than 15–20% of total health care spending (WHO, 2010a). Assuming that the sample is representative of the situation observed in other high-, middle- and low-income countries, the authors estimate that 150 million people incur catastrophic health expenditures every year. More than 90% of these people live in low-income countries.

Another option is to produce gap measures of catastrophic spending. In this case, the interest lies in the *intensity* of the lack of financial protection in a given health system. This can be assessed by examining the catastrophic payment gap, defined as the amount (in monetary terms) by which households cross the catastrophic threshold. The catastrophic payment gap across all households is then summed to give an aggregate picture of the lack of financial protection in a health system. Alternatively, an average figure for the catastrophic payment gap across households can be calculated to make within- and cross-country comparisons over time.

Both count and gap metrics can be extended to give insights into the distribution of financial protection. A simple way of doing this is to examine the incidence and intensity of catastrophic health care spending by levels of pre-payment income. For example, using household survey data from Vietnam and alternative income aggregates and thresholds, Wagstaff and van Doorslaer (2003) find that both the incidence and the intensity of catastrophic spending decreased between 1993 and 1998, in particular becoming less concentrated among the poorest individuals in the sample.

Impoverishing spending on health care

This measure relates out-of-pocket health care spending to a minimum acceptable level of living standards, so that the threshold is defined in terms of a poverty line. Impoverishing spending occurs if health care payments push the household's disposable income below the poverty line. Theoretically, this approach should provide a broader picture of financial protection than catastrophic spending measures: from a policy perspective, interest in financial protection ultimately stems from the objective of avoiding financial hardship caused by illness or injury, and measures of impoverishing spending more directly address this issue.

Defining the poverty line

Data on household income and health spending aggregates are normally obtained from the same sources as in catastrophic spending studies (expenditure or multipurpose household surveys). To aid cross-country comparison of living standards before and after health care payments, a common approach has been to use the World Bank's one- (or two-) dollar-a-day poverty line (World Bank, 1990). This global poverty threshold was initially constructed using figures adjusted for purchasing power parity (PPP), based on a survey of national poverty lines in 33 developing and developed countries during the 1970s and 1980s. Analysis of more recent data has led the World Bank to propose an update of the international poverty line to US$1.25 a day at 2005 PPP household consumption levels (Ravallion, Chen & Sangraula, 2009).

Although the use of this poverty line goes some way toward enhancing international comparability, cross-country differences in consumption patterns (basic baskets of goods and services) and the lack of PPP figures for most countries and years can introduce unknown biases when the poverty line is converted into local currency. Recent comparative studies have opted instead to construct country-specific poverty lines based on the share of total household expenditures spent on food. Food-based poverty lines indicate the amount of income needed for a household to purchase a basic-needs food basket and nothing more in a given country, minimizing the influence of different cross-country consumption patterns and accounting for different prices and household sizes. For example, Xu et al. (2003a) set a country's poverty line as the average food expenditure of households whose food share (relative to total spending) was in the 45th to 55th percentile range, thus also accounting for the fact that poorer households tend to spend a higher share of their income on food.

Measuring the extent of impoverishing spending in a health system

The analyst can obtain a simple count measure of the incidence of impoverishing health care spending by comparing the number of households with pre-payment income below the poverty line to the number of households with post-payment income below the poverty line. For example, van Doorslaer et al. (2006) used survey data to measure poverty in 11 low- and middle-income countries in Asia before and after out-of-pocket spending on health care. When calculating the number of people living on less than US$1 a day before and after incurring health care payments, the authors found that health care payments pushed an additional 2.7% of individuals in the sample below the one-dollar poverty line. The largest incidences of impoverishing health care spending were measured in Bangladesh, China, India, Nepal and Viet Nam, countries that also exhibited the largest shares of health care costs funded out-of-pocket. In Bangladesh, impoverishing spending in health care was estimated to affect 3.8% of individuals.

Analysts can also construct measures of the degree of hardship imposed by health care payments by estimating the aggregate or average (monetary) distance from the poverty line, for the households' pre-payment and post-payment situations. This gap measure has two advantages: it allows an estimation of the intensity of financial hardship caused by health care spending and it accounts for impoverishment among those who were already below the poverty line before making any health care payments. Following this approach, and using the one-dollar-a-day poverty line, van Doorslaer et al. (2006) found an increase of around 18% in the population-weighted average poverty gap for their sample of countries, compared to the situation without health care payments.

The main limitations of catastrophic and impoverishing health spending as measures of financial protection

The interpretation of catastrophic and impoverishing spending metrics hinges on two important assumptions. First, all out-of-pocket health care spending is regarded as involuntary – a response to a health shock – and is therefore considered to impose an opportunity cost in terms of foregone consumption of other goods and services. Unlike the things a household foregoes in order to pay for health care, spending on health care is assumed not to contribute to welfare. Second, it is assumed that all resources spent on health care reported by a given household would have been spent on non-health items in the absence of any health shock. These assumptions, combined with a focus on measuring out-of-pocket payments, are at the root of the four main criticisms directed at financial protection metrics:

1. The construction of the indicators depends crucially on accurately defining and measuring households' capacity to pay for health care, which is not straightforward.
2. The indicators only account for the short-term effects of financial hardship and ignore longer-term consequences for household welfare.

3. They do not account for the impact of lost earnings caused by illness.
4. They do not tell us about unmet need created by financial barriers to accessing health care.

Some of these issues have been discussed at length elsewhere (see, for example, Flores et al. (2008) and Wagstaff (2009)). Others have received little – if any – attention in the literature.

Assessing household capacity to pay: distinguishing between 'essential' and 'discretionary' health spending

On the face of it, defining all out-of-pocket health expenditures as involuntary consumption that does not contribute to household welfare may seem far-fetched. It is possible that some individuals choose to spend part of their income on treatment that is not the result of an unforeseen episode of illness or injury. However, from a more theoretical perspective, it is very difficult to draw a clear line between 'essential' and 'discretionary' spending. Even if theoretically possible, in practice it is difficult to measure only essential out-of-pocket health care spending because household surveys do not allow the analyst to distinguish spending genuinely driven by a health shock from more discretionary medical outlays. This has forced studies to focus on all out-of-pocket spending and to assume all of it is non-discretionary. As a result, it is doubtful whether existing research provides an accurate assessment of capacity to pay. In fact, it may underestimate the extent of financial protection, particularly for richer groups, who are more likely to engage in discretionary spending.

Assessing household capacity to pay: accounting for coping strategies

The assumption that all spending on health care would have been spent on non-health consumption had the household not experienced a health shock has also been disputed. It is tantamount to assuming that the household funds health care purely by foregoing current consumption of other things. However, there is growing evidence to suggest that many households finance health care by resorting to coping strategies such as selling assets, drawing on savings (dissaving) and borrowing, which temporarily raises their observed income when health care payments are necessary. For example, Gotsadze et al. (2005) found that, in Georgia, lack of capacity to fund outpatient care from current earnings frequently forced households to borrow from a friend or relative (70% of users), or sell household valuables (10%) or household-produced goods (10%). Flores et al. (2008) found similar results in India, where coping strategies financed around three-quarters of inpatient care spending. Because household survey data overestimate total current income for these households, catastrophic and impoverishment spending indicators do not identify the 'hidden poor' (people not conventionally identified as poor) and may therefore overestimate the extent of financial protection in a health system.

Accounting for the longer-term financial consequences of health spending

Catastrophic and impoverishing spending indicators often reflect only short-term impacts occurring over a few months or a year. They do not capture the long-run consequences of health care spending caused, for instance, by interest payments on loans taken out to pay for current health expenses. These consequences are likely to differ according to the type of coping strategy a household employs. For example, under high interest rates, households that have to rely on loans to fund health expenses will tend to suffer more financially in the future compared to those that can use savings or sell assets. The longer-term costs of health care payments can be particularly significant for poorer households (see Wagstaff (2009) for an illustration), who may not be able to recover sufficiently (financially) from an initial health shock, thus undermining further their ability to cope with subsequent shocks. Because longer-term effects are currently overlooked in financial protection analyses, the extent of financial protection in a health system may be overestimated.

Accounting for loss of earnings

As noted in section 8.1, the need for financial protection may be linked to income losses resulting from illness or injury, particularly when ill health prevents people from working or affects their productivity at work. However, current indicators focus on health care payments alone and do not account for foregone earnings. This is partly because available datasets do not contain information sufficiently detailed to permit calculation of the income an individual would have received had he or she not fallen ill.

The lack of attention to current and future loss of earnings in measuring financial protection has also been justified on policy grounds. Some commentators argue that, essential as it is, protection against health-related income loss is not strictly within the remit of the health system, representing instead an activity for which the more general social protection system should take responsibility (for example, Wagstaff (2009)). As a result, the dominant view has been not to focus on attempting to capture the magnitude of foregone earnings, since measures of financial protection are primarily intended to serve as indicators of health system performance.

However, health systems have been defined as "comprising all the organizations, institutions and resources that are devoted to producing health actions (. . .) [which are understood as] any effort, whether in personal health care, public health services or through intersectoral initiatives, whose primary purpose is to improve health" (WHO, 2000). Under this broad, multisectoral definition, protection against lost earnings due to illness arguably *does* represent a 'health action' and hence a useful parameter to gauge the performance of a health system. After all, inadequate protection against loss of earnings – stemming from a poorly designed social security system – might drive households to incur higher health expenditures *because* of the imperative to get back to work (perhaps even before full recovery from illness has been achieved). In contrast, in a country with better social security, the need to spend on health care to facilitate a rapid return to work might not be so pressing.

Insufficient social security provision for lost earnings can affect the estimated incidence of catastrophic and impoverishing spending. While this is more likely to be the case in poorer country contexts, consistency would seem to require the issue to be dealt with explicitly in analysing financial protection in any setting. Nevertheless, practical limitations imposed by data availability are likely to represent a major hurdle to making the necessary adjustments to current metrics.

Accounting for unmet need

The exclusive focus of catastrophic and impoverishing spending metrics on out-of-pocket payments for health care poses a major obstacle to assessing the extent to which people are protected from the financial consequences of illness. These measures do not acknowledge that lack of capacity to pay may actually prevent people from accessing needed health care, resulting in very low or no reported health expenditures. If lack of capacity to pay for health care does lead people to forego treatment, to self-treat or to substitute lower quality care, the adverse consequences of inadequate financial protection may be manifested in terms of worsening health rather than merely in short-term catastrophic or impoverishing spending.

Financial protection measurement focusing on health care payments cannot capture unmet need caused by financial barriers to access. As a result, performance assessment based on catastrophic and impoverishing metrics alone would give a highly misleading picture of the actual situation with regard to financial protection. For example, two countries may have low levels of catastrophic spending for very different reasons. In the first country most citizens may spend little out-of-pocket because health care is mainly free at the point of use, but in the second country observed out-of-pocket expenditures may be low because citizens cannot afford to pay existing user charges and therefore under-use or forego health services when they need them. Despite similar performance in terms of the incidence of catastrophic health spending, it is likely that policy-makers would consider financial protection to be worse in the second country.

The fact that current financial protection measures do not account for differences in financial barriers to health care use across population groups seems to be at least partially responsible for some unexpected empirical results. For instance, Wagstaff (2007) finds very small reductions in the incidence of catastrophic spending in Viet Nam due to the introduction of social health insurance and the expansion of tax-funded insurance for the poor, with still high rates of catastrophic spending even among the insured. As the author acknowledges, part of the explanation seems to be that health care use increased due to insurance. If any part of this additional demand was due to individuals who were previously deterred from seeking care by high user fees (reporting zero, or close to zero, medical expenditures in the baseline survey) now spending non-catastrophic amounts on health care, there is some gain from the policies in terms of improved financial protection that is not captured by catastrophic spending measures.

Accounting for distributional effects

Analysts have attempted to gain some understanding of the distributional aspects of financial protection by looking at the incidence and intensity of catastrophic and impoverishing spending by levels of household income. This practice treats the incidence of financial hardship as proportional across income levels, since the same catastrophic or impoverishing threshold is applied to all households irrespective of their position in the overall income distribution. Yet, having a constant threshold may be seen as problematic, not least because richer households usually have a larger proportion of discretionary total and health care spending. Poorer households tend to spend a higher share of their income on non-discretionary consumption of items such as housing, clothing and food, but also on non-discretionary health care. For instance, in their analysis of catastrophic health care spending in Estonia, Võrk and colleagues (2009) found medicines to be a far more important share of out-of-pocket payments for the poorest quintile than for the richest quintile (84% vs 33% in 2007), whereas (more discretionary) adult dental care was considerably less relevant as a share of out-of-pocket expenses for the poor than for the rich (7% vs 32%) (Võrk, Saluse & Habicht, 2009). Given the observed differences in discretionary health care spending found in this and other studies, it may be argued that the catastrophic spending threshold itself should be adjusted according to household income levels. Such an adjustment could take the form of 'progressive' thresholds which are lower for poorer than for richer households (Ataguba, 2011). This issue highlights the importance of examining the structure of catastrophic and impoverishing spending in order to obtain a more complete picture of financial protection in a health system.

8.3 Developing better indicators of financial protection: methodological challenges, research priorities and data issues

From the discussion so far, it seems clear that catastrophic and impoverishing spending indicators should continue to play a major role in assessing financial protection. Yet it is also clear that these metrics are subject to important criticisms, revealing multiple methodological challenges in the development and application of more accurate and informative measures. Some of these challenges are not unique to analysis of financial protection. For example, it is well known that comparisons of spending magnitudes across health systems need PPP adjustments to be accurate (Gerdtham & Jönsson, 2000). The focus of this section is on key methodological issues pertaining specifically to the construction and comparison of financial protection indicators.

Challenges to accurate measurement of capacity to pay, subsistence expenditures, health care payments and the long-run financial consequences of ill health

Capacity to pay

The burden of health care payments on household welfare ought to be calculated based on household capacity to pay. Ideally, this should correspond to a measure of permanent income (over the household's life-cycle) so as to include, for instance, the household's ability to cope with health shocks through asset sales and borrowing. Such an approach requires detailed information on household wealth, ability to obtain loans and future earnings. It is therefore difficult to measure permanent income within a country, let alone across countries. Most studies deal with this obstacle by using a measure of the household's non-subsistence *spending* (see below) as a proxy for permanent income. There are two main reasons for this choice. First, spending figures are likely to be more smoothed over time than reported income, in part due to the role of credit mechanisms. In this respect, spending figures are better suited to reflect a household's ability to cope with health shocks through borrowing. Since the aim is to get as close as possible to estimating permanent income, it is essential to minimize the effect of random shocks. Moreover, as a general rule, reported expenditures tend to be more reliable than income figures in household surveys (Deaton, 1997; Xu et al., 2003b).

Second, the use of non-subsistence expenditures acknowledges households' need to meet their basic needs before paying for health care.

Subsistence spending

Calculating household subsistence spending also presents significant challenges. Spending on food may include both essential and non-essential goods. Disaggregated figures on food spending can permit the exclusion of non-essential food consumption from subsistence expenditure, although much depends on the level of detail provided by a given survey and, importantly for comparative purposes, on the compatibility of consumption items across surveys in different countries. In addition, spending on food as a share of total household expenditures tends to be inversely related to income, even though richer households usually spend more on food in absolute terms and incur greater discretionary spending in general. This leads to an underestimation of richer households' capacity to pay for health care in financial protection analyses (Xu et al., 2003b).

Health care payments

In deciding *which* health expenditures to consider, the general approach in the literature has been to focus on out-of-pocket spending on health care and to exclude spending through pre-paid contributions to (public and private) health insurance schemes or medical savings accounts. One reason for this is that it conforms more closely to the idea that financial protection concerns financial hardship caused by *unexpected* health spending. Since pre-paid spending is usually anticipated, it does not strictly represent a health shock. Another reason for excluding compulsory or voluntary pre-paid spending is that it may be seen as providing valued protection against the uncertainty of health care need and any associated expenses, thus *contributing* to household welfare. In contrast, out-of-pocket payments are usually regarded as having a detrimental effect on household welfare by reducing the consumption of welfare-enhancing goods such as food. Of course, it is also possible for pre-payment to reduce spending on food and other necessities for generally poorer households, particularly following a health shock. Where this is a concern, analysts can include pre-paid spending in their estimate of health-related expenditures.

Long-term financial consequences

Discussion of the main criticisms of catastrophic and impoverishing spending metrics in section 8.2 highlighted the potentially distorting role of coping strategies (such as asset sales, borrowing or depleting savings) in calculating, from survey data, household capacity to pay for health care. It seems important to adjust for coping strategies so as to account for the resulting transitory increases in income and their long-term financial consequences for household welfare (for example, through interest payments and access to credit). However, the construction of the necessary counterfactual – the household's income had it not needed to incur health care payments – is not straightforward. Most survey data provide very limited information on how health care payments are financed, adding to the problem of frequent under-declaration of income in household surveys, especially in low-income countries (Deaton, 1997).

The practical implication of these shortcomings is that the financial protection metrics routinely constructed in the literature do not account for income derived from coping strategies, or for the likely possibility that some households incur expenses every year in the form of interest payments on health care-related loans. Furthermore, the simple adjustments suggested in the literature may introduce other unknown biases (Flores et al., 2008; Wagstaff, 2009). The distorting effect of coping strategies is likely to depend, among other things, on differences in the degree of access to formal and informal credit mechanisms across countries. Additional research is clearly warranted to permit the development of financial protection metrics – and relevant data sources – better suited to capturing the intertemporal financial consequences of illness.

Financial barriers to access and unmet need for health care: the elephant in the room

Current financial protection indicators do not consider financial barriers to accessing health care. The main argument for this, presented in Wagstaff (2009), is based on the notion that private health spending represents the single focal variable belonging to the financial protection domain, and is therefore the one observable quantity policy-makers should try to influence within such a domain. The argument states that access issues, including financial barriers to access, involve focal variables pertaining to other domains, notably equity.[8] Wagstaff (2009) suggests that financial barriers to access and other elements of health care use go beyond what should be measured under the domain of financial protection. Rather, they should be included in a broader framework of policy analysis alongside factors such as health services availability and provider payment methods. Policy instruments, such as the elimination of user fees for publicly financed health care, will therefore potentially affect two focal variables pertaining to different domains: out-of-pocket payments (financial protection) and the number of people able to afford to use needed health services (equity).

The apparently clear line between financial protection and broader policy aspects drawn in the argument above seems to be more blurred in practice. Even though financial barriers to access are linked to the equity domain, we argue that they are also important indicators of the extent of financial protection in a health system. As we noted in section 8.2, in most countries, people whose health expenditures are very low (or non-existent) because they cannot afford to pay for health care when ill would *not* be considered to be adequately protected against the financial consequences of ill health. To be relevant for policy, assessment of financial protection should attempt to capture this broader dimension. It should not be limited to focusing on observed expenditure alone, since the incidence of catastrophic or impoverishing spending only tells us about one aspect of financial protection.

There is extensive quantitative and qualitative evidence pointing to the importance of financial factors in deterring access to health care in a wide range of countries, including high-income countries (see, for example, Ensor & Cooper, 2004; Falkingham, 2004; Gotsadze et al., 2005; Schoen et al., 2010). This evidence makes it clear that relying on catastrophic and impoverishing spending metrics to assess financial protection is of limited value both for measuring performance and developing policy guidance. Figures 8.2 and 8.3 illustrate this point. They present international comparisons of catastrophic spending incidence[9] and national coverage levels for two selected interventions used as proxies for access: diphtheria-tetanus-pertussis (DTP3) immunization among 1-year-olds and births attended by skilled personnel. The figures show that the relationship between catastrophic spending and health care coverage is highly variable. For a given level of financial catastrophe, there are remarkable discrepancies in coverage levels, suggesting important differences in the presence of financial and other barriers to access across health systems. Lack of attention to the influence of barriers to access might lead an observer to conclude that people in Uganda enjoy a similar level of financial protection to their counterparts in Greece and Portugal, despite the much better breadth and depth of health coverage in the two richer countries, when this is not at all the case (Mossialos et al., 2002). In fact, evidence from Uganda strongly suggests that a large share of its population has to forego necessary health care due to cost and, as a result, incurs very low or no health expenditures (Kiwanuka et al., 2008).

The same discrepancies can be found within groups of countries with similar income levels, including high-income countries. The study by Schoen et al. (2010) indicates that financial barriers to access have different effects among

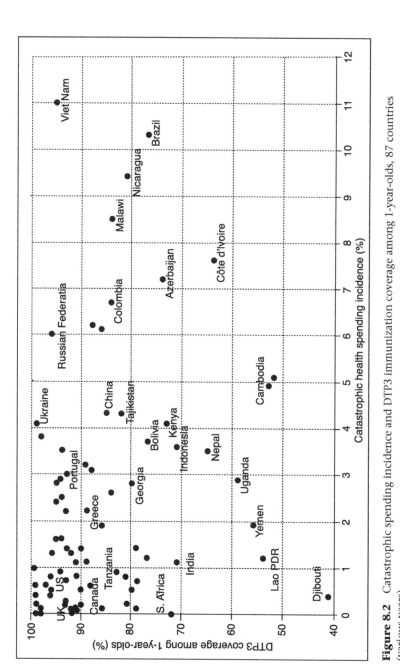

Figure 8.2 Catastrophic spending incidence and DTP3 immunization coverage among 1-year-olds, 87 countries (various years)

Source: WHO, 2010b. (Catastrophic spending incidence data from Xu et al., 2007. Financial catastrophe is defined as out-of-pocket payments for health reaching at least 40% of a household's non-subsistence income.)

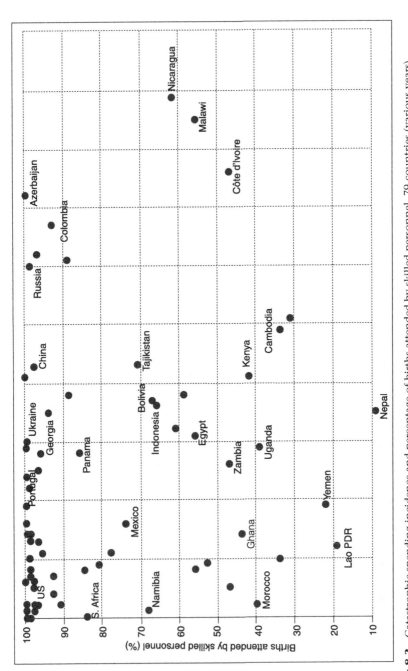

Figure 8.3 Catastrophic spending incidence and percentage of births attended by skilled personnel, 79 countries (various years)

Source: WHO, 2010b. (Catastrophic spending incidence data from Xu et al., 2007. Financial catastrophe is defined as out-of-pocket payments for health reaching at least 40% of a household's non-subsistence income.)

OECD countries with very low estimated incidence of financial catastrophe (0.5% or less). For example, it found that 33% and 25% of individuals in the US and Germany (respectively) reported having been deterred from seeking necessary health care due to costs, against 10% in Sweden and only 5% in the United Kingdom. This suggests that people living in these high-income countries are not equally or adequately protected against the financial consequences of ill health, in spite of negligible estimated levels of catastrophic spending. It strengthens the case for including analysis of financial barriers to access when assessing financial protection.

Accounting for financial barriers to access

Very few studies have tried to account for financial barriers to accessing health care when estimating the incidence of catastrophic or impoverishing spending. One way forward is for financial protection studies to build on the widely applied approach adopted when measuring equity in health service use, i.e. to adjust for need (see Wagstaff & van Doorslaer (2000b) for an early discussion). Pradhan and Prescott (2002) do this by estimating the distribution of needed health expenditures from survey data to simulate the impact of different price subsidy regimes on catastrophic spending incidence in Indonesia. Through simulations,[10] the authors obtain expected household expenditures for self-treatment, outpatient and inpatient care. The resulting need-adjusted distribution for total health expenditures is then used to compute the incidence of catastrophic spending in the sample (using a 10% threshold in terms of total household consumption) for different pricing policies. An interesting extension of the analysis would have been to compare the catastrophic incidence of the need-adjusted health spending to the incidence based on reported health expenditures. Given the high frequency of zero health expenditures in the Indonesian data, and the major differences in health care use between rich and poor households (with the latter using far fewer services), the conclusions reached and resulting policy guidance might have been markedly different had unadjusted spending figures been used instead.

In future, many more analysts are likely to adopt a similar approach. A starting point would be to estimate a two-part econometric model of the predicted probability of any health care use through a binary choice model (probit or logit), and the amount spent on health care conditional on positive use through (for example) a truncated ordinary least-squares estimator. The first part of the model should include a set of household- and individual-level regressors capturing the need for health care, including age, gender and any other available objective and subjective indicators. The second part of the empirical model should also include the need regressors, with the two-part model estimated in the whole sample. Expected need-adjusted health spending for each individual can then be obtained by taking the product of the predicted individual probability of positive health spending and the expected amount of health spending conditional on positive expenses.[11]

This methodology allows the researcher to measure the need-adjusted incidence of catastrophic and impoverishing spending within a health system and to compare performance across countries. It also allows an assessment of the gap between expected and reported health expenditures in household surveys, indicating the extent to which barriers to access have a bearing on reported out-of-pocket spending. However, some important methodological challenges remain; two in particular stand out. First, in the equity literature, need-adjusted health spending figures for a given individual are estimated based on the amount of health care they would have received had they been treated as others with the same need characteristics in the sample were, *on average*, treated. For financial protection assessments, actual health care use for a given individual should ideally be compared not to the average but to the 'best' amount of care received by people with the same need characteristics, so as to indicate how much of that 'ideal' amount of care the person foregoes due to inability to pay. Even though it seems logical to equate best care to the health care expenses necessary to restore an individual to full health after illness, obtaining a distribution of best care from the observed data seems less straightforward. Research is needed to investigate how the empirical tools described above can be adapted to construct, using survey data, the distribution of best care and foregone health care expenditures, while accounting for capacity to pay.

Second, analysis based on estimating expected health care expenditures assumes that any barriers to access are related to ability to pay. Yet the large literature on barriers to access highlights the important role of non-financial factors in determining individual demand for health services, including education levels, information issues, and cultural and social barriers (Ensor & Cooper, 2004). In financial protection analyses, the influence of non-price barriers should be netted out so that need-adjusted health spending figures only reflect the effect of financial barriers to access. The challenge here is to find informative (and internationally comparative) data on individual, household and health system characteristics that can serve as proxies for non-price barriers to access in econometric regressions.

In spite of these challenges, there is emerging consensus on the need for practical alternatives to account for financial barriers to access in analysing financial protection. The 2010 World Health Report (WHO, 2010a) suggests a set of indicators to monitor financial protection, based both on whether people have access to needed health services and on whether they risk financial hardship in paying for them. For example, it proposes complementing catastrophic and impoverishing spending metrics with information on coverage levels for key health care interventions, such as immunization, as a way of acknowledging barriers to access.

Data issues

Minimum requirements

The two key elements for measuring financial protection are household out-of-pocket payments for health care and household capacity to pay. As noted above, the most basic information required to calculate catastrophic and impoverishing expenditures comes from household surveys and includes total household consumption expenditure, food expenditure (not including tobacco, alcohol or eating in a restaurant), out-of-pocket health expenditure and household size. This information exists for most countries. The availability of household socioeconomic characteristics allows a more comprehensive analysis.

Sources of data

Few research projects can afford to conduct a nationally representative household survey to analyse and measure financial protection. Consequently, most studies rely on existing household surveys that include the basic required variables, such as the *Living Standard Measurement Study* (LSMS), income and expenditure surveys, socioeconomic surveys and health surveys. Although available for many countries, these surveys have different focuses and use different instruments for data collection.

The Living Standards Measurement Study (LSMS)

The LSMS surveys were designed by the World Bank and widely implemented in low- and low–middle-income countries by the late 1990s. The LSMS surveys cover national populations and have been repeated on a regular basis in most countries, collecting information at both the individual and household levels, including detailed household income and consumption data, household characteristics, individual health needs and service utilization. Other surveys, such as the *Priority Survey*, *Poverty Survey* and *Integrated Survey* are under different programmes of the World Bank but use similar questionnaires as the LSMS.

The LSMS is a good data source for analyses of financial protection as well as health service utilization. The cross-sectional LSMS data can be used to perform comparisons over time. The fact that the data collection instruments are similar also allows the possibility of cross-country comparison. Micro-level LSMS data are published for most countries and can be downloaded free of charge in some cases, while in others the access to data requires national government approval and is subject to certain fees.

European Union Household Budget Survey (HBS) and Survey on Income and Living Conditions (EU-SILC)

The HBS and EU-SILC are conducted in European Union countries with technical support from Eurostat. The HBS collects very detailed information on household expenditure and consumption. It has collected data for decades, and in most countries data collection is a continuous process year round. Micro-level data are published annually or quarterly. Although countries are allowed to modify the questionnaires, the framework is quite similar overall and cross-country comparisons are possible in most cases.

The EU-SILC is the continuation of the European Community Household Panel (ECHP), and is being implemented by most EU countries. The EU-SILC includes more socioeconomic indicators than the HBS, as well as detailed information on income and expenditures. Its longitudinal nature allows more in-depth statistical analyses to be carried out. Access to the micro-level data of HBS and EU-SILC is subject to approval by the national officials.

The World Health Survey (WHS)

The WHS was launched by the World Health Organization with the aim of strengthening national capacity to monitor critical health inputs, outputs and outcomes (Üstün et al., 2003). Seventy-two countries implemented the WHS during 2002 and 2003 using standard questionnaires. They collected information on total household expenditure with a breakdown that included health expenditures, together with a wide range of indicators on health status, health service utilization, risk factors, and the perceived responsiveness of the health system. Among the 72 countries, 50 used the so-called long version household questionnaire (applied only in low- and middle-income countries), which provides a more detailed breakdown of total household expenditure and out-of-pocket health expenditure.

The uniform questionnaires make the WHS appealing for cross-country comparisons. However, when compared with the information derived from other types of surveys (such as the ones mentioned above), the WHS gives higher estimates of out-of-pocket payments and lower total household consumption, resulting in higher estimated percentages of catastrophic expenditure (Xu et al., 2009). Moreover, the application of the WHS is a one-time event, which limits the possibility of over-time comparisons. The micro-level data are in the public domain and accessible free of charge (WHO, 2011).

The Commonwealth Fund International Health Policy Survey (IHPS)

The IHPS is carried out by the Commonwealth Fund, a philanthropic organiz-ation based in the United States. It aims at providing information on health policy in various high-income countries with a focus on access, cost and perceived quality. Data collection is based on telephone interviews of nationally representative samples of adults aged 18 and older. The survey has been implemented since 1998 and is intended to run at regular intervals of three years. The sample of countries has varied over the years, starting with five in 1998 and reaching eleven countries in 2010 (Australia, Canada, France, Germany, Netherlands, New Zealand, Norway, Sweden, Switzerland, United Kingdom and the United States). Other surveys conducted by the Commonwealth Fund have collected similar data specifically for some sub-populations, such as chronically ill adults.

The IHPS collects valuable individual-level information for financial protec-tion assessments, including financial burden of medical payments; utilization and access; health needs; insurance coverage; and demographics. Unfortunately, the breakdown levels of expenditure and income data, based on intervals of total amounts, is less conducive to in-depth analyses than those of the surveys mentioned previously. On the plus side, the IHPS provides information on financial barriers to access, such as whether individuals have been deterred from using health services due to costs (separated into categories, e.g. drugs). Since the basic questionnaire applied is the same across countries, IHPS data can be used for cross-country comparisons and, to a certain extent, time-series analyses (there have been some changes over time in the basic questionnaire). Access to the micro-level data needs to be requested from the Commonwealth Fund (Commonwealth Fund, 2011).

Other household surveys

Apart from the major survey groups cited above, there are other nationally representative household surveys that can be used for financial protection analyses, including income and expenditure surveys, socioeconomic surveys and health service surveys. The International Household Survey Network enables analysts to search easily for household survey data in a specific country (IHSN, 2011).

Availability

Access to timely and up-to-date information is a challenge. Data collection for most surveys occurs only every three to five years and the time between data collection and publication can be a year or more. Most income expenditure surveys do not include the data required to provide a more complete picture of financial protection, such as health care need and use, and household coping strategies. Addressing household coping strategies and the long-term impacts of health care payments requires panel data, which are often unavailable. There is an urgent need for new data collection procedures specifically designed to address these issues using standardized instruments to allow cross-country comparison.

Quality

Differences in data quality are significant over time and across countries. In addition to the general principles of quality control, data collection methods (diary vs interview), recall period and the number of breakdown items used are especially important when collecting expenditure data. In general, the diary method provides more accurate estimates of household expenditure than interviews. However, when the diary lasts more than two weeks, the quality of the record falls significantly (Silberstein, 1991). More breakdown items often yield a higher estimate of expenses (Grosh & Glewwe, 2000). A shorter recall period can better capture frequent spending items, while a longer recall period better captures infrequent spending items (Lu et al., 2009). There is a trade-off between memory loss and telescoping (misdating events) when choosing the recall period. Currently, there are not enough studies to be able to say which instrument collects the most valid expenditure data.

Comparability

Time-series data are critical for health policy monitoring and evaluation. This requires data collection to be repeated using the same instrument. The interval between surveys is determined by many factors, but cost is a major consideration. It is therefore difficult for low-income countries to collect data regularly without external funding. LSMS surveys are the main time-series data source for financial protection analysis in low-income countries. Cross-country analysis presents even more challenges. Current instruments vary widely and, even within the same type of survey, questions often differ from country to country. Most surveys are designed to provide information for specific national needs. The common ground for both national use and cross-country comparison is to obtain valid expenditure data. As there is no gold standard in data collection, some suggest adopting a standardized questionnaire based on current methods until a better alternative emerges. Others argue that this may discourage further exploration of the best survey instruments and compromise within-country, over-time comparison.

Feasibility in low- and middle-income countries

Financial protection indicators have been widely used in low- and low–middle-income countries. The data required to compute the indicators already exist in many developing countries and, as national information systems improve, more and more countries are able to conduct this analysis. However, carrying out an independent national household survey solely to measure financial protection is not a realistic option.

8.4 Policy uses and abuses: what financial protection indicators can and cannot tell us about system performance

In light of the many methodological issues surrounding the construction of financial protection measures, it may be useful to provide a clear summary of what the main indicators – catastrophic and impoverishing spending metrics – *can* and *cannot* tell us about health system performance. What the indicators do is provide a picture of the extent to which people suffer financial hardship due to the cost of using health services, as well as the intensity of this hardship. Distributional analysis – examining the incidence of catastrophic or impoverishing spending by income group and, for example, applying different thresholds for rich and poor households – helps to identify the groups of people most affected by financial hardship. Additionally (and depending on the data available), analysing the structure of catastrophic or impoverishing spending can help to identify potential sources of financial hardship. Knowing who is most affected by out-of-pocket spending on health care, and which types of services incur the heaviest financial burden, can contribute to the development of appropriate policy responses.

Valuable as they are for performance assessment, catastrophic and impoverishing spending metrics have limitations that must be clearly understood in order to avoid 'policy abuses' arising from their uncritical use to guide (and justify) health policy-making. These metrics can only provide partial insight into the major determinants of inadequate financial protection in a given context. They also say very little about the role and magnitude of financial barriers to accessing health care, or which people are most affected by such barriers. Consequently, they should be accompanied by complementary analyses, including studies of financial barriers to access, or health service coverage levels across socioeconomic groups. These types of further analysis are more likely to provide policy-relevant information.

A high incidence of catastrophic or impoverishing health spending is likely to correspond to a similarly high reliance on out-of-pocket payments in a given health system. So the policy prescription of moving away from out-of-pocket payments towards pre-payment mechanisms to enhance financial protection follows naturally. The converse is not necessarily true, however. As we have already noted, low incidence of catastrophic or impoverishing health spending *cannot* be interpreted as unequivocally indicating low reliance on out-of-pocket spending or an adequate level of financial protection. A health system might exhibit low levels of catastrophic and impoverishing spending precisely because of substantial reliance on out-of-pocket payments, which prevent many people from seeking needed care because of their cost. Furthermore, levels of financial protection may look adequate in the present period due to households engaging in coping strategies (selling assets and taking out loans) to enable them to pay for health care. These coping strategies temporarily increase income and may therefore mask the true share of households suffering financial hardship now and in the future.

The misuse of conventional catastrophic and impoverishing spending indicators can end up serving as (misleading) justifications for 'quick fixes' in health policy. Governments may try to reduce the overall incidence of impoverishing spending by subsidizing the health care use only of those poor individuals close to the poverty line, so as to bring them just above the poverty threshold. However, this would ignore the intensity of poverty in the country – that is, the (potentially large) group of individuals who are further away from the poverty line and whose situation might deteriorate.

Similar policy 'abuses' of financial protection indicators may arise if the distributional issues raised by their exclusive focus on *observed* payment for health care are not understood and made explicit in performance assessment. For example, van Doorslaer et al. (2007) found the incidence of catastrophic spending to be concentrated among better-off individuals, probably due at least in part to the lower capacity to pay for necessary health services (and therefore lower utilization figures) among the poorest individuals. Based on Indonesian survey data, Pradhan and Prescott (2002) also found a lower incidence of catastrophic spending in the poorest quintile than in the richest quintile. In these cases, the quickest way to lower the incidence of catastrophic spending would be to reduce out-of-pocket health spending among the rich. Yet doing so would not address the generally higher financial barriers to access that the poor face, resulting in worse health outcomes among the poor and, ultimately, a failure to enhance efficiency.

8.5 Conclusion

It is widely accepted that protecting people from incurring financial hardship through the use of needed health care should be a central objective of any health system, mainly to secure efficiency gains, but also to avoid inequities (WHO, 2010a). Devising effective policies to enhance financial protection requires accurate and informative measures to assess performance within and across countries. This chapter has discussed in detail the construction of current financial protection indicators and their usefulness for health system performance assessment and international comparisons. A summary of this discussion is presented in Table 8.1. The growing use of catastrophic and impoverishing health spending metrics in recent years has significantly enlarged the evidence base in this area, providing ever-accumulating information about the devastating effect on household welfare of income and wealth losses associated with the use of health care. Nevertheless, conventional financial protection indicators suffer from a number of limitations, which should be well understood and fully taken into consideration when drawing implications for policy.

Careful analysis of these metrics as they are currently used highlights how they are likely to understate the adverse effects of inadequate financial protection in most national settings, possibly to a considerable extent. Because the metrics rely on spending figures taken directly from household surveys, they ignore cases in which inability to pay deters access to necessary health care, resulting in very low or no reported health expenditures. A country may therefore perform well in terms of catastrophic spending incidence, but only because the high prevalence of financial barriers to access means most of its people are unable to use needed health services. Although financial barriers to access are traditionally associated with the equity domain, they are also primary indicators of the extent to which people are protected from the financial consequences of paying for health care when ill. Additionally, current metrics do not account for earnings lost through ill health or for any longer-term effects on household welfare, including the impact of coping strategies, such as depleting savings, selling assets and borrowing. Finally, the construction of more accurate and informative financial protection indicators depends crucially on the availability of reliable data to determine household capacity to pay for health care and actual outlays on health care. Performance assessment requires such data to be collected regularly and in a comparable manner within and across countries over time.

Notwithstanding these limitations, the evidence strongly suggests that the way in which a health system is financed – in particular the relative importance of out-of-pocket payments used to finance health care – constitutes a key determinant of financial protection levels, as measured by any of the indicators discussed here. The higher the share of out-of-pocket payments in total health expenditures, the more exposed citizens are to financial catastrophe and impoverishment due to illnesses. Since there is little evidence of the influence of other health system functions on levels of financial protection, one clear implication for policy is that efforts to enhance financial protection should focus on lowering financial barriers to access, especially for poorer people and

Table 8.1 Main indicators of financial protection in health systems

Measurement category	Indicators	Data and methodological issues	Policy uses
Financial protection	Out-of-pocket spending as share of total health spending	• Expenditure may refer to essential and non-essential health care • Financial protection assessment requires comparison of households' out-of-pocket spending with some measure of their living standards • Does not account for the effect of financial barriers to health care access	Financial protection performance should consider differences in the extent of financial barriers to access. Performance in this area may be better understood within a country by considering the extent of financial protection across population groups. It seems important for performance comparison to consider differences in broader determinants of financial protection (e.g. social security system), financing mechanisms (e.g. extent of cost-sharing and provider payment arrangements) and fiscal capacity constraints.
	Catastrophic health spending: incidence and gap measures	• Expenditure may refer to essential and non-essential health care • Need informative data to measure households' capacity to pay • Do not account for long-term impacts of financial hardship (e.g. coping strategies) • Do not account for lost earnings due to illness • Do not account for the effect of financial barriers to health care access	
	Impoverishing health spending: incidence and gap measures		
	Coverage levels of key interventions	• Proxy for financial barriers to access • Difficult to make system performance comparisons if set of interventions varies across countries • Actual coverage may reflect non-financial barriers to access (e.g. cultural, information, services availability)	
	Proportion of individuals unable to access needed health services due to costs (unmet need)	• Proxy for financial barriers to access • Need to improve frequency of and consistency of data on unmet need across countries	

those with greater health care needs. Attention should be paid not just to who is covered by pooled pre-paid resources, but also to the range of benefits and the proportion of benefit costs covered.

As a way forward for performance assessment and policy development, in addition to collecting better data more frequently, analysts can adopt complementary strategies to help overcome the limited ability of current metrics to isolate the sources of inadequate financial protection. WHO's recommendation to use information on coverage levels for selected health interventions, while not free from caveats, represents a way of shedding further light on gaps in financial protection (WHO, 2010a). In a similar vein, household surveys with questions on unmet health needs (that is, patterns of and reasons for foregone health care), have great potential to help assess the importance of financial barriers to access in undermining financial protection. These surveys have been used in many countries and can provide highly policy-relevant information. The challenge lies in ensuring regular data collection and applying a standard approach across countries.

The use of catastrophic and impoverishing spending indicators to assist countries in identifying the best policy levers to improve financial protection also calls for a broader understanding of the interaction between health care demand and supply. Without this, it is difficult to predict the knock-on effects of policies to promote financial protection. For example, user fee caps or coverage extensions may result in greater use of health services, which might increase out-of-pocket spending (e.g. on prescription medicines), pushing up the incidence of catastrophic spending. Other unintended consequences include: the overstretching of the public sector (potentially lowering quality); price increases for other non-subsidized services; and growth in informal payments (particularly if providers attempt to make up for revenue losses from user fees). The latter could, in turn, result in more people foregoing the use of needed non-subsidized services due to lack of capacity to pay, generating a counterbalancing effect on the overall extent of financial protection.

One final word of caution: it may be wise for judgements about a health system's financial protection performance to be made against the benchmark of what can *realistically* be achieved given the very different constraints countries face in terms of their ability to generate financial and other resources for health care. As Kutzin and Jakab (2010) note, the relative importance of public and private finance to total health spending depends on two related factors. The first is the country's overall *fiscal capacity*, referring to the national current and (expected) future capacity to spend, often assessed by total public expenditures (i.e. the government budget) as a proportion of GDP. The second corresponds to social preferences as reflected by the share of the total government budget spent on health or, in other words, the *fiscal priorities* arising from the political process. Fiscal capacity is usually highly correlated with the share of total health spending that is publicly funded: poor countries tend to rely more heavily on private sources of health financing than do richer countries (see WHO, 2000; Kutzin & Jakab, 2010). The high prevalence of out-of-pocket payments in many low-income countries increases the risk of financial catastrophe and, at the same time, limits the range of interventions available to policy-makers, as well as their potential achievement in promoting financial protection. Other things equal, there is little scope under a tight public budget constraint for implementing sustainable policies of user fee waivers for large population groups or for significantly enlarging the range of benefits available.

Variations in public capacity to spend imply different prospects for reducing reliance on out-of-pocket payments and improving financial protection across countries. However, the evidence suggests that fiscal capacity should not be automatically regarded as the main determinant of the prevalence of out-of-pocket payments or catastrophic spending in a health system. For a given level of national income, there can be remarkable discrepancies in the amount of public resources allocated to health. In 2007, Germany devoted over 18% of total government spending to the health sector compared to less than 13% in Finland, despite both countries having an annual per capita income (in international dollars) of around US$36,000 (WHO, 2010b). And although higher per capita income is often associated with a lower expected risk of financial catastrophe, there is no robust evidence confirming this link when other characteristics, such as the share of total health spending based on pre-payment and the proportion of GDP spent on health care, are controlled for (Xu et al., 2007). Resource allocation decisions made in a particular country are therefore likely to matter as much (if not more than) fiscal capacity in reducing reliance on out-of-pocket payments and increasing pre-payment, with inevitable consequences for the degree of financial protection.

Notes

1 The others are improving health equitably and improving responsiveness equitably.
2 We refer to these unexpected adverse events as 'health shocks'.
3 In general terms, efficiency gains in a health system arise when more (e.g. better health outcomes or more extensive health services coverage) is achieved with the same amount of resources, or when a given level of health output (outcomes or services) is obtained at a lower cost.
4 See Chapter 7 for definitions of these concepts.
5 These include formal and informal payments for provider consultations, laboratory tests and diagnostic expenses, medicines (traditional or alternative) and hospital care. They typically exclude reimbursements from statutory or voluntary health insurance (see e.g., Xu et al., 2007).
6 A publicly financed insurance scheme for older or disabled people.
7 As in the poverty measurement literature; see Atkinson (1987) for a review.
8 See the vast literature on demand-side barriers to health care access (for example, Ensor & Cooper, 2004). This literature examines the role of factors such as user fees and informal charges in determining patterns of health care use within an equity framework, alongside non-cost factors that are also usually associated with demand for health care. These include: differences in education levels across individuals (and thus in the ability to promote one's own and one's family's health, assimilate health messages and so on); information issues (ability to identify available and better places to seek care); and cultural/social barriers, such as intra-household preferences (for instance, concerning the allocation of resources across family members according to gender).
9 As reported in the appendix to Xu et al. (2007) and defined as out-of-pocket payments for health care of at least 40% of a household's non-subsistence income.

10 Accounting for the income dependence of patterns of use, the authors derive the stochastic distribution of needed health care spending from the estimated actual distribution standardized at the median income level in the sample, using age and gender to predict need. Their Monte Carlo simulations are based on per capita consumption fixed at the median value.

11 For a more detailed explanation of the econometric techniques involved in the estimation of two-part models, see, for example, Cameron and Trivedi (2005).

References

Ataguba, J. (2011) Reassessing catastrophic health care payments with a Nigerian case study, *Health Economics, Policy and Law*, (Epub ahead of print: http://journals. cambridge.org/action/displayAbstract?fromPage=online&aid=8019656, accessed 8 June 2012).

Atkinson, A. (1987) On the measurement of poverty, *Econometrica*, 55(4): 749–64.

Backman, G. et al. (2008) Health systems and the right to health: an assessment of 194 countries, *The Lancet*, 372(9655): 2047–85.

Baeza, C. and Packard, T.G. (2006) *Beyond survival: Protecting households from health shocks in Latin America*. Washington, DC: The World Bank.

Barr, N. (2004) *The Economics of the Welfare State*, 4th edn. Oxford: Oxford University Press.

Cameron, A. and Trivedi, P. (2005) *Microeconometrics: Methods and applications*. New York: Cambridge University Press.

Commission on Macroeconomics and Health (2001) *Macroeconomics and Health: Investing in health for economic development*. Geneva: World Health Organization.

Commonwealth Fund (2011) *Commonwealth Fund International Health Policy Survey*. (http://www.commonwealthfund.org/Surveys/View-All.aspx?topic=International+Health+Policy, accessed 8 June 2012).

Deaton, A. (1997) *The analysis of household surveys: a microeconometric approach to development policy*. Baltimore, MD: Johns Hopkins University Press.

Ensor, T. and Cooper, S. (2004) *Overcoming barriers to health service access and influencing the demand side through purchasing*. HNP Discussion Paper, September. Washington, DC: The World Bank.

Falkingham, J. (2004) Poverty, out-of-pocket payments and access to health care: evidence from Tajikistan, *Social Science and Medicine*, 58(2): 247–58.

Finkelstein, A. and McKnight, R. (2008) What did Medicare do? The initial impact of Medicare on mortality and out of pocket medical spending, *Journal of Public Economics*, 92(7): 1644–68.

Flores, G. et al. (2008) Coping with health care costs: implications for the measurement of catastrophic expenditures and poverty, *Health Economics*, 17(12): 1393–412.

Gerdtham, U-G. and Jönsson, B. (2000) International comparisons of health expenditure, in A. Culyer and J. Newhouse (eds) *Handbook of Health Economics*. New York: Elsevier.

Gotsadze, G. et al. (2005) Health care-seeking behaviour and out-of-pocket payments in Tbilisi, Georgia, *Health Policy and Planning*, 20(4): 232–42.

Grosh, M. and Glewwe, P. (2000) *Designing household survey questionnaires for developing countries: Lessons from 15 years of the living standards measurement study*. Washington, DC: The World Bank.

IHSN (2011) *International Household Survey Network* (http://www.international surveynetwork.org, accessed 8 June 2012).

Kiwanuka, S. et al. (2008) Access to and utilization of health services for the poor in Uganda: a systematic review of available evidence, *Transactions of the Royal Society of Tropical Medicine and Hygiene*, 102(11): 1067–74.

Knight, F.H. (1921) *Risk, uncertainty, and profit.* New York: Houghton-Mifflin.

Kutzin, J. and Jakab, M. (2010) Fiscal context and health expenditure patterns, in J. Kutzin et al. (eds) *Implementing health financing reform: lessons from countries in transition.* Copenhagen: WHO Regional Office for Europe (European Observatory on Health Systems and Policies).

Lu, C. et al. (2009) Limitations of methods for measuring out-of-pocket and catastrophic private health expenditures, *Bulletin of the World Health Organization*, 87(3): 238–44.

McIntyre, D. (2010) WHR 2000 to WHR 2010: what progress in health care financing? *Health Policy and Planning*, 25(5): 349–51.

Millett, C. et al. (2010) Impact of Medicare Part D on seniors' out-of-pocket expenditures on medications, *Archives of Internal Medicine*, 170(15):1325–30.

Mossialos, E. et al. (eds) (2002) *Funding health care: Options for Europe.* Buckingham: Open University Press.

Pradhan, M. and Prescott, N. (2002) Social risk management options for medical care in Indonesia, *Health Economics*, 11(5): 431–46.

Preker, A., Langenbrunner, J. and Jakab, M. (2002) Rich-poor differences in health care financing, in D. Dror and A. Preker (eds) *Social re-insurance – a new approach to sustainable community health care financing.* Washington, DC: The World Bank.

Ravallion, M., Chen, S. and Sangraula, P. (2009) Dollar a day revisited, *World Bank Economic Review*, 23(2): 163–84.

Schoen, C. et al. (2010) How health insurance design affects access to care and costs, by income, in eleven countries, *Health Affairs*, 29(12): 2323–34.

Sepehri, A., Sarma, S. and Simpson, W. (2006) Does non-profit health insurance reduce financial burden? Evidence from the Vietnam living standards survey panel, *Health Economics*, 15(6): 603–16.

Silberstein, A. (1991) *Response performance in the Consumer Expenditure Diary survey.* Washington, DC: Bureau of Labor Statistics.

Üstün, B. et al. (2003) WHO Multi-country Survey Study on Health and Responsiveness 2000–2001, in C.J.L. Murray and D.B. Evans (eds) *Health Systems Performance Assessment: Debates, methods and empiricism.* Geneva: World Health Organization.

van Doorslaer, E. et al. (2006) Effect of payments for health care on poverty estimates in 11 countries in Asia: an analysis of household survey data, *The Lancet*, 368(9544): 1357–64.

van Doorslaer, E. et al. (2007) Catastrophic payments for health care in Asia, *Health Economics*, 16(11): 1159–84.

Võrk, A., Saluse, J. and Habicht, J. (2009) *Income-related inequality in health care financing and utilization in Estonia 2000–2007.* Copenhagen: World Health Organization Regional Office for Europe (Health Financing Technical Report).

Wagstaff, A. (2007) *Health insurance for the poor: initial impacts of Vietnam's health care fund for the poor.* Washington, DC: The World Bank (Policy Research Working Paper, no. 4134).

Wagstaff, A. (2009) Measuring financial protection in health, in P.C. Smith et al. (eds) *Performance measurement for health system improvement: Experiences, challenges and prospects.* Cambridge: Cambridge University Press.

Wagstaff, A. and van Doorslaer, E. (2000a) Equity in health care financing and delivery, in A. Culyer and J. Newhouse (eds) *Handbook of Health Economics.* Amsterdam: Elsevier.

Wagstaff, A. and van Doorslaer, E. (2000b) Measuring and testing for inequity in the delivery of health care, *Journal of Human Resources*, 35(4): 716–33.

Wagstaff, A. and van Doorslaer, E. (2003) Catastrophe and impoverishment in paying for health care: with applications to Vietnam 1993–1998, *Health Economics*, 12(11): 921–34.

WHO (2000) *World Health Report 2000 – Health systems: improving performance.* Geneva: World Health Organization.

WHO (2010a) *The World Health Report 2010. Health systems financing: the path to universal coverage*. Geneva: World Health Organization.

WHO (2010b) *World Health Statistics 2010* (http://www.who.int/whosis/whostat/2010/en/index.html, accessed 8 June 2012).

WHO (2011) *World Health Survey* (http://www.who.int/healthinfo/survey/en/index.html, accessed 8 June 2012).

World Bank (1990) *World Development Report: Poverty*. New York: Oxford University Press.

Xu, K. et al. (2003a) Household catastrophic health expenditure: a multicountry analysis, *The Lancet*, 362(9378): 111–17.

Xu, K., et al. (2003b) Household health system contributions and capacity to pay: definitional, empirical and technical challenges, in C.J.L. Murray and D.B. Evans (eds) *Health Systems Performance Assessment: Debates, methods and empiricism*. Geneva: World Health Organization.

Xu, K. et al. (2007) Protecting households from catastrophic health spending, *Health Affairs (Millwood)*, 26(4): 972–83.

Xu, K. et al. (2009) Assessing the reliability of household expenditure data: results of the World Health Survey, *Health Policy*, 91(3): 297–305.

chapter nine

Understanding Satisfaction, Responsiveness and Experience with the Health System

Reinhard Busse

9.1 Introduction

The World Health Report 2000 (*WHR2000*) on the performance of health systems posited responsiveness to citizens' expectations as a central and particular goal. It pushed forward a debate that framed responsiveness as a valued and desired outcome of health system interventions regardless of the extent to which those interventions lead to health improvement (WHO, 2000). Health services reforms in many countries thus place ever-increasing emphasis on meeting citizens' expectations, improving responsiveness to patients, and increasing both population and patient satisfaction.

This text first explores the basic concepts behind patient and citizen experience, namely *satisfaction, responsiveness, experience* and related terms. The following sections consider the major approaches and actors to measure these, and discuss possible indicators and available data.

9.2 Conceptual and measurement issues

Satisfaction and responsiveness are terms that aim to capture the degree to which health systems, or their components, are successful in responding to the expectations of the general population or a population subgroup of patients.

According to WHO, responsiveness is limited "to the legitimate expectations of the population for their interaction with the health system". This has at least two major implications: (1) Unlike similar measures in the quality-of-life and satisfaction domains, responsiveness requires self-reports to be based on one (or several) actual experience(s) with health services in the respondents' recent past (previous year). Usually these experiences are based on some type of interaction with the health system – with a specific person, a communication campaign or another type of event or action that did not entail direct personal interactions; (2) There can be illegitimate or unjustified expectations too, but the instrument used to measure responsiveness should only capture those that are regarded as legitimate. The "satisfaction of the overall population with the health system", as well as the satisfaction of patients with particular providers, may be influenced by other expectations (which experts or policy-makers may consider illegitimate) and factors outside the direct control of the health care system (such as government in general). Thus, satisfaction is likely to be more dependent on expectations than responsiveness surveys – the lower the expectations, the higher the satisfaction with the actual system and vice versa. WHO initially used a vignette approach in its responsiveness methodology in order to correct for different expectations but this approach was dropped due to the complex data requirements. It is extremely difficult to adjust for variations in expectations between countries and this has not been achieved with any approach to date. As a response, questions in such surveys aim to capture the actual patient experience (e.g. waiting time) rather than a judgement on its appropriateness.

Related – but not identical – to the differences in terminology and concepts is the issue of the persons surveyed. In brief, three approaches can be differentiated: (1) the whole population; (2) persons with any health care encounter and thus experience; and (3) a subgroup of these, e.g. defined by a certain degree of illness or particular diagnosis. Thus, the last group encompasses regular users of the health care system (e.g. those with chronic illness, termed 'sicker adults' in the Commonwealth Fund surveys); the second includes regular as well as irregular users of the health care system; while the first group includes, in addition to these two groups, those persons who do not utilize the system (but still pay for it).

A wide range of methods has been used to attempt to measure responsiveness and/or satisfaction over the last decades, most visibly work by population satisfaction questions in *Eurobarometer* surveys since 1996 (European Commission, 1996, 1998, 1999, 2000, 2002); the Picker Institute's development of patient experience surveys (Coulter & Cleary, 2001; Jenkinson, Coulter & Bruster, 2002); the EUROPEP instrument to assess general practice (Grol et al., 2000; Wensing et al., 2004; Petek et al., 2011); *WHR2000* (WHO, 2000); and work by the Commonwealth Fund (Schoen et al., 2007, 2009, 2010, 2011).

Measurement instruments, available data sources, the selection of indicators and the dimensions they cover are discussed in turn in the following section (including some results to highlight certain issues). More information about the international patient experience surveys, as well as national patient survey programmes, can be found in Garratt et al. (2008).

9.3 Measurement approaches, actors, indicators and data

Population satisfaction in Eurobarometer and other surveys

In principle, the concept of population satisfaction with the whole health system is straightforward. In fact, it is difficult to measure satisfaction, as the answers to all questionnaires depend on the specific wording of the question asked as well as the answer categories provided. The answers depend particularly on factors not yet well understood, i.e. (1) the context in which a survey takes place, e.g. coloured by recent media coverage of scandals, fraud or underprovision of services; (2) no differentiation between the system as a whole and certain subsectors about which the respondent may be more knowledgeable; or (3) the inability to differentiate between the health care system and government in general.

These caveats need to be kept in mind when drawing international comparisons. Comparisons of absolute levels of satisfaction should be treated with caution. Cultural and locally temporal differences in the expression of satisfaction and its dynamics make this a complex tool. Busse et al. (2012) provide a complete overview of different population surveys over the last decades (updated results for the period since 1996 in Table 9.1).

All but one of these surveys share a common focus on the broader health system, but the actual questions – and therefore the range of answers that can be considered positive or negative – differ between surveys. One survey focuses on the local area of the respondents. In the International Health Policy surveys of the Commonwealth Fund, satisfaction with the health care system is only one item, while the others focus on domains of responsiveness and an assessment of actual care in terms of care coordination, quality, medical errors, and so on (see below).

The actual percentages of those answering that they are satisfied are – besides expectations and the assessment of the situation at any given point in time – dependent on: (a) the exact phrasing of the question; and (b) the number of answer categories. Regarding the former, Denmark provides a good example. In 1998, 91% were satisfied "with the way health care runs" (European Commission, 1998), while only 48% were satisfied "with health services" (European Commission, 1999); apparently Danes make a distinct difference between these terms. Regarding the latter, the relatively high 2008 Gallup results (Brown & Khoury, 2009) should be treated with caution, as only two answer categories were possible (positive and negative), while all other surveys presented at least three possibilities. Given such semantic and methodological complexities, the main attention should be devoted to the relative position of countries within the particular surveys.

9.4 Responsiveness to legitimate expectations

In preparation for *WHR2000*, an extensive literature review covered disciplines including sociology, anthropology, ethics, health economics and management, in order to elicit what people value most in their interactions with the health system (De Silva, 2000). This was used to select a common set of seven dimensions (or domains) that characterize the concept of responsiveness. Four were grouped under 'client orientation' and three under 'respect for persons' (dignity, confidentiality and autonomy).

The data presented in *WHR2000* were based on expert opinions but WHO consequently undertook two large population surveys in a number of countries. The *Multi-Country Survey* study in 2000/01 (MCS) (Üstün et al., 2001) and the

Table 9.1 Satisfaction with country's health care system or availability of quality health care in city/area in EU15 countries plus Switzerland and Norway (in %), various surveys 1996–2011; countries sorted according to results of 2008 survey

	Country's health care system												Health care in city or area
	1996 (A)	1998 (B)	1998 (C)	1999 (D)	2002 (E)	2004 (F)	2007 (G)	2008 (H)	2008 (I)	2008 (J)	2010 (K)	2011 (L)	2008 (M)
Luxembourg	71	67	50	72	58					90			90
Belgium	70	63	57	77	65					88			91
Finland	86	81	78	74	73					85			66
Austria	63	73	71	83	67					84			93
France	65	65	59	78	64	65		23	41	83	42	40	83
Sweden	67	58	46	59	48					79	44	40	77
Netherlands	73	70	70	73	46		42		42	77	51	46	89
Denmark	90	91	48	76	52			37		77			86
Spain	36	43	31	38	46	42				73			74
UK	48	57	49	56	31	32	26	17	38	73	62	51	85
Portugal	20	16	6	24	14					58			64
Germany	66	58	43	50	47	28	20	20	21	54	38	32	87
Italy	16	20	15	26	31	21		13		53			57
Greece	18	16	11	19	19					45			52
Ireland	50	58	23	48	20					40			64
Switzerland											46	69	
Norway											40	32	

Note: (A) & (B) "In general, would you say you are very satisfied, fairly satisfied, neither satisfied nor dissatisfied, fairly dissatisfied or very dissatisfied with the way health care runs in (our country)?": *very or fairly satisfied*; (C) "And, on a scale from 1 to 10, how satisfied are you with health services in (our country)?":

answers 7, 8, 9 or 10; (D): "Please tell me whether you are very satisfied, fairly satisfied, not very satisfied or not at all satisfied with each of the following?" *(our country's health care system in general": very or fairly satisfied*; (E), (G), (I), (K) & (L) *"On the whole the system works pretty well, and only minor changes are necessary to make it work better"* (as opposed to *"There are some good things in our health care system, but fundamental changes are needed to make it work better"* and *"Our health care system has so much wrong with it that we need to completely rebuild it."*); (F) *"feel positively about health care system (in my country)"*; (H) "How do you think (country) is doing in regard to health care?": *very well, well or neither well nor badly* (as opposed to *"badly"* and *"very badly"*); (J) *"have confidence in (own) national health care or medical system"* (as opposed to *"no confidence"*); (M) *"satisfied with the availability of quality health care in (own) city or area"* (as opposed to *"dissatisfied"*).

Sources: (A) *Eurobarometer 44.3* (conducted February–April 1996): European Commission, 1996; (B) *Eurobarometer 49* (conducted April–May 1998): European Commission, 1998; (C) *Eurobarometer 50.1* (conducted November–December 1998): European Commission, 1999; (D) *Eurobarometer 52.1* (conducted November–December 1999): European Commission, 2000; (E) *Eurobarometer 57.2* (conducted April–June 2002): European Commission, 2002: (F) The Harris Poll (conducted in June 2004): Taylor, 2004; (G) Commonwealth Fund International Health Policy Survey 2007 (conducted March–May): Schoen et al., 2007; (H) The Harris Poll (conducted in January 2008): Taylor, 2008; (I) Commonwealth Fund International Health Policy Survey 2008 (conducted March–May): Schoen et al., 2009; (J) & (K) Gallup World Poll 2008: Brown & Khoury, 2009; (K) Commonwealth Fund International Health Policy Survey 2010 (conducted March–June): unpublished data; (L) Commonwealth Fund International Health Policy Survey, 2011 (conducted March–June): unpublished data.

World Health Survey (WHS) in 2002 (Üstün et al., 2003) both worked mainly via interviews and partly by postal surveys (in the MCS study). Both WHO surveys include two major categories (inpatient and ambulatory care) for responsiveness, each including a total of eight domains, as 'communication' was added as an eighth dimension (most closely related to the 'respect for persons' group).

The detailed labels of the dimensions, the weighing of each dimension in the *WHR2000*, and the number of questions used in the two surveys are given in Table 9.2, while the exact wording of the questions is presented in Table 9.3. Both WHO instruments focus on what happened during actual contacts rather than eliciting respondents' satisfaction with, or expectations of, the health system in general. Thus, they have much in common with patient experience surveys, such as those developed earlier by the Picker Institute (see below).

Inerviewees in the MCS study were asked to rate their experiences over the past 12 months. While Interviewees in the MCS study were asked to rate their experiences over the past 12 months. While the questions regarding six of the eight domains were relevant for both inpatient and ambulatory care, only inpatients were asked about social support and only outpatients about the quality of basic amenities. All domains included a summary rating question (scaled 1–5, from very good to very bad). In addition, several domains included

Table 9.2 Definition, grouping and weights of responsiveness dimensions in *WHR2000* and number of questions used to measure it in two subsequent population surveys

Dimension	WHR 2000: grouping and weighting	Multi-Country Survey study 2000–01	World Health Survey 2002
Client-orientation			
Choice of health care provider	5%	3 questions	1 question
Prompt attention: Convenient travel and short waiting times	20%	2 questions	2 questions
Quality of basic amenities: Surroundings	15%	3 questions	2 questions
Access to family and community support: Contact with outside world and maintenance of regular activities	10%	3 questions	2 questions
Respect for persons			
Dignity: Respectful treatment and communication	16.7%	4 questions	2 questions
Confidentiality of personal information	16.7%	2 questions	2 questions
Autonomy: Involvement in decisions	16.7%	3 questions	2 questions
Clarity of **communication**	Not included	4 questions	2 questions

Source: Author's own compilation based on: WHO, 2000; Valentine et al., 2003.

Table 9.3 WHO dimensions of responsiveness and questions used to measure it in two population surveys

Dimension	MCS study 2000/2001: questions used	WHS 2002: questions used
Choice	How big a problem, if any, was it to get a health care provider you were happy with? How big a problem, if any, was it to get to use other health services other than the one you usually went to? How would you rate your experience of being able to use a health care provider or service of your choice?	How would you rate the freedom you had to choose the health care providers that attended to you?
Prompt attention	How often did you get care as soon as you wanted? How would you rate your experience of getting prompt attention at the health services?	How would you rate: – the travelling time? – the amount of time you waited before being attended to?
Quality of basic amenities	How would you rate the basic quality of the waiting room, for example, space, seating and fresh air? How would you rate the cleanliness of the place? How would you rate the quality of the surroundings, for example, space, seating, fresh air and cleanliness of the health services?	How would you rate: – the cleanliness of the rooms inside the facility, including toilets? – the amount of space you had?
Access to family and community support	How big a problem, if any, was it to get the hospital to allow your family and friends to take care of your personal needs, such as bringing in your favourite food, soap etc.? How big a problem, if any, was it to have the hospital allow you to practise religious or traditional observances if you wanted to? How would you rate your experience of how the hospital allowed you to interact with family, friends and to continue your social and/or religious customs?	How would you rate: – the ease of having family and friends visit you? – your [child's] experience of staying in contact with the outside world when you [your child] were in hospital?
Dignity	How often did doctors, nurses or other health care providers treat you with respect? How often did the office staff, such as receptionists or clerks there, treat you with respect? How often were your physical examinations and treatments done in such a way that your privacy was respected? How would you rate your experience of being treated with dignity?	How would you rate: – your experience of being greeted and talked to respectfully? – the way your privacy was respected during physical examinations and treatments?

(Continued)

Table 9.3 WHO dimensions of responsiveness and questions used to measure it in two population surveys (*Continued*)

Dimension	MCS study 2000/2001: questions used	WHS 2002: questions used
Confidentiality	How often were talks with your doctor, nurse or other health care provider done privately so other people, who you did not want to hear, could not overhear what was said? How often did your doctor, nurse or other health care provider keep your personal information confidential? This means that anyone whom you did not want to be informed could not find out about your medical conditions.	How would you rate: – the way the health services ensured you could talk privately to health care providers? – the way your personal information was kept confidential?
Autonomy	How often did doctors, nurses or other health care providers involve you in deciding about the care, treatment or tests? How often did doctors, nurses or other health care providers ask your permission before starting the treatment or tests?. Rate your experience of getting involved in making decisions about your care or treatment.	How would you rate: – your experience of being involved in making decisions about your health care or treatment? – your experience of getting information about other types of treatments or tests?
Communication	How often did doctors, nurses or other health care providers listen carefully to you? How often did doctors, nurses or other health care providers explain things in a way you could understand? How often did doctors, nurses or other health care providers give you time to ask questions about your health problem or treatment? Rate your experience of how well health care providers communicated with you in the last 12 months.	How would you rate: – the experience of how clearly health care providers explained things to you? – your experience of getting enough time to ask questions about your health problem or treatment?

Source: Author's own compilation based on: WHO, 2000; Valentine et al., 2003.

report questions on how often a particular experience had occurred during encounters with the health system (scaled 1–4, from always to never).

The WHS 2002 collected data on responsiveness, among other aspects related to health systems performance. Data were collected from 69 countries globally, including 29 in the WHO European Region. Respondents were asked to rate their last encounter with the (ambulatory or inpatient) health care system on a five-point scale across eight domains. In addition, the survey contained vignettes depicting a variety of situations that may arise in people's interactions with the health care system. Respondents were asked to rate these hypothetical experiences on a five-point scale ranging from very bad to very good. Five vignettes were used for choice and ten vignettes for every other domain. These have recently been analysed to examine how they can be used to adjust for threshold effects across countries and enhance comparability in this area (Rice, Robone & Smith, 2012). Available data on both responsiveness and expectations are given in Busse et al. (2012).

Expectations and responsiveness

Austria showed both the lowest (overall) expectation scores and the highest responsiveness score. The country with the lowest responsiveness score (Ukraine) had comparatively high expectation scores. This led to the hypothesis that people with different expectations rate similar experiences differently. For example, those with low expectations may rate their last experience as good while those with higher expectations may rate an experience with similar characteristics and quality as only moderate. As shown in Busse et al. (2012), the responsiveness score (not adjusted for expectations) decreases as the population expectations increase for both ambulatory and inpatient care. Also, the t-test for equality of means reveals that the average responsiveness scores for countries with high expectations are significantly different from those for countries with low expectations. Some intercountry variations in responsiveness may thus be explained by differences in population expectations. This indicates that expectations-based adjustment to the scores may be necessary before meaningful intercountry comparisons can be made. This was especially the case for 'choice', 'prompt attention' and 'communication'.

Especially for 'choice', this was further underscored in a survey conducted by the Picker Institute around the same time (Coulter & Jenkinson, 2005). Respondents in eight countries – drawn from the general population, with patient experience-related questions limited to those with health care encounters – were interviewed about the choice of provider, their involvement in treatment decisions (autonomy), and communication with their physician (Table 9.4).

Table 9.5 shows that Swedes expected very little choice of specialist (only 31%), while almost all Germans expected such a choice (97%). Spaniards ranged in between but were the most satisfied regarding their actual opportunities to make choices (even though they were not satisfied that they were provided with sufficient information to enable them to do so); both Swedes and Germans were only moderately satisfied in this regard. Polish respondents' expectations were as high as those of the Germans, but were met to a much smaller extent.

Table 9.4 Questions used in Picker responsiveness survey, sorted according to WHO responsiveness domains and whether they address expectations or patient experience

	Expectations and values (whole population)	Patient experience
Choice	In general, if you need to [consult a primary care doctor/consult a specialist doctor/go to hospital] do you think that you should have a free choice?	
	Do you feel you have sufficient information about [primary care doctors/specialist doctors/hospitals] to choose the best one?	
	Overall, how would you rate the opportunities for patients in this country to make choices about their health care?	
Autonomy	In general, when you need medical treatment and more than one treatment is available, who do you think should make the decision about which treatment is best for you?	How often did the doctor involve you as much as you wanted to be in deciding about your care, treatment or tests?
Communication		How often did the doctor: – listen to you carefully? – give you time to ask questions? – explain things in a way you could understand? Overall how would you rate how well health care providers communicated with you?

Source: Author's own compilation based on: Coulter & Jenkinson, 2005.

Table 9.5 Expectations for and rating of choice of different types of providers in eight European countries, 2002; countries sorted from left to right by responsiveness rating

	Spain	Switzerland	Germany	Italy	Sweden	Slovenia	UK	Poland
Expectation: In general, if you need to [consult a primary care doctor/consult a specialist doctor/go to hospital] do you think you should have a free choice? (answering yes)								
Primary care doctor	89%	93%	98%	86%	86%	98%	87%	98%
Specialist	86%	84%	97%	83%	31%	87%	79%	95%
Hospital	78%	85%	94%	85%	54%	86%	80%	94%
Information to support choice of provider: Do you feel you have sufficient information about [primary care doctors/specialist doctors/hospitals] to choose the best one for you? (answering yes)								
Primary care doctor	30%	52%	52%	53%	31%	45%	40%	43%
Specialist	23%	41%	42%	53%	23%	25%	28%	32%
Hospital	32%	52%	42%	54%	36%	30%	35%	35%
Rating: Overall, how would you rate the opportunities for patients in this country to make choices about their health care? Average of answer categories 1–5 (very bad, bad, moderate, good, very good)								
	3.93	3.86	3.35	3.28	3.19	3.05	3.05	2.67

Source: Busse et al., 2012, based on: Coulter & Jenkinson, 2005.

Expectations regarding autonomy also differed considerably, e.g. Spaniards expected significantly less patient autonomy than Germans.

Health care expenditure and responsiveness

Keeping all other factors constant, well-resourced health system environments should be able to afford better quality care and receive better responsiveness ratings. A simple correlation for each responsiveness domain result (keeping development contexts constant by looking at correlations within World Bank country-income groups) was used to analyse whether higher health expenditures are associated with higher responsiveness (Valentine et al., 2009). In general, the results show a positive association across many of the domains for most country-income groupings. Especially for high-income countries, there are clear correlations between total health care expenditure and levels of responsiveness. If public expenditure alone is taken into account, there are correlations for even more domains. This suggests a more direct impact on levels of responsiveness – in other words, that private expenditure does not (or only marginally) contributes to higher levels of responsiveness. However, increasing levels of health expenditures are no guarantee that responsiveness will improve automatically. Conversely, lower responsiveness is associated with lower coverage and greater inequity in access.

9.5 Patient experience surveys

As mentioned previously, patient surveys of their experience of treatment by particular providers constitute a third pillar of data. Usually, these relate more to responsiveness than to satisfaction as they are based on: (1) predetermined domains; and (2) patients' actual health service encounters. Surveys are mainly available within countries but also sometimes across countries, especially for inpatient care (see below), general practitioners (see below), and mental health care (comparative study across five countries with a total of 404 patients: Becker et al., 2000); as well as for specific groups of patients, for example, those with diabetes (comparative survey across 13 countries with a total of 5104 patients: Peyrot et al., 2006) or cancer (comparative survey across six countries with a total of 762 patients: Brédart et al., 2007).

Inpatient care

While patient experience surveys among inpatients have become regular features in many countries of the European Region (e.g. in Denmark, Ireland, the Netherlands, Norway and the United Kingdom), they are seldom comparable across countries. The Picker Institute questionnaire is an exception (Coulter & Cleary, 2001; Jenkinson, Coulter & Bruster, 2002), but unfortunately this was only published once and was limited to a small number of countries. The survey asks inpatients to describe a range of aspects of their care upon discharge. It distinguished seven dimensions of patient-centred care, which largely overlap with the areas of responsiveness, but drawing different boundaries between them:

1. Physical comfort – including pain management; help with activities of daily living; surroundings and hospital environment.
2. Coordination and integration of care – including clinical care; ancillary and support services; front-line care.
3. Involvement of family and friends – including social and emotional support; involvement in decision-making; support for caregiving; impact on family dynamics and functioning.
4. Respect for patients' values, preferences and expressed needs – including impact of illness and treatment on quality of life; involvement in decision-making; dignity; needs; and autonomy.
5. Information, communication and education – including clinical status; progress and prognosis; processes of care; facilitation of autonomy; self-care; and health promotion.
6. Emotional support and alleviation of fear and anxiety – including clinical status; treatment and prognosis; impact of illness on self and family; financial impact of illness.
7. Transition and continuity – including information about medication and danger signals to look out for after leaving hospital; coordination and discharge planning; clinical, social, physical and financial support.

Available results across four European countries are summarized in Table 9.6.

Table 9.6 Patients reporting problems with hospital, 1998–2000 (%); available countries sorted by overall evaluation from left to right, dimension sorted by average percentage from low to high

	Switzerland	Germany	Sweden	UK
Overall level of care NOT GOOD	4	7	7	9
Problems with:				
– physical comfort	3	7	4	8
– coordination of care	13	17	NA	22
– involvement of family and friends	12	17	15	28
– respect for patients' preferences	16	18	21	31
– information and education	17	20	23	29
– emotional support	15	22	26	27
– continuity and transition	30	41	40	45
Would not recommend this hospital to friends/family	4	5	3	8

Source: Figueras et al., 2004, based on data from: Coulter & Cleary, 2001.

9.6 Care by general practitioners

The measurement of patient experience with general practitioners has developed separately from other areas. The most developed instrument in this area is the EUROPEP one, produced by the European Task Force on Patient Evaluations of General Practice Care (Grol et al., 2000). This contains 23 questions, which cover issues relating to five of the eight responsiveness domains (prompt attention, dignity, confidentiality, autonomy and communication), as well as certain issues regarding processes during the physician–patient encounter, e.g. thoroughness, and patient-reported outcomes ("helping you to feel well so that you can perform your normal daily activities"). For a full list of the items see Table 9.8.

This survey was first applied in 17 countries in 1998 (Wensing et al., 2004; Table 9.7); detailed data on the 23 items were published for 10 countries only, involving more than 17 000 patients (Grol et al., 2000). The data on outpatient care responsiveness from the WHS in 2002 (Üstün et al., 2003; Busse et al. 2012; Table 9.7) are partly contradictory however; for example, Slovenia rated comparatively high in EUROPEP, but low in the WHS, while the opposite can be observed for Denmark. This may be due to the sampling strategy, i.e. the EUROPEP was only used by patients in a limited number of practices (around 36 per country), or due to the more specific questions asked. Kerssens et al. (2004) used yet another instrument to measure responsiveness in ambulatory care in 12 countries (Table 9.7; average results per country are not available).

The EUROPEP survey was repeated in 2009, this time in eight countries. In contrast to 1998, the surveyed patients either had a high risk for cardiovascular disease or established coronary disease, i.e. were not selected irrespective of health status as in 1998. Table 9.8 presents the data for all 23 items for those six countries for which results were reported for both 1998 and 2009. As can be

Table 9.7 Evaluations of general practice care in four different surveys; countries sorted from top to bottom by rating in 2009

Instrument	1998 EUROPEP (% positive answers across 23 items)	2002 World Health Survey (score)	Not reported (early 2000s) Quote (quality of care through patients' eyes)	2009 EUROPEP (% positive answers across 23 items)
Surveyed population	25 052 patients in 17 countries; selected in GP practices irrespective of health status; avg. age ca. 50, 2/3 women	General population with GP encounter	5133 patients in 12 countries; different selection in each country*; age and sex not reported	7472 patients in 8 countries; selected in GP practices either due to high risk for cardiovascular disease or established coronary disease; avg. age ca. 67, 1/3 women
Switzerland	91.4#	–	–	93.0#
Belgium	87.2#	90.2	–	92.0#
France	63.9	85.6	–	88.4
Slovenia	88.4#	77.8	–	87.9#
Austria	89.7	90.6	–	87.5
Germany	88.2#	83.9	–	84.7#
Spain	84.6	79.2	–	–
Netherlands	79.9#	84.3	X	83.5#
Israel	79.4	81.8	X	–
Sweden	78.5	77.6	–	–
Portugal	78.3	73.2	X	–
Norway	76.5	76.9	X	–

Denmark	73.3	85.9	X	–
UK	72.8#	82.5	–	82.1#
Finland	70.1	81.7	X	–
Other European countries	Iceland, Turkey	Luxembourg, Greece, Ireland, Czech Rep., Georgia, Bosnia and Herzegovina, Hungary, Slovakia, Estonia, Italy, Latvia, Kazakhstan, Croatia, Russian Federation, Ukraine	Belarus, Greece, Ireland, Italy, Ukraine	–

Notes: * X = included, – = not included; # detailed breakdown of results by question (see Table 9.8).

Source: Author's own compilation based on: Üstün et al., 2003; Wensing et al., 2004; Kerssens et al., 2004; Petek et al., 2011.

Table 9.8 Evaluation of general practice care in six European countries with data for 1998 and 2009 (% with positive rating); countries sorted from left to right by overall evaluation in 2009, items from top to bottom by average across countries in 2009

	Switzerland		Belgium		Slovenia		Germany		Netherlands		UK		Max difference	
	1998	2009	1998	2009	1998	2009	1998	2009	1998	2009	1998	2009	1998	2009
Overall evaluation	91	93	87	92	89	88	88	85	80	84	72	82	19	11
1. Keeping records and data confidential	96	97	97	95	97	97	94	91	95	92	91	95	6	6
2. Providing quick services for urgent health problems	96	98	93	96	89	90	95	93	85	88	71	84	25	14
3. Listening to you	96	95	93	95	95	94	92	88	89	89	83	90	13	7
4. Helpfulness of the staff (other than the doctor)	93	95	83	90	89	92	92	93	84	86	70	84	23	11
5. Thoroughness	90	94	89	95	92	92	91	85	81	87	78	88	14	10
6. Explaining the purpose of tests and treatments	92	94	89	94	89	90	89	86	83	87	79	86	13	8
7. Making you feel you had time during consultations	96	95	92	95	92	88	90	86	88	88	80	89	16	9
8. Making it easy for you to tell him/her about your problems	94	94	88	93	87	85	89	87	83	85	81	89	13	9
9. Telling you what you wanted to know about symptoms/illness	93	96	90	93	92	89	90	85	83	88	79	83	14	13
10. Physical examination	93	94	88	94	90	91	91	82	82	87	76	85	17	12
11. Getting an appointment to suit you	97	97	88	91	85	90	93	90	78	84	62	76	35	21
12. Helping you to feel well so that you can perform your normal daily activities	91	94	89	94	93	90	88	83	79	85	69	85	24	11
13. Interest in your personal situation	95	95	90	94	79	77	90	88	82	83	78	86	17	18

14. Helping you to understand the importance of his/her advice	89	92	86	93	91	90	86	84	80	83	76	82	15	10
15. Involving you in decisions about medical care	91	93	87	94	89	84	87	83	81	85	76	83	15	11
16. Offering you services for preventing disease	84	90	77	87	85	87	85	83	76	88	74	87	11	7
17. Quick relief of your symptoms	85	89	84	92	94	93	83	75	75	84	67	87	27	18
18. Getting through to the practice on the telephone	96	95	93	96	92	83	95	95	71	73	62	86	34	23
19. Knowing what he/she has done or told you during previous contacts	89	91	84	91	90	89	85	78	76	82	72	86	18	13
20. Preparing you for what to expect from specialists or hospital care	89	90	85	88	88	86	85	80	75	79	72	83	17	11
21. Help in dealing with emotional problems related to health status	90	91	85	90	87	83	85	80	76	78	71	83	19	13
22. Being able to speak to the GP on the telephone	91	88	90	94	93	88	87	84	72	71	51	83	40	23
23. Waiting time in the waiting room	79	83	66	73	60	75	70	67	61	72	50	72	29	16

Source: Author's own compilation based on data from: Grol et al., 2000 and Petek et al., 2011.

seen from the table, the average rating improved in four of the six countries over that period, especially the United Kingdom and, in general, differences across countries decreased. Regarding individual items, 'providing quick services for urgent health problems', 'offering you services for preventing disease', 'getting through to the practice on the phone', 'waiting time in the waiting room' and 'getting an appointment to suit you' improved most across countries. Whether this is an effect of improved responsiveness over time or whether it is largely due to the different patient populations is unclear.

9.7 International Health Policy Survey

The Commonwealth Fund, a New York-based foundation has been conducting international surveys for a number of years, originally limited to five English-speaking countries (among them only one European country, namely the United Kingdom). Since the inclusion of six more European countries over the years (France, Germany, the Netherlands, Norway, Sweden and Switzerland), it has included eleven countries since 2010, among them seven from Europe. There are three distinct surveys, two of them population surveys (and the other focused on physicians), which are used in turn every three years. The general adult population was last surveyed in 2007 and 2010 (next survey planned for 2013), while 'sicker adults' were surveyed in 2008 and 2011, with 'sicker' operationalized as follows: 'fair or poor health'; 'had surgery or been hospitalized in past two years'; or 'received care for serious or chronic illness, injury, or disability in past year'.

Both types of population surveys by the Commonwealth Fund contain a question on satisfaction with the health care system (see above). The others focus on domains of responsiveness (especially access and communication) and an assessment of actual care in terms of care coordination, quality, medical errors and so on. Table 9.9 presents a selection of questions and results from the 2010 and 2011 surveys.

Comparative methodology

All the satisfaction, responsiveness and experience surveys mentioned so far are based on surveys among health system users and/or the general population rather than (for example) expert opinion or facility audits. This differentiates them from approaches based on an expert assessment of published data and health system characteristics. The most high profile of these approaches is the annual *Euro Health Consumer Index* produced by the Health Consumer Powerhouse.

Table 9.10 demonstrates that the questions on the population's satisfaction with the health system in general (or the need to reform it) are in a separate category in the *Eurobarometer*, Commonwealth Fund and Gallup surveys and do not overlap directly with any of the WHO responsiveness domains. The more recent *Euro Health Consumer Index* (which was published annually between 2006 and 2009) only partially overlaps with the WHO responsiveness domains; its overlap with the 'respect for persons' domains is especially weak as only

Table 9.9 Example questions and results from the Commonwealth Fund's International Health Policy Surveys, 2010 (adults with health care encounter) and 2011 ('sicker adults')

	France	Germany	Netherlands	Norway	Sweden	Switzerland	UK
Did not fill a prescription for medicine or skipped doses – Answer 'no'							
2010	88	93	90	93	88	90	95
2011	89	86	92	92	93	91	95
Had a specific medical problem but did not visit a doctor – Answer 'no'							
2010	90	82	91	94	91	89	95
2011	90	88	93	92	94	88	93
Skipped or did not get a medical test, treatment, or follow-up that was recommended by a doctor – Answer 'no'							
2010	90	89	89	93	92	89	94
2011	91	86	92	92	96	89	96
If seriously ill, confident to receive the most effective treatment, including drugs and diagnostic tests – Answers 'very confident' or 'confident'							
2010	85	82	88	81	67	89	92
If seriously ill, confident to be able to afford needed care – Answers 'very confident' or 'confident'							
2010	73	70	81	69	70	78	90
Overall, how do you rate the quality of medical care that you have received in the past 12 months? – Answers 'excellent' or 'very good'							
2011	43	31	34	50	50	68	81

Source: Author's own compilation, based on: Schoen et al., 2010 and 2011.

aspects of autonomy are covered (for details of its subcategories, weighing and data sources, see Busse et al., 2012). The table also demonstrates that the EUROPEP instrument on patient experience in general practice, as well as the Commonwealth Fund's survey, expand beyond responsiveness into asking patients about: medical processes during the physician–patient encounter; quality and medical errors; and patient-reported outcomes – i.e. a patient questionnaire can be used for different dimensions of performance assessment.

Table 9.10 also includes information on the data sources, i.e. whether the results are based on a survey (general population; patients (recruited at random or within specific providers); or 'sicker' patients), routine data or expert judgement.

Methodological considerations

The questions of how satisfied patients are with their health care system; whether they have choice and access to providers; and whether they had a good (or bad) experience with the care from the provider, are important dimensions when assessing a health system's performance. However, the terminology in this area is not yet consistent, and different terms for similar concepts have

Table 9.10 Important questionnaires/studies/surveys/rankings with questions on patients' and citizens' experience; sorted by date of first use

	Eurobaro-meter^a	Picker inpatient survey^b	EUROPEP GP practice evaluation^c	WHR 2000^d	MCS study, WHS^e	Euro Health Consumer Index^f	Common-wealth Funds^g	Gallup Poll^h
Data sources used*	A	B	B	C, D	E	C, D	E, F	A
Satisfaction								
– with country's health system	X						X	X
– with local availability of health care								X
Client orientation								
Choice of care provider				X	X	X	X	
Access/travel/waiting			X	X	X	X	X	
Basic amenities				X	X			
Access to social support networks		X		X	X			
Respect for persons								
Respect for dignity		X	X	X	X			
Respect for confidentiality		X	X	X	X			
Respect for autonomy		X	X	X	X	X	X	
Communication		X	X		X		X	

Other issues related to responsiveness

Patients' rights and information		X	X
Range of benefit basket		X	X
Access to pharmaceuticals		X (system level)	X (patient level)
Care coordination			X

Processes and patient-reported outcomes

Processes	X		
Errors and quality		X	
Patient-reported outcomes	X		

Notes: *A: randomly selected population; B: patients recruited within specific providers; C: routine data; D: experts; E: randomly selected adult population with health care encounter; F: randomly selected 'sicker' adults with health care encounter.

Source: Modified and expanded from Busse et al., 2012, based on: [a]European Commission, 1996, 1998, 1999, 2000, 2002; [b]Jenkinson, Coulter & Bruster, 2002; [c]Grol et al., 2000; [d]WHO, 2000; [e]Üstün et al., 2001, 2003; [f]Health Consumer Powerhouse, 2006, 2007, 2008, 2009; [g]Schoen et al., 2007, 2009, 2010, 2011; [h]Brown & Khoury, 2009.

contributed to confusion and have hindered the establishment of the area as a firm indicator of health systems' performance.

Often, the interpretation of differences in data is complicated by: different definitions of domains and indicators; differences in the methodology of surveyed populations (general population, patients with any health care encounter, or sicker patients) and data collection (e.g. sampling); and the calculation of average scores. In addition, sample sizes are often too small to produce any valid values for the population in question. Only careful consideration of both the dimensions included and the population surveyed will enable potential gaps to be identified, for example, while it is necessary to base a rating of most dimensions of responsiveness on actual patient encounters, such a methodology will not identify those persons who could not access the system due to its poor responsiveness.

The results of these assessments are therefore often inconsistent or contradictory and difficult to interpret. As Garratt et al. (2008) note:

"the difficulties in making such international comparisons are well documented and consideration must be given to methods of questionnaire translation, consistency in survey design and sampling processes, and differences in patient characteristics (Coulter & Cleary, 2001). For valid comparisons to be made across countries, questionnaires must demonstrate cross-cultural equivalence, that is similar levels of data quality, reliability and validity. In the absence of such equivalence, it is difficult to ascertain whether any differences found between countries is related to real differences in health care quality or differences in questionnaire performance.

The forward–backwards translation methodology is designed to promote cross-cultural equivalence (Leplege & Verdier, 1995). However, there is variation in the reporting of the results of such translation procedures, the focus often being on the results of cross-national comparisons rather than underpinning methodology. The sampling and recruitment of patients and survey administration including use of reminders and incentives, must also be consistent across countries so as to ensure representative samples. Comparisons must also control for potential confounders (Coulter & Cleary, 2001). The results of a systematic review found that a number of patient characteristics were consistently associated with patient satisfaction, including age, education and health status (Crow et al., 2002). Hence it is important that these variables are controlled for when reporting the results of cross-national comparisons."

As a result, it is often possible to "demonstrate" that a particular health system is "better" or "worse" than another one. If confronted with data of international comparative surveys, the recipient is well advised to carefully check the basic underlying definitions, assumptions, database and results, before accepting any conclusions based on the latter.

9.8 Conclusions and priorities for development

Overall, no individual survey currently enables any clear conclusions to be drawn about the differences in the degree of satisfaction, responsiveness and patient experience across health systems and even less about the health system strategies that may explain them. All currently existing surveys contain different items, leading to different results. In some instances, such differences have large impacts on potential rankings. All methodologies are therefore rightly subject to further extensive critical debate. As there is currently no consistent source providing population and/or patient-derived measures of responsiveness and/or satisfaction, it will be necessary to establish such a source. Considering experience and regularity of surveys, the Commonwealth Fund's surveys are best suited to form the basis for such a development.

References

Becker, T. et al. (2000) Aims, outcome measures, study sites and patient sample. EPSILON Study 1. European Psychiatric Services: Inputs linked to outcome domains and needs, *British Journal of Psychiatry*, 39(Suppl): s1–7.

Brédart, A. et al. (2007) Determinants of patient satisfaction in oncology settings from European and Asian countries: preliminary results based on the EORTC IN-PATSAT32 questionnaire, *European Journal of Cancer*, 43(2): 323–30.

Brown, I.T. and Khoury, C. (2009) *In OECD countries, universal healthcare gets high marks* (http://www.gallup.com/poll/122393/oecd-countries-universal-healthcare-gets-high-marks.aspx, accessed 8 June 2012).

Busse, R. et al. (2012) Being responsive to citizens' expectations: the role of health services in responsiveness and satisfaction, in M. McKee and J. Figueras (eds) *Health Systems: Health, wealth and societal well-being*. Maidenhead: Open University Press/McGraw-Hill.

Coulter, A. and Cleary, P.D. (2001) Patients' experiences with hospital care in five countries, *Health Affairs (Millwood)*, 20(3): 244–52.

Coulter, A. and Jenkinson, C. (2005) European patients' views on the responsiveness of health systems and healthcare providers, *European Journal of Public Health*, 15(4): 355–60.

Crow, R. et al. (2002) The measurement of satisfaction with healthcare: implications for practice from a systematic review of the literature, *Health Technology Assessment*, 6(32): 1–244.

De Silva, A. (2000) *A framework for measuring responsiveness*. Geneva: World Health Organization (GPE Discussion Paper 32) (http://www.who.int/responsiveness/papers/paper32.pdf, accessed 8 June 2012).

European Commission (1996) Eurobarometer, 44.3. Brussels: European Commission.

European Commission (1998) Eurobarometer, 49. Brussels: European Commission.

European Commission (1999) Eurobarometer, 50.1. Brussels: European Commission.

European Commission (2000) Eurobarometer, 52.1. Brussels: European Commission.

European Commission (2002) Eurobarometer, 57.2. Brussels: European Commission.

Figueras, J. et al. (2004) Patterns and performance in social insurance systems, in R.B. Saltman, R. Busse and J. Figueras (eds) *Social Health Insurance Systems in Western Europe*. Buckingham: Open University Press.

Garratt, A.M., Solheim, E. and Danielsen, K. (2008) *National and cross-national surveys of patient experiences: a structured review*. Rapport nr 7-2008. Oslo: Nasjonalt kunnskapssenter for helsejenesten.

Grol, R. et al. (2000) Patients in Europe evaluate general practice care: an international comparison, *British Journal of General Practice*, 50(460): 882–7.

HCP (2006) *Euro Health Consumer Index 2006*. Brussels: Health Consumer Powerhouse (http://www.healthpowerhouse.com/media/RaportEHCI2006en.pdf, accessed 8 June 2012).

HCP (2007) *Euro Health Consumer Index 2007*. Brussels: Health Consumer Powerhouse (http://www.healthpowerhouse.com/media/Rapport_EHCI_2007.pdf, accessed 8 June 2012).

HCP (2008) *Euro Health Consumer Index 2008*. Brussels: Health Consumer Powerhouse (http://www.healthpowerhouse.com/files/2008-EHCI/EHCI-2008-report.pdf, accessed 8 June 2012).

HCP (2009) *Euro Health Consumer Index 2009*. Brussels: Health Consumer Powerhouse (http://www.healthpowerhouse.com/files/Report%20EHCI%202009%20091005%20final%20with%20cover.pdf, accessed 8 June 2012).

Jenkinson, C., Coulter, A. and Bruster, S. (2002) The Picker Patient Experience Questionnaire: development and validation using data from in-patient surveys in five countries, *International Journal for Quality in Health Care*, 14(5): 353–8.

Kerssens, J.J. et al. (2004) Comparison of patient evaluations of health care quality in relation to WHO measures of achievement in 12 European countries, *Bulletin of the World Health Organization*, 82(2) (http://www.scielosp.org/scielo.php?pid=S0042-96862004000200007&script=sci_arttext, accessed 17 October 2012).

Leplege, A. and Verdier, A. (1995) The adaptation of health status measures: methodological aspects of the translation procedure, in S. Schumaker and B. Berzon (eds) *International Assessment of Quality of Life: Theory, translation, measurement and analysis*. Oxford: Rapid Communications.

Petek, D. et al. (2011) Patients' evaluation of European general practice – revisited after 11 years, *International Journal for Quality in Health Care*, 23(6): 621–8.

Peyrot, M. et al. (2006) Patient and provider perceptions of care for diabetes: results of the cross-national DAWN Study, *Diabetologia*, 49(2): 279–88.

Rice, N., Robone, S. and Smith, P. (2012) Vignettes and health systems responsiveness in cross-country comparative analyses, *Journal of the Royal Statistical Society*, 175(2): 1–21.

Schoen, C. et al. (2007) Toward higher-performance health systems: adults' health care experiences in seven countries, 2007, *Health Affairs (Millwood)*, 26(6): w717–734.

Schoen, C. et al. (2009) In chronic condition: experiences of patients with complex health care needs, in eight countries, 2008, *Health Affairs (Millwood)*, 28(1): w1–16.

Schoen, C. et al. (2010) How health insurance design affects access to care and costs, by income, in eleven countries, *Health Affairs (Millwood)*, 29(12): 2323–34.

Schoen, C. et al. (2011) New 2011 survey of patients with complex care needs in eleven countries finds that care is often poorly coordinated, *Health Affairs (Millwood)*, 30(12): 2437–48.

Taylor, H. (2008) Majorities in United States and three of five largest European countries believe healthcare is doing badly in their countries, *Healthcare News*, 8(3) (http://www.harrisinteractive.com/vault/HI_HealthCareNews2008Vol8_Iss03.pdf, accessed 26 September 2012).

Üstün, T.B. et al. (2001) *WHO Multi-country Survey Study on Health and Responsiveness 2000–2001*. Geneva: World Health Organization (GPE Discussion Paper 37). (http://www.who.int/responsiveness/papers/gpediscpaper37.pdf, accessed 8 June 2012).

Üstün, T.B. et al. (2003) The World Health Surveys, in C.J.L. Murray and D.B. Evans (eds) *Health Systems Performance Assessment: Debates, methods and empiricism*. Geneva: World Health Organization.

Valentine, N.B. et al. (2003) Health system responsiveness: concepts, domains and operationalization, in C.J.L. Murray and D.B. Evans (eds) *Health Systems Performance Assessment: Debates, methods and empiricism.* Geneva: World Health Organization.

Valentine, N.B. et al. (2009) Health systems responsiveness: a measure of the acceptability of health care processes and systems from the user's perspective, in P.C. Smith et al. (eds) *Performance measurement for health system improvement: Experiences, challenges and prospects.* Cambridge: Cambridge University Press.

Wensing, M. et al (2004) Impact of national health care systems on patient evaluations of general practice in Europe, *Health Policy*, 68(3): 353–7.

WHO (2000) *The World Health Report 2000 – Health systems: improving performance.* Geneva: World Health Organization.

chapter ten

Comparative Measures of Health System Efficiency

Jonathan Cylus and Peter C. Smith

10.1 Introduction

The concept of health system efficiency is beguilingly simple, represented at its most simple as a ratio of some measure of valued health system outputs to the associated inputs. Efficiency indicators serve as a summary measure of the extent to which the inputs to the health system, in the form of expenditures and other resources, are used to secure the goals of the health system. Few would argue that pursuit of such measurement is not important. Inefficient use of health system resources imposes a cost to society, perhaps in the form of a loss of potential health gain, or of a loss of consumption opportunities somewhere else in the economy. The main reasons for an interest in efficiency therefore relate to accountability: to reassure payers that their money is being spent wisely, and to reassure patients, caregivers and the general population that their claims on the health system are being treated fairly and consistently. Comparative efficiency indicators can help decision-makers pinpoint which parts of the health system are not performing as well as they should be, based on the experiences of other health systems.

The interest in efficiency has been heightened by the apparently inexorable growth in health system expenditure in most countries, and the widespread belief that major improvements in efficiency can be made (Aaron, 2008; Bentley et al., 2008; OECD, 2010b). However, although it is one of the most fundamental health system performance metrics for researchers and policy-makers (WHO, 2000), the concept of health system efficiency is in practice heavily contested and its accurate measurement across countries difficult to realize (Reinhardt, Hussey & Anderson, 2002). It has proved challenging to develop robust measures of comparative efficiency that are feasible to collect or estimate, that offer consistent insight into comparative health system performance and that can be usable in guiding policy reforms (Hussey et al., 2009). This chapter first discusses the concept of efficiency. It then discusses some of the various approaches to measurement that currently exist. The chapter summarizes the issues and debates that have arisen, and concludes with the research priorities.

10.2 Transforming inputs into outcomes

The intention in any analysis of comparative efficiency is to offer insight into the success with which health system resources are transformed into outputs, or (more ambitiously) into valued outcomes. Economists conceive this transformation as a 'production function', which for a given set of inputs indicates the maximum level of output or outcome. Any failure to attain that maximum is an indication of inefficiency (Jacobs et al., 2006). The concept of a production function can be applied to the functioning of very detailed micro units (such as a physician's office) through to huge macro units (such as the entire health system). However, almost all efficiency analysis relies on comparison of performance, so it is important to ensure that the entities under scrutiny are genuinely comparable. A great deal of efficiency analysis is concerned with securing such comparability.

For health production processes of any complexity, there are usually a number of stages in the transformation of resources to outcomes, and much of the confusion in discussing efficiency arises because commentators are discussing different parts of that process. As an example, Figure 10.1 illustrates a typical (but simplified) process associated with the treatment of hospital patients.[1] The overarching concern is with cost–effectiveness – which summarizes the transformation of costs (on the left hand side) into valued health outcomes (the right hand side). However, the data demands of a full system cost–effectiveness analysis are often prohibitive, and the results of such endeavours may in any case not provide policy-makers with relevant information on where to improve efficiency. In order to take remedial action, decision-makers may often require more detailed diagnostic indicators of just part of the transformation process.

Inefficiency might occur at any stage of this transformation process. Take first the transformation of money into physical inputs. There are two questions related to assessing the efficiency of this process. First, are inputs purchased at minimum cost (sometimes referred to as 'economy')? For example, is the organization paying wage rates in excess of local market rates? And second, is the correct mix of inputs being put in place? For example, is the organization

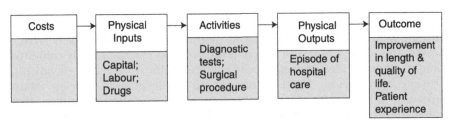

Figure 10.1 The production process in hospital care

employing the right mix of doctors, other professionals and administrators, thereby perhaps avoiding wasteful use of funds as a result of employing skilled personnel that remain idle or work on prosaic tasks?

The production process now moves to the creation of activities produced from those physical inputs, such as diagnostic tests or surgical procedures. Possible sources of waste here may include the use of highly skilled (and therefore costly) workers to produce activities that could be done by less specialized workers, or using excessive hours of labour or other physical inputs in the creation of a particular activity.

Next, physical outputs are created by aggregating activities for a particular service user. In a hospital setting, this usually refers to single episodes of patient care. There is great scope for waste in this process in the form, for example, of duplicated or unnecessary diagnostic tests, the use of branded rather than generic medicines, or unnecessarily long lengths of stay. Much depends on how the internal processes of the hospital are organized so as to maximize outputs using the given inputs.

The final stage of the health system production process is the quality of the outputs produced. There is great scope for variation in effectiveness, even when employing the same physical inputs, activities or physical outputs. The notion of quality in health care has a number of connotations. This book refers to two broad concepts: the clinical outcomes achieved (usually measured in terms of the gain in the length and quality of life (Chapter 6) and the patient experience (a multidimensional concept, discussed further in Chapter 9). So, for example, even though two hospitals produce identical numbers of hip replacements, because of variations in clinical practice and competence, the value they confer on patients (in the form of length and quality of life, as well as the patient experience) can vary considerably. Quality-adjusted output is usually referred to as the outcome of care in the literature. The quality of care has become a central concern of policy-makers, and its measurement, while contentious, is usually essential if a comprehensive picture of efficiency is to be secured.

The holy grail of value for money is the notion of cost–effectiveness, the ratio of valued health outcomes to the costs incurred, which embraces the entire production process, and therefore all the separate efficiency concepts mentioned above. Much analytic effort has gone into estimating production functions for the entire care pathway (Hollingsworth, 2003). However, although informative from a macro perspective, such analysis does not in general provide decision-makers with usable information on which to act because it does not identify the detailed sources of inefficiencies.

Efficiency measures of just part of the production process therefore give important complementary diagnostic information because they allow one to pinpoint where inefficiencies are arising. For example, measurement at each of the stages of the hospital transformation process offers a range of comparative performance metrics casting light on some parts of the process. Most measures of efficiency do not reflect the entire production process but, rather, encompass one or more segments that provide partial insight into some aspect of the transformation process.

For example, the familiar length of inpatient stay metric offers an insight into the relationship between a physical output (an episode of hospital care) and one specific input: the use of a hospital bed (a proxy for capital consumed). This is partial in two senses: (1) it does not embrace all of the transformation process (ignoring outcomes and costs); and (2) it does not include all of the resources used. It will nevertheless often offer a useful insight into some aspects of comparative hospital efficiency.

Finally, in addition to the efficiency of the production process, note that we have not considered whether the intervention under scrutiny was a sensible use of health system resources, even assuming perfectly efficient use of those resources. In short, was the intervention *appropriate*, given current technology and the priorities of the health system? Appropriateness is related to the notion of 'allocative' efficiency discussed in the next section and is central to the science of health technology assessment. Overall health system efficiency may therefore be undermined if a significant proportion of resources are devoted to inappropriate interventions. Even if each stage of the production process is undertaken efficiently, the system may be inefficient if it is producing the 'wrong' treatments.

In summary, efficiency can be examined in a number of ways, including:

- the economy with which physical inputs are purchased;
- the extent to which the chosen physical inputs are combined in an optimal mix to produce activities;
- the efficiency with which activities are converted into physical outputs;
- the quality of the care provided (its effectiveness);
- the appropriateness of the interventions provided.

The efficiency metrics described in this chapter seek to offer insights into these concepts.

10.3 Allocative and technical efficiency

Economists often make a distinction between two types of efficiency: allocative efficiency and technical efficiency. Allocative efficiency indicates the extent to which limited resources are directed towards producing the correct mix of health care outputs in line with the preferences of payers who supply the necessary inputs. It is central to the work of health technology assessment agencies, which often use expected gains in quality-adjusted life years (QALYs) as the central measure of the benefits of a treatment, and 'cost per QALY' as a prime cost–effectiveness criterion for whether or not to mandate adoption of a treatment. The assumption underlying this approach is that payers wish to see their financial contributions used to maximize health gain. Under these circumstances, a provider would not be allocatively efficient if it produced treatments with low levels of cost–effectiveness, because the inputs used could be better deployed producing outputs with higher potential health gain.

To illustrate this, Table 10.1 gives an example of a 'cost per QALY' ranking, which indicates the relative value of a set of treatments based on conventional estimates of cost–effectiveness. For a given budget, a producer can maximize health by concentrating on delivering treatments with the lowest cost per

Table 10.1 An example of an incremental cost per QALY league table

Pacemaker for atrioventricular heart block	£700
Hip replacement	£750
Valve replacement for aortic stenosis	£900
CABG (severe angina; left main disease)	£1 040
CABG (severe angina; triple vessel disease)	£1 270
CABG (moderate angina; left main disease)	£1 330
CABG (severe angina; left main disease)	£2 280
CABG (moderate angina; triple vessel disease)	£2 400
CABG (mild angina; left main disease)	£2 520
Kidney transplantation (cadaver)	£3 000
CABG (moderate angina; double vessel disease)	£4 000
Heart transplantation	£5 000
CABG (mild angina; triple vessel disease)	£6 300
Haemodialysis at home	£11 000
CABG (mild angina; double vessel disease)	£12 600
Haemodialysis in hospital	£14 000

Source: Briggs & Gray, 2000, adapted from Williams, 1985.

QALY. Of course, the volume of expenditure consumed by each intervention will depend on the incidence of the associated disease.

Discussion of allocative efficiency need not be confined to the use of such micro-level cost–effectiveness indicators. At a macro level, allocative efficiency is concerned with ensuring that the appropriate level of resources (i.e. share of GDP or government budget) is dedicated to health care relative to other sectors of the economy, given prevailing societal values. That is, an allocatively efficient country is spending an appropriate amount of its resources on health care, and society would not find itself better off by redirecting more resources towards health and away from other sectors of the economy (or away from health and towards other sectors).

Allocative efficiency can also be considered within the health care system at an intermediate level to examine whether the correct mix of services is funded, such that, at a given aggregate level of expenditures, health outcomes will be maximized. For example, an allocatively efficient health system dedicates the share of its funds between areas like prevention, hospital care and long-term care in such a way that the maximum level of health-related outcomes in line with societal preferences is secured. Allocative efficiency indicators at this intermediate level should indicate whether a health system is performing poorly because of a misallocation of resources between health system subsectors.

Whereas allocative efficiency assesses whether the system is producing an appropriate mix of outputs, technical efficiency makes no judgement on how much the outputs are valued by society. Technical efficiency indicates the extent to which the system is minimizing costs in producing its chosen outputs, regardless of the value placed on those outputs. An alternative but equivalent formulation is to say that it is maximizing its outputs given its level of inputs. In either case, the theoretical optimum is indicated by the production function, and any variation in performance from that optimum is an indication of technical inefficiency. The prime interest in technical efficiency is therefore in the operational performance of the entity, rather than its strategic choices relating to what outputs it produces.

As an example, although they may be deployed with great technical efficiency, a hospital may be producing outputs that are not much valued by society (e.g. treatment of glue ear), in relation to alternative outputs that it could be producing with the same resources. The extent to which the outputs of the organization are maximized in line with society's valuations of their characteristics is measured using the concept of allocative efficiency, while the extent to which the quantity of output is maximized (given the hospital's inputs) is measured using the concept of technical efficiency.

Finally, it is important to note other concepts of efficiency that can be employed, notably the ideal of 'scale' efficiency. If the relationship indicated by the production function between inputs and outputs is non-linear, then there exist variable returns to scale. This implies that – if parts of a health system cannot operate at an optimal scale, perhaps because they are serving a remote rural area – they cannot be expected to secure the same ratio of outputs to inputs as other less constrained providers. Efficiency analysis often seeks to take account of constraints such as scale limitations when they are clearly beyond the control of the systems under scrutiny.

10.4 Related concepts

It is important to make a distinction between efficiency and two related concepts: performance and productivity. Health system performance is a general term that seeks to describe how successfully health care is delivered. It might take efficiency into consideration, but can also encompass other facets of a health system assessment. It is perhaps unfortunate that in its World Health Report 2000 (*WHR2000*) the WHO used the term 'performance' interchangeably with efficiency.

Productivity is a concept that is closely related to efficiency. It is concerned with the ratio of an input (or aggregation of inputs) to an output (or aggregation of outputs) (Cylus & Dickensheets, 2007). For example, in much of the literature, there is a concern with *labour* productivity (such as patients treated per physician). Productivity measures like this usually take no account of whether the observed variations in output can be attributed solely to the entity under scrutiny. That is, labour productivity measures the amount of total output per worker, but does not take into consideration the level of other non-labour inputs, such as capital, that were used in producing that output. In contrast, efficiency indicators seek to indicate the extent to which output variations are directly attributable to the entity. Productivity measures are therefore usually more simplistic than efficiency measures.

To take another example, one of the reasons why a provider exhibits low productivity may be because it is operating at a small scale and cannot secure the economies of scale enjoyed by larger entities. The small-scale provider may therefore offer low productivity, even though its efficiency is high, given its size. Relative efficiency indicators measure the output that producers *actually* produce relative to the maximum possible output that they *could* produce, given their external circumstances over which they have no control. In health services, as well as the scale of operations, those external circumstances might include the demography, epidemiology and socioeconomic circumstances of the population served by the provider, or regulatory constraints not affecting other providers.

10.5 Measuring efficiency

Efficiency is almost always a comparative indicator because it assesses the production process of an entity relative to what has been produced by similar entities. Key questions to be addressed are: what individuals, organizations or systems are to be compared? And what aspects of their operations are to be compared? To begin, we review the most commonly used internationally comparable data sources. We then discuss some examples of existing indicators that measure comparative efficiency at the system level, disease level and sector level (as categorized by Häkkinen & Joumard, 2007), comment on their usability, and categorize them as either total efficiency indicators or one of three types of partial indicators based on the scope of the entity and the extent to which the entire production process is captured. We then rehearse some of the most important analytic techniques used to compare efficiency.

Common data

Comparative efficiency indicators are constructed using health care system data from the various stages of production processes, such as the hospital transformation process discussed earlier, although the precise types of data used depend on availability and the scope of the entity under scrutiny. Examples of data from the various stages include:

- Costs: sometimes disaggregated into categories, with or without overheads allocated.
- Physical inputs: such as measures of labour (staff employed, by category) or capital (e.g. hospital beds).
- Activities: such as procedures undertaken, days of care provided, diagnostic tests ordered, community visits made.
- Physical outputs: such as episodes of care or patients cared for.
- Outcomes: such as QALYs, avoidable deaths, or other health status data.

Almost all efficiency indicators are constructed as a ratio of one of these measures (for example, costs) to another (such as some activities), offering an indication of the extent to which resources have been used efficiently along some or all of the production pathway.

The nature and usefulness of data sources for comparing efficiency indicators depend largely on the purpose of the analysis. For some purposes, indicators using national health statistics, such as national health accounts (NHA) data, may be perfectly adequate for analyses at an aggregate level. In other circumstances, more micro-level indicators may require data such as patient-level claims files or country-specific surveys. In particular, those metrics that necessitate the tracking of an individual through the health system depend on highly detailed patient records, which are available only in certain datasets and for certain countries.

Reasonably comparable macro-level data are available from international organizations such as the OECD or WHO, though individual countries will often have more detailed data available than those provided to those international organizations. The OECD Health Data (OECD, 2012) offers comparable data at a system level for OECD member and accession countries along much of the production pathway, such as health care expenditures, resources, utilization and health status. In addition, the WHO Global Health Observatory and the WHO Health For All databases report data on a range of topics, including health care expenditures, mortality, health workforce and infrastructure (WHO, 2011; WHO Regional Office for Europe, 2011). Specific EU research projects, such as the HealthBasket project and Euro-DRG, have also collected cost data for specific types of care in a number of European countries (Busse, Schreyögg & Smith, 2008; Street et al., 2010).

To create truly comparable efficiency measures, data must often be adjusted to account for differences in the populations for which each health system is responsible. For example, different hospital systems will in general handle different case-mixes of patients, and it is usually inappropriate to compare the efficiency of treating patients without controlling for case-mix. There are a number of methods that can be used to make this sort of modification, referred to variously as standardization, case-mix adjustment or – most generally – risk adjustment.

Risk adjustment is a requirement for most of the types of comparison described in this book, so we offer only the briefest treatment. The simplest approach is to compare only similar types of service user (for example, as used in the HealthBasket project, which sought to compare costs of a small subset of health care treatments across nine countries. This method is however, by construction, limited in scope.

A more general method seeks to compare the observed level of a variable (say, costs) with the expected level if the provider were to operate at some standard level of efficiency (usually the sample mean). The celebrated system of diagnosis-related groups (DRGs) was originally designed for just this purpose (Fetter, 1991). It works by aggregating patients into a limited number of groups with similar clinical and resource utilization needs. The groups can be weighted and subsequently aggregated to determine the expected costs of a given group of service users, which can then be compared with observed costs. For example, in a recent study, Halsteinli and colleagues case-mix-adjusted the total number of patients by grouping patients by characteristics such as age, gender or reason for referral, and found that case-mix adjustment has a significant impact on the results of productivity analysis (Halsteinli, Kittelsen & Magnussen, 2010).

Data from discrete stages of the production process are combined in ratio form to create simple efficiency measures. For example, unit costs are constructed from cost estimates (numerator) and an associated measure of physical outputs (denominator). A data item used as a denominator in one indicator of efficiency (e.g. number of staff in an indicator such as labour costs per full-time member of staff) may become a numerator in another indicator (patients treated per member of staff). Both are valid efficiency indicators referring to different stages of the production process, and their product yields a new indicator (labour cost per patient treated).

Multiple data items may sometimes be incorporated in either the numerator or denominator of any efficiency indicator. For example, a measure of physical outputs may include different categories of hospital episode, defined by the patient's diagnosis. These different categories are often combined according to a weighting system that reflects the relative 'importance' of each category. Determining the weights to be used will be discussed later (section 10.7, Analytic techniques). Developing a persuasive set of weights is often challenging, although sometimes a natural weighting system arises. For example, when aggregating measures of labour inputs of different categories of staff, it is natural to use the relative wages of each category as a weighting mechanism.

Finally, it is important to note that many factors that affect health system efficiency cannot be handled in the conventional 'risk adjustment' methods noted above. For example, exogenous factors, such as education, environment or diet, are known to have a powerful influence on the ability of the health system to produce health outputs for a given level of resources. They are therefore often included as additional explanatory inputs when developing indicators of efficiency. By including exogenous factors in this way, the intention is to offer an indication of efficiency that acknowledges certain uncontrollable influences on health system performance.

There are numerous combinations of data that can be used as numerators or denominators to generate efficiency measures. A generic sample of efficiency indicator types is presented in Table 10.2.

Examples of efficiency indicators

A major decision in comparative efficiency analyses is whether to develop a comprehensive measure of efficiency, embracing all the major inputs or outputs of the whole system, or to resort to partial efficiency indicators. The attraction of comprehensive measures is obvious and is the ideal pursued by WHO in *WHR2000*. Yet there is a powerful argument that partial efficiency measures also offer useful insights, especially when seeking to diagnose the reasons for poor efficiency. This section considers the various approaches, but note that for many purposes it will be helpful to have available both comprehensive and partial metrics.

To illustrate this, Table 10.3 categorizes the various types of completeness available for health system comparisons. At the top left, analysis might assess

Table 10.2 Sample of efficiency indicators

Indicator	What is it?	What are the assumptions and what does it ignore?
Cost-effectiveness of certain intervention	Cost per QALY	Assumes average costs of providing intervention do not change with scale; major data constraints
Emergency department visits that could have been seen in less invasive settings	The proportion of ED visits that could have been seen in a different, less costly setting	Ignores quality of care Depends on definitions
Average length of stay	The number of days per hospital inpatient stay	Cases are identical, both in terms of outcomes and in terms of intensity
Unit costs	Estimates of costs	Assume uniform treatment, uniform accounting methods, ignore quality
Case-mix adjusted cost per episode of care	The average costs for treating a certain type of condition	Cases are identical, both in terms of outcomes and in terms of intensity; assumes uniform treatment, uniform accounting methods
Duplicate medical tests	The number of tests that are done more than once for the same patient	Assumes any duplicate test is an inefficiency regardless of situation
Share of total expenditures spent on administration	The percentage of total health expenditures dedicated to administration	Assumes that greater share of admin expenditure is inefficient without accounting for scale; highly dependent on accounting methods used
Labour hours per episode of care	The number of hours per case-mix adjusted episode of care	Assumes patients require the same intensity of care; difficult to accurately measure across a large sample; affected by health system design as well as efficiency
Share of health worker hours spent treating patients	The percentage of health worker hours spent treating patients	Assumes patients require the same intensity of care; difficult to accurately measure across a large sample; assumes time not spent with patients is unproductive
Disease costs	The average cost per case of treating a certain disease	Can be difficult to calculate without linking patient data across providers; assumes uniform case-mix; highly dependent on accounting methods used
Effective coverage	The share of actual health gains achieved relative to maximum potential health gains for an intervention	Difficult to measure need and quality

Table 10.3 Categorization and examples of total and partial indicators

	Total efficiency	Partial efficiency
Whole entity	Box D WHO health system performance assessment	Box C Case-mix-adjusted cost per episode of care
Part of the entity	Box B Cost–effectiveness measures for selected treatments	Box A Average length of inpatient stay for selected treatment

all the health system outcomes and all costs to develop comparative measures of whole-system cost–effectiveness, as in *WHR2000*. In practice, data limitations make it very challenging to implement satisfactorily. More modest ambitions might be to compare, say, hospitals' productivity based on case-mix-adjusted costs (top right hand cell) without reference to quality, thereby omitting an important element of cost–effectiveness (quality), but nevertheless offering useful insights into some aspects of performance. Alternatively, the comparison might seek to retain the comprehensive principle of cost–effectiveness as a basis for comparison, but only for a selected disease or treatment (bottom left hand cell). Finally, the most modest analysis offers an incomplete indication of efficiency, for only part of the system's activity (bottom right hand cell). We consider examples from these four categories, referred to simply as Box A, B, C and D indicators.

Box A – Part of the entity/part of production process

The simplest and most commonly used types of comparative efficiency indicators are those described in Box A, which measure only part of the production process for just a segment of the system. So, referring again to Figure 10.1, Box A partial indicators evaluate any portion of the production process other than the full production process (cash to health outcomes) for parts of a health care system, such as an inpatient ward of a hospital. For example, the hospital performance assessment tool PATH compared average lengths of hospital stay for selected types of care (Veillard et al., 2005). This type of study assumes that output – a completed hospital stay – is of the same quality and complexity across countries and that the indication of inefficiency is the greater time needed to produce that output. The Commonwealth Fund also assessed comparative efficiency using Box A partial indicators by looking at metrics such as the incidence of visits to emergency departments that could have been dealt with in less costly and invasive settings, and whether patients were sent for duplicate tests in the previous two years (Figure 10.2) (Davis, Schoen & Schoenbaum, 2007).

Likewise, the OECD Ageing-Related Diseases (ARD) study collected data on costs and outcomes for a selection of diseases (Moise et al., 2003; OECD, 2003). Although data on the entire production process were reviewed, some indicators only revealed the efficiency of parts of that process. For example, special attention was paid to the availability of mammography machines, as

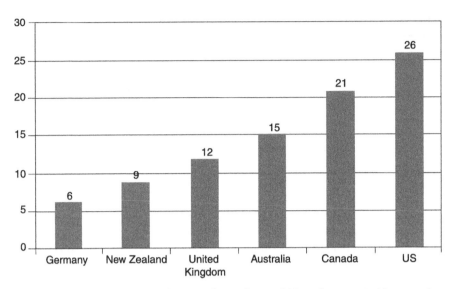

Figure 10.2 Went to the ER for a condition that could have been treated by a regular doctor, among sick adults, 2005

Source: Davis, Schoen & Schoenbaum, 2007.

shown in Figure 10.3, to try to gauge whether a greater number is an efficient tool for increasing breast cancer survival rates. In principle, such studies can offer information on comparative efficiency, by indicating systems that secure good outcomes relative to the inputs consumed. However, as they focus on only a small part of the production process, they can offer a misleading picture, for example, if other resources also contribute to the good results found in some countries.

Some national-level studies that compare inter-regional efficiency use similar indicators that could be applied in international settings. The Canadian Institute for Health Information examined the comparative efficiency of hospitals across Canadian provinces using indicators including staff hours per inpatient case, costs per inpatient case, the share of health worker hours spent treating patients, and the shares of total expenses that go to administration versus patient care (CIHI, 2010). Such indicators often ignore case-mix and assume that output quality does not vary and that organizations that require more inputs are wasteful.

A collection of related studies has looked into differences in the costs of providing an episode of care in different countries, irrespective of outcome. The HealthBasket and EuroDRG projects have sought to compare 'case vignettes' across Europe to determine reasons why hospital costs differ across European countries for certain types of case (Busse, Schreyögg & Smith, 2008; Street et al., 2010). These studies look into differences in the way in which treatments are delivered and the reasons for variations in the costs for those treatments by examining 'vignettes' of similar types of patients across countries. These projects therefore tackle the case-mix issue by constraining case studies to a small group of similar types of patients (Figure 10.4). Whilst ensuring some

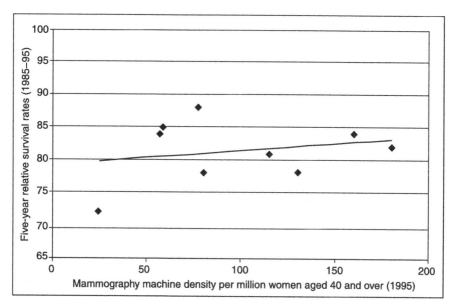

Figure 10.3 Five-year relative survival rate and availability of mammography machines in a recent year

Source: OECD, 2003.

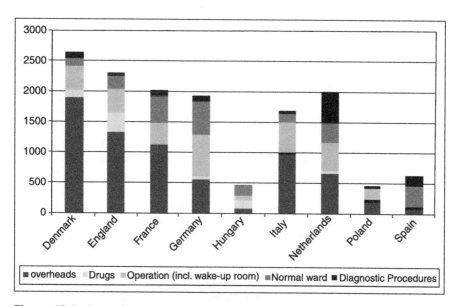

Figure 10.4 Appendectomy: comparison of costs by country

Source: Mason et al., 2007.

comparability, this methodology, like all Box A indicators, does not allow full comparison of health system efficiency.

The HealthBasket project highlighted a number of challenges that occur when seeking to compare unit costs across countries, including:

- securing access to comparable micro-data across countries;
- differences in the organization of services across countries;
- variations in accounting practice, including the measurement of clinical time with patients, the treatment of overheads and measurement of the cost of capital; and
- methodologies for currency conversion.

Generally, Box A indicators may reveal patterns that are indicative of efficient health care systems, and offer useful diagnostic information. However, they offer only an incomplete picture, and care should be taken in extrapolating findings from such indicators to other unmeasured aspects of the health system.

Box B – Part of the entity/entire production process

Some indicators examine only parts of the system, but make attempts to measure the efficiency of full production processes, from cash to health outcomes (Box B). For example, a handful of studies have sought to measure the comparative efficiency with which countries treat a selection of diseases. Disease-level indicators require measurable outcome data such as estimates of life years or QALYs lost, although such data exist only for certain diseases and in certain countries. Furthermore, cross-country comparisons in general suffer from the absence of a universally agreed categorization of diseases, or framework for the measurement of associated inputs and outcomes. It is particularly challenging to develop estimates of 'whole disease' costs in countries without linkage of the care patients receive from multiple providers. It is then often impossible to disaggregate the contribution, and subsequently measure the efficiency, of different types of providers (i.e. outpatient versus inpatient) in treating the disease in question (Häkkinen & Joumard, 2007).

The ARD study mentioned in the previous section compared treatments and health outcomes for a selection of diseases, including ischaemic heart disease, breast cancer and stroke, to determine which health systems offer the best value for money (Moise et al., 2003; OECD, 2003). To this end, the ARD study amassed information on health policy, epidemiology, treatments, costs and outcomes in an attempt to assess which countries address these diseases most efficiently. While some indicators presented in the study were partial indicators, the study itself provided insight into the entire production process for treating the aforementioned diseases.

A study by the McKinsey Global Institute assessed differences in "productive efficiency" at the disease level for Germany, United Kingdom and United States for four diseases: breast cancer, lung cancer, diabetes and gall stones (McKinsey Global Institute, 1996). This study defined output as health status (using the most appropriate metrics and timeframes for each disease). Inputs were measured by the relative cost-weighted units of labour, capital and supplies, rather than expenditure, a means of avoiding the currency conversion difficulties encountered in international efficiency comparison. In the same vein, Technological Change in Health Care (TECH) Global Research Network (McClellan & Kessler,1999; Technological Change in Health Care (TECH) Research Network, 2001) concentrated on the contribution of technology to improvements in outcomes for AMI in selected countries. Their approach was to use national representative micro-level hospital discharge records to directly link treatments and outcomes, although they found that a lack of linked patient records in many countries made it difficult to track care by multiple providers for the same patient.

Studies comparing the cost–effectiveness of certain types of public health or prevention programmes can also be categorized under Box B. Many of these indicators have difficulties accounting for outcomes (in the form of QALYs) because the benefits of public health programmes or preventive interventions must be assessed over the long term; nonetheless, comparative efficiency studies do exist. A study by Horton et al. compared the cost–effectiveness of different breastfeeding promotion programmes in Brazil, Honduras and Mexico (Horton et al., 1996). This study compared similar hospitals with and without breastfeeding promotion programmes and estimated differences in mortality, morbidity and DALYs to infer cost–effectiveness. Similarly, a number of studies have examined the relative cost–effectiveness of malaria prevention programmes in African countries (Goodman & Mills, 1999). These studies typically account for outputs such as deaths averted or discounted years of life gained. While these approaches can compare efficiency within a fraction of the health care system, their results cannot be extrapolated to draw conclusions about system-level efficiency. They also have to be treated with some caution as the fragment of the health system being evaluated may benefit from unmeasured inputs from other parts of the health system (for example, if there economies of scope exist).

Finally, a Box B indicator that to date has not received much attention for country comparisons is effective coverage (Murray & Evans, 2003). Effective coverage measures the extent to which those who need health care services are able to obtain them, and seeks to indicate whether those services have achieved their expected health gains. On a health system level, it is an indicator of the share of potential health gain that is actually realized. For example, if a certain procedure is expected to provide an average of three QALYs to the population but in the end provides only two QALYs, its effective coverage would be 66%; each intervention's effective coverage can be aggregated to the system level. Low effective coverage could be due to issues accessing health care, low-quality services or some other cause of unmet need. Although offering a useful potential tool, because of data constraints, very few countries have begun to measure effective coverage.

Box C – Entire entity/part of production process

Box C indicators measure whole entities (e.g. the health system or providers in their entirety), but for only part of the production process. For example, a Box C partial indicator on a provider level could measure costs per episode of care for entire hospitals but neglect to incorporate outcomes. Similarly, health care spending as a share of gross domestic product (GDP) could be an example of a system-level Box C indicator if it is assumed that generally equivalent quality care is provided (i.e. epidemiology, outcomes and quality are considered equal). It seeks to indicate which countries are able to provide some unspecified level of health care using a comparatively smaller share of their own resources (Davis, Schoen & Schoenbaum, 2007).

The majority of Box C comparative efficiency studies have taken a provider or subsector level approach, with the overwhelming majority focused on the hospital sector. The key issue is often securing a satisfactory case-mix adjustment to ensure comparability of entities. A study by Stakes/CHESS in conjunction with researchers in Norway compared hospital cost efficiency in Norway and Finland (Linna, Häkkinen & Magnussen, 2006). This study utilized case-mix-adjusted outputs such as DRG-adjusted admissions, weighted outpatient visits, day care and inpatient days. Inputs were defined as net operating costs from hospital accounting systems, adjusted for exchange rates. Using data envelopment analysis (DEA, described in detail in section 10.6, Descriptive methods), the average level of cost efficiency was found to be higher overall in Finnish hospitals.

Mobley and Magnussen compared efficiency among public regulated hospitals in Norway to private unregulated hospitals in California, also using DEA models (Mobley & Magnussen, 1998). They defined output as the number of inpatient days, outpatient visits and a case-mix index; inputs were measured using a measure of the quantity of health care workers and the number of beds as a proxy for capital. The use of physical rather than monetary inputs eliminated concerns over currency conversions, but cannot account for any differences in the quality of inputs.

Box C indicators, particularly those on the sector level, have tended to focus on hospitals, probably because it is easier to obtain data for full episodes of care within a hospital, rather than attempt to track patients across other providers. Box C measures can avoid problematic issues like quantifying changes in health status that are needed for measuring efficiency of the full production process. However, if the indicator does not make efforts to account for differences in case-mix, cross-country efficiency comparisons will often be biased against comparators with comparatively sicker or older populations. Furthermore, a methodology often has to be found for aggregating a variety of outputs measured in incommensurate units.

Box D – Entire entity/entire production process

Metrics that can be categorized within Box D seek to capture the full production process for an entire health system. If undertaken properly, the main advantage of such system-level indicators is that they can account for the possibility that otherwise identical patients might be treated in different settings in different systems. Even if all individual providers are technically efficient, if the system is using the wrong mix of services, the system as a whole may be allocatively inefficient (Häkkinen & Joumard, 2007). System-level Box D indicators are the most ambitious approaches to efficiency measurement, and are therefore very challenging. Most fundamentally, these types of indicators must account for all inputs responsible for healthy patient outcomes, and adjust for the potentially large number of uncontrollable influences on outcomes – such as, diet, environment, demography, tobacco and drug use – that lie outside the influence of the health system.

In *WHR2000*, WHO attempted to measure whole health system efficiency by looking at the relationships between resources and a composite measure of health system attainment based on five weighted components: level of health; distribution of health; level of responsiveness; distribution of responsiveness; and fairness of financial contribution (WHO, 2000). This measure of attainment was modelled as a function of health expenditure and years of schooling, with the intention that years of schooling would act as a proxy for factors such as social capital that affect outcomes but are beyond the control of the health care system. Each country's distance from the estimated production frontier was used to infer their level of inefficiency and countries were subsequently ranked. The indicator therefore provided an estimate of health system attainment relative to expenditures (Murray & Evans, 2003). Whilst based on a coherent intellectual framework, the WHO study attracted widespread criticism, and prompted a debate about the feasibility and desirability of producing such efficiency rankings (Murray & Evans, 2003).

Joumard and colleagues measured health system efficiency in OECD countries using both panel data regressions and DEA to estimate the contribution of the health system to life expectancy (not adjusted for morbidity or quality of life) (Joumard et al., 2008; OECD, 2010a). The studies took other exogenous factors into account, including lifestyle, education, pollution and income, although the research ultimately suggested that health care spending was the most important factor for explaining differences in life expectancy. The methods produced reasonably consistent results (Figure 10.5), with the most efficient countries offering the least scope for further gains in life expectancy. The contributions of the main explanatory variables used in the analysis can be found in Table 10.4.

Retzlaff-Roberts and colleagues developed a DEA approach using both an output-oriented model (maximizing output while maintaining levels of inputs and exogenous environmental factors) and an input-oriented model (minimizing inputs while maintaining levels of output and environmental difficulty) to measure comparative efficiency in OECD countries (Retzlaff-Roberts, Chang & Rubin, 2004). They defined outputs as infant mortality and life expectancy at birth; inputs were represented by proxy variables for three general areas: the social environment and demographics; lifestyle characteristics; and access to medical care services and health expenditures. This study found that inefficient OECD countries should be able to reduce infant mortality by an average of 14.5% or increase life expectancy by an average of 2.1% without adding more resources. From an input perspective, inefficient countries should be able to reduce inputs by an average of 14.0% without increasing infant mortality, or reduce inputs by an average of 21% without lowering life expectancy.

10.6 Analytic methods

While efficiency is in principle a simple construct, representing the ratio of outputs to inputs, the preceding sections suggest that there are numerous

Table 10.4 Contributions of main explanatory variables to cross-country differences. Differences in life expectancy at birth between countries and the OECD average for each variable, expressed in years, 2003

	Determinants								
	Life expectancy at birth	Spending	Education	Tobacco	Alcohol	Diet	Pollution	GDP	Country-specific effect
Australia	2.2	0.7	-0.3	0.1	-0.1	0	-0.9	0.2	2.5
Austria	0.8	1	0.2	0	-0.2	0	0.1	0.3	-0.7
Belgium	0.8	0.8	-0.3	0	-0.2	0	0.1	0.2	0.2
Canada	1.8	0.9	0.4	0.1	0.1	0	-0.8	0.3	0.9
Czech Republic	-2.7	-1.8	0.5	-0.1	-0.3	-0.1	0	-0.6	-0.3
Denmark	-0.5	0.7	0.3	0	-0.2	0	-0.2	0.3	-1.5
Finland	0.5	-0.2	0.1	0.2	0	-0.1	-0.3	0.2	0.5
France	1.3	0.9	-0.2	0	-0.3	0	0.4	0.2	0.4
Germany	0.6	0.8	0.4	-0.1	-0.1	0	0.5	0.1	-1
Greece	0.9	0.3	-0.7	-0.2	0	0.2	0	0	1.3
Hungary	-5.6	-2	0.1	0	-0.3	0	0.5	-0.8	-3.1
Iceland	3.1	1.1	-0.2	0	0.3	-0.1	-1	0.3	2.6
Ireland	0.3	0.3	-0.3	0	-0.4	0	0.1	0.4	0.2
Netherlands	0.6	0.6	-0.2	-0.1	-0.1	0	0.3	0.3	-0.3
New Zealand	1.5	-0.6	0.2	0.1	0	0	-0.5	-0.1	2.3
Norway	1.5	1.8	0.5	0.1	0.3	0	-0.3	0.7	-1.5
Poland	-3.4	-3.5	0.3	0	0.1	-0.1	0.4	-1.1	0.5
Republic of Korea	-0.6	-2.4	0.1	0	0	0.1	0.3	-0.4	1.7

Sweden	2.1	0.6	0.3	0	0.2	0	0.3	0.2	0.5
Switzerland	2.5	1.5	0.4	-0.1	-0.2	0	0.9	0.3	-0.4
Turkey	-7.4	-4.5	-2.3	-0.1	1.5	0.1	0.7	-1.9	-1
United Kingdom	0.5	-0.1	0.4	0.1	-0.2	0	0.1	0.2	0
United States	-0.5	2.9	0.5	0	0	0	-0.6	0.6	-4
Memorandum items:									
Maximum range	10.5	7.4	2.8	0.4	1.8	0.3	1.8	2.5	6.6
Estimated coefficients	0.041	0.03	-0.004		-0.011	0.004	-0.012	0.019	

Note: The country-specific effect is calculated as the sum of the country fixed-effect plus the residual of the equation.

Source: Joumard et al., 2008.

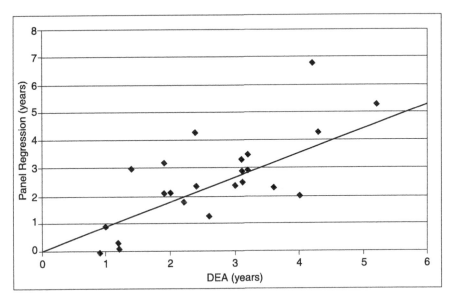

Figure 10.5   Comparing DEA and panel data regression results

Source: Joumard et al., 2008.

difficulties involved in converting the *principle of efficiency* into an operationally satisfactory *measure of efficiency*. Reasons include issues attaching weights with which to value outputs and the need to adjust for environmental factors that may cause production possibilities to differ across producers. In parallel with the piecemeal analysis of individual performance measures, which say nothing about maximum potential levels of production, a great deal of research effort has also gone into developing 'single number' measures of organizational efficiency, under the general banner of productivity analysis (Fried, Lovell & Shelton, 1993; Coelli, Rao & Battese, 1998). The objective of productivity analysis is to secure a measure of the technical efficiency of an organization, confusingly referred to almost universally as a measure of efficiency. Whatever the terminology, the measure of organizational attainment is nonetheless still defined as a ratio of weighted outputs to organizational inputs, adjusted where necessary for environmental constraints.

The key contribution of productivity analysis models to measuring efficiency is: (a) to adjust for the external environmental influences on performance; and (b) to handle the problem of attaching relative valuations to diverse outputs. Two approaches have dominated the productivity literature: econometric methods, pre-eminently various forms of statistical methods such as stochastic frontier analysis (SFA); and descriptive methods, known as data envelopment analysis (DEA) (Jacobs, Smith & Street, 2006). Although these methods approach the task in radically different fashions, they have the common intention of using the observed behaviour of all organizations to infer the maximum feasible level of attainment (the production function), and offering estimates of the extent to which each individual organization falls short of that optimum. The methods are technically challenging, and a full treatment is beyond the scope of this chapter. Here, we merely seek to give an intuitive description of each of the approaches.

Statistical methods

Traditional statistical models of health care performance usually take the form of a cost function, under which an organization's costs are modelled as a function of a range of organizational outputs.[2] The simplest statistical approach to developing a cost function is to use conventional multivariate regression analysis, in which costs are modelled as a function of a range of outputs, the organizational environment, and an unexplained error term. This yields an empirical model that predicts an organization's expenditure, given its current levels of outputs and environmental circumstances.[3] The deviation from this prediction (the difference between actual and model predicted costs) can be used as a basis for estimating the organization's overall efficiency. That is, all unexplained variation from the statistical model is assumed to be due to inefficiency.

Various refinements of the conventional regression model have been developed to examine organizational efficiency, including a suite of methods known collectively as stochastic frontier analysis (SFA) (Kumbhakar & Lovell, 2000). These retain the basic principles of regression analysis, but seek to decompose unexplained cost variations into random statistical 'noise' and inefficiency, the issue of interest from a value for money perspective. However, SFA requires very restrictive modelling assumptions that are highly contested, leading some commentators to question the usefulness of SFA (Smith & Street, 2005).

Some of the difficulties brought about by applying statistical methods to a single cross-section of observations can be obviated by using panel data (that is, a time series of observations for each organization, rather than a single measure). The important gain offered by panel data is the vastly increased ability to distinguish transient (random) variations in performance measures from persistent (systematic) variations that can form the basis for estimates of inefficiency. However, important technical assumptions must still be made, for example, about how inefficiency is assumed to change over time, and there is a risk that any model is estimating historical rather than contemporary levels of inefficiency.

For example, Jacobs, Smith and Street (2006) present an application of cost function analysis to 171 acute English hospitals. They model hospital costs as a function of a range of outputs, including inpatient episodes, outpatient episodes, accident & emergency attendances, teaching and research, and a number of environmental factors.[4] Using a conventional regression analysis, which treats all the unexplained variation as 'inefficiency', they find that the average level of efficiency is 70.4%. However, when they use SFA (which treats some of the unexplained variation as random), the average efficiency levels increase to 90.4%.

Descriptive methods

Data envelopment analysis is based on similar economic principles to SFA, but uses very different estimation techniques, based on linear programming models (Thanassoulis, 2001). In summary, it searches for the organizations that 'envelope' all other organizations on the basis of a composite estimate of efficiency. For each organization, it looks for all other organizations that secure the same (or better) outputs at lowest use of inputs. Or conversely, it can be used to search for the other organizations that use the same (or lower) inputs to secure the highest level of outputs. For each organization, the ratio of actual to optimal performance is referred to as inefficiency.

Compared to SFA, DEA has some attractive features. It requires none of the restrictive assumptions required to undertake regression methods. It can handle multiple inputs and multiple outputs simultaneously, and requires none of the stringent model testing that is required of statistical techniques. However, it also suffers from a number of drawbacks. It can be vulnerable to data errors, because the DEA 'best practice' frontier is composed of a small number of highly performing organizations, and the performance of all other units is judged in relation to that frontier. Therefore, if the measurement of one key 'best practice' organization is incorrect, it can result in excessively negative judgements on many of the inefficient units.

Moreover, from the point of view of ranking organizations, DEA has the profound drawback that it permits flexibility in the valuation weights attached to each output. The method is agnostic about the valuation of outputs in the sense that it allows each organization to be judged using valuations that show it in the best possible light. So each organization can, in principle, be compared to the frontier according to an entirely different set of output weights. That is, DEA measures technical efficiency, and ignores allocative efficiency or overall cost–effectiveness. In particular, this means that an organization might be deemed efficient using DEA, but only if a zero weight is placed on an important output. This appears to contradict the principle that organizations should be evaluated on a consistent basis, and has also exposed the technique to fierce criticism (Stone, 2002). For this reason, many commentators advocate the use of DEA as a useful tool for exploring large and complex datasets and making preliminary comparisons, but not as a device for passing judgements or setting efficiency targets. Those seeking comparisons would normally want to apply to all organizations a consistent set of weights, in line with regulatory priorities.

Jacobs, Smith and Street (2006) present an application of DEA to 171 acute English hospitals. In the simplest specification, they use total costs as a measure of inputs; and inpatient episodes, outpatient episodes and accident & emergency attendances as outputs. They find that 14 hospitals are 100% efficient (lie on the best practice frontier). The average level of efficiency amongst all hospitals is 74.4%, and 5 hospitals have an efficiency level of less than 50%. They then progressively refine the model to include outputs such as teaching and research, and include a number of environmental factors. This leads to a dramatic increase in the number of 100% efficient hospitals (to 150 of the 171), and an increase in the average level of efficiency to 98.8%.

This example demonstrates a number of characteristics of 'comprehensive' efficiency measurement, most notably its sensitivity to the underlying modelling assumptions, and the critical importance of value weights. If more outputs are included, then it becomes increasingly difficult to identify 'best practice' organizations without assigning valuations to the outputs produced. And, other things equal, the inclusion of more environmental factors offers organizations more 'excuses' for lower levels of performance. This may be appropriate, but requires careful scrutiny. In practice, any analysis should examine a range of modelling perspectives, in order to identify the sensitivity of judgements to different technical choices.

Steinmann also compared hospitals in Germany and Switzerland using DEA (Steinmann et al., 2004). This study considered the number of patient days in separate analyses to be either an input or an output, illustrating the flexibility in constructing efficiency indicators so long as they encompass any segment of the production process highlighted in Figure 10.1. Other inputs included the quantity of different types of staff, beds and other expenses. Outputs were most often defined as the aggregate number of certain types of cases. Efficiency was compared by first developing a production frontier that consisted of output for hospitals from both countries. Then, production frontiers were constructed using data from each country separately and the frontiers were compared relative to the productivity of hospitals from the other country. The study also looked to see whether hospitals are subject to differing returns to scale. Steinmann et al. found German hospitals to be roughly twice as large as Swiss hospitals and on average more efficient.

10.7 Issues, gaps and debates

In a review of published efficiency measures, Hussey et al. (2009) note:

> Efficiency measures have been subjected to few rigorous evaluations of reliability and validity, and methods of accounting for quality of care in efficiency measurement are not well developed at this time. Use of these measures without greater understanding of these issues is likely to engender resistance from providers and could lead to unintended consequences (Hussey et al., 2009).

While we have characterized comparative efficiency measures as the ratio of some aspect of resources consumed to some aspect of valued services or outcomes, our discussion has noted weaknesses in the measurement of the numerator, the denominator and the alignment of the two. In this section we discuss some of the key issues, gaps and debates that have arisen in constructing comparative efficiency measures. In doing so, we largely set aside the problems of measuring outputs and outcomes, which are treated in other chapters in this volume. Instead, we focus on the following key issues: conceptual models of efficiency; analytic techniques; and data issues.

Conceptual models

The many different concepts of efficiency encountered in the literature is a serious weakness that has given rise to confusion and the unsatisfactory development of efficiency measures. Many indicators in use reflect the administrative convenience of collecting information rather than an effort to produce meaningful evidence that can help managers, regulators, governments and citizens understand how the resources they provide are being used, and how improvements can be secured.

Somewhat paradoxically, most conceptual thinking has been devoted to whole system efficiency, the most challenging aspect of efficiency measurement (Jacobs, Smith & Street, 2006). Conventional models from the general productivity literature have been applied to the health sector, for example, informing *WHR2000* as well as the Atkinson review of productivity growth being developed in the UK (WHO, 2000; Atkinson, 2005). This conceptual thinking has undoubtedly heightened awareness of efficiency issues and helped to focus the debate on the broad approach to comparison. However, it has been less helpful in promoting better understanding of the partial, operational measures of efficiency that can have more immediate relevance for understanding health system weaknesses and guiding the development of reforms.

In this respect, some of the most important conceptual thinking occurred some time ago, for example, in the development of DRGs and other episode-related measures of efficiency. These seek to cluster health system outputs into homogeneous groups that facilitate like-for-like comparison. Whilst in widespread use within countries, projects such as EuroDRG have found very little evidence of convergence between countries, a serious weakness in the pursuit of international comparison. Some movement towards an international standard of DRG development and definition is an urgent priority for cross-country comparison.

The majority of existing comparative efficiency indicators have sought to measure technical efficiency. This makes sense from a feasibility standpoint because it is conceptually simpler to measure output production at given input levels rather than to assess whether the most valued output possible has been produced. The act of valuing health system outputs, or outcomes, is highly problematic. The one exception is for disease-level indicators, for which QALYs and their DALY counterparts have been accepted as a measure of outcome; however, such data are not consistently available across countries. Nevertheless, allocative efficiency indicators may provide policy-makers with helpful information on how to reorganize services so as to achieve better value for money.

In contrast, the consistent accounting of expenditures has received considerable attention through the development of the international *System of Health Accounts*. While it does suffer from some weaknesses, notably in the non-hospital setting, and the boundary between health and long-term care, the SHA initiative offers a forum for further debate and refinement, and might serve as a model for the development of international standards in other areas, such as output measurement. However, it should be noted that, due to the extensive data demands of SHA, many low- and middle-income countries will continue to have difficulties capturing internationally comparable expenditure and efficiency data.

Finally, it is important to note that many outputs are the result of years of health system interventions and cannot be attributed to inputs in a specific period, while some of today's endeavours will affect outcomes only at some time in the future. This is true for a large segment of public health and prevention activities, where current expenditures on activities like vaccinations are responsible for improved health status over the duration of the activities' impact, which may well last a patient's lifetime. When analysing the efficiency of some services, it is therefore in principle necessary to adopt a longer time horizon, and there may be a strong case for treating some preventive activity as a capital expenditure. Any comparison over time may be further complicated by the need to take account of input price changes. We are not aware of any significant advances in handling these dynamic aspects of efficiency.

Analytic techniques

There have been considerable efforts to apply the methods of productivity analysis (regression analysis, SFA and DEA) to infer comparative efficiency of various aspects of health systems. Such techniques seek to build production functions by explaining justifiable variations in performance between the entities under scrutiny, and to characterize the unexplained residual as 'inefficiency'. Although conceptually attractive, there are few examples of such methods being used in earnest by decision-makers.

Efficiency is intrinsically unmeasurable, as it focuses on the variation in performance that cannot be explained by levels of inputs and uncontrollable influences on outcomes. A central analytic task is therefore to partition the residual, or unexplained 'error' found in any statistical model, between inefficiency and other unmeasured causes of variation in attainment. Hence, there is a central concern with the residual for each unit of observation. These preoccupations are in sharp contrast to traditional statistical modelling, which emphasizes parameter estimation. Yet, most efficiency analysis continues to use traditional model-building principles. Most notably, inadequate attention is given to model specification and testing in a context where standard statistical tests do not apply (Smith & Street, 2005).

Productivity analysis yields a ratio of (weighted) outputs to inputs. As demonstrated above, there is often no need to deploy analytic techniques to develop such a simple calculation. The key analytic issue is rather: how should various outputs be combined into a composite measure of the value produced? (There is also an analogous concern about aggregating physical inputs, but this is often more straightforward using the input prices as a weighting system). The creation of composite indicators requires identification of the relative value of an extra unit of each output. Weaknesses in this respect were a key criticism of *WHR2000*, and there has been only modest progress since then in informing the creation of composite indicators. One of the contributions of the formal models of productivity analysis is to inform weighting systems. However, the solicitation of values attached to different outputs remains a key area for future research.

A particular issue for composite measures is how to place a value on the reduction of inequalities in health and inequalities in access to health services relative to aggregate improvements in health. There are two broad schools of thought on how to handle equity issues in efficiency measurement. One is simply to treat some measure of equity, based, for example, on divergence of outcomes for different social groups, as a distinct output. The other approach uses a single measure of output or outcome (such as health gain), but weights the gains more heavily for disadvantaged groups. Although the latter approach is probably more promising, quantification of differential weights is in its infancy (Dolan, 2008).

A significant element of health outcomes is attributable not to health system interventions, but to external factors. Different health service organizations work in the context of different external constraints, such as the health characteristics of the local population, local transport, geography and economic conditions, and the activities of other agencies both inside and outside the health sector. A great deal of analytic effort has gone into developing methods of adjusting for environmental differences, with the simplest approach comparing only organizations working in similar environments, using methods such as cluster analysis (Retzlaff-Roberts, Chang & Rubin, 2004; Smith, 2009). However, these are crude expedients, and researchers have developed more subtle methods of risk adjustment to address some aspects of environmental variation. These enjoy wide acceptance in some domains (such as the use of DRGs for hospital cost comparison), but are less advanced in many other areas of the health system.

An important contribution of productivity analysis is to adjust measures of efficiency for variations in the uncontrollable circumstances of organizations, such as population characteristics, often by including measures of uncontrollable factors as additional inputs into the production process. This is also a key problem for many of the comparative measures discussed in other chapters, and there remains a great deal of uncertainty regarding how best to adjust for legitimate external influences on performance for which health systems cannot be held accountable. In practice, many studies introduce indicators of such influences into efficiency models without much justification or conceptual clarity, and this remains an area requiring further development.

Data issues

In developing health care comparative efficiency indicators, inputs are often represented as expenditures on resources like labour, capital and intermediate inputs. There are a number of unresolved challenges associated with costing methodology to obtain comparable expenditure data (Mogyorosy & Smith, 2005). For instance, inputs can often be readily identified if the units are discrete organizations such as hospitals, which are discrete accounting entities. However, they can be much more difficult to identify if the unit of analysis is smaller, such as a hospital department, as it becomes difficult to estimate what fraction of the hospital's resources are devoted to producing the outputs of that department (Smith, 2009). Also, many health services are the product of different teams of health workers working together, who may or may not be drawing on joint resources; appropriate attribution is again a major concern. The HealthBasket project identified major discrepancies in accounting practices across countries, for example, in the treatment of overhead costs. Standardization of accounting practices across providers and countries is of utmost importance to ensure comparability across countries.

There are particular difficulties measuring capital inputs because the use of capital is by definition spread over the long term. Assigning a capital input value for a single period – the portion of the capital investment that is 'used up' in the period – is therefore problematic. Moreover, as the value of capital depreciates over time, it becomes even harder to measure the true value of capital consumed in a single accounting period. Again, a standardized approach to measuring and attributing capital costs is needed.

A health system also creates and uses up important capital endowments that are not physical, for example, in the form of education and training, or disease prevention programmes. Such investments create value that is consumed in future periods, and should in principle be treated like other capital investments, rather than revenue expenditure. However, we are not aware of any major initiatives adopting such an approach.

To conduct efficiency analysis across countries using expenditures as inputs it is necessary to normalize national currencies and price levels to create a common base, as exchange rate adjusted currencies (or identical currencies, in the case of the euro) may purchase different quantities of the same good in different countries. Some researchers believe that current methods of adjusting expenditures using PPP indexes are ineffective because PPPs do not reflect prices of health-related goods and services alone (Schreyögg et al., 2008). If the PPP index does not accurately reflect variations in health care system prices, this will bias the comparability of currencies. The OECD is working to develop output-based PPPs, which are intended to more accurately reflect the prices of health system output (OECD, 2007).

10.8 Concluding comments

Clearly, the production of health outcomes is a dynamic, complex process, not nearly as straightforward as the production process presented in Figure 10.1. A fundamental challenge in developing an efficiency measure is ensuring that the output that is being captured is directly and fully dependent on the inputs that are included in the measurement. This is particularly true when trying to account for the inputs responsible for health outcomes. Environmental factors, policy constraints, population characteristics and other factors may be largely responsible for determining health outcomes, yet it is difficult to incorporate all possible determinants appropriately into an efficiency assessment. From an accounting perspective, the assignment of inputs and associated costs to specific health system activities is fundamentally problematic, often relying on arbitrary accounting rules or other questionable assignments.

Figure 10.6 summarizes the considerations raised in this chapter relating to the measurement of health system efficiency. In addition to standard current year health system inputs, certain system constraints and other exogenous risk factors have a role in determining what the health system is able to produce. The health system today may also be affected by endowments in previous years, such as investments in medical technology or infrastructure; conversely, investments

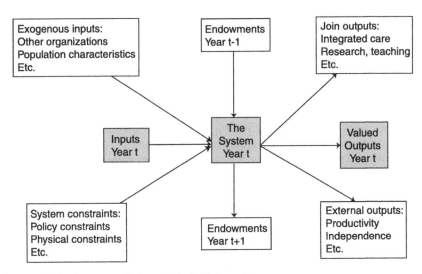

Figure 10.6 A more realistic model of efficiency?

today may have impacts on future health system production. Indirect outputs of the health system are often produced and should be accounted for as health system output. For example, inputs into the health system may lead to medical research or teaching with implicit societal value as this can lead to better future health outcomes. Improvements in health status may also lead to increased labour productivity, happiness or wellbeing, and may reduce burdens on other sectors such as social care. There is value in accounting for all of these elements of the production process. However, it is not feasible to address all these issues, and they are largely absent from health system efficiency indicators.

Many health system policy-makers rely on comparative efficiency measures to guide regulation, reorganization and reform. Although researchers have developed indicators that seek to measure full production processes, these measures are often not the most informative for policy-makers looking to identify and address inefficiencies. This review has indicated that many existing measures are practical and have useful policy information, but they are often partial and rely on weak data or analytic methods. In general, current measures of comparative efficiency can offer some information, but require careful interpretation and commentary.

Comparative efficiency indicators should be usable in policy to identify systems, sectors, interventions and providers that provide the greatest value for money. In turn, policy-makers must take advantage of any efficiency assessments by subsequently dedicating greater resources to those elements of their health system that are demonstrated to perform efficiently and reforming elements that are shown to be wasteful. Efficiency indicators have the capacity to provide insight into all the common elements of health system architecture. For example, an indicator like labour hours per episode of care can suggest whether certain organizational settings inefficiently use human resources or whether inappropriate levels of resources have been allocated although, of course, a complete picture will need measures of the associated health outcomes. In terms of financing or resource generation, efficiency indicators enable policy-makers to recognize if they are achieving minimum costs and, if not, to identify whether a particular part of the production process may be at fault.

In making comparisons of health systems, the measurement of comparative efficiency is probably the single most powerful lever for securing political attention and encouraging system change. *WHR2000* would not have attracted a fraction of the policy attention if it had merely reported outputs (say, adjusted life expectancy) or inputs (say, expenditure). It was the attempt to link the two that generated the policy interest. In the same way, attempts by the UK Office for National Statistics to track trends in UK health system productivity have generated political interest and debate in a way that the long series of mortality and expenditure data have never remotely stimulated (UK Centre for the Measurement of Government Activity, 2008).

The apparently simple concept of efficiency is nevertheless difficult to measure. Existing efficiency measures can be useful so long as decision-makers do not draw unfounded conclusions about entire systems or production processes as a result of them. We have identified the following difficulties with existing methodologies.

- The production process underlying health systems is intrinsically complex and poorly understood. Most measures make simplifying assumptions that may sometimes lead to misleading data.
- Outputs are generally multidimensional and therefore preference weights are needed if they are aggregated into a single measure of attainment. The choice of such weights is intrinsically political and contentious.
- A significant element of many outputs is attributable not to health system interventions, but to external factors (environment or the work of other agencies).
- Many outputs are the results of years of health system endeavour, and cannot be attributed to inputs in a single period.
- The assignment of inputs and the associated costs to specific health system activities is fundamentally problematic. It often relies on arbitrary accounting rules or other questionable assignments.
- Comparison over time is often complicated by the need to take account of input price changes.
- Comparison between nations is often complicated by the need to adjust for currency movements.
- Equity and distributional issues are not well handled in efficiency analysis.
- Efficiency measures have not been rigorously tested for reliability and validity.

We take it as axiomatic that decision-makers require authoritative and analytically satisfactory measures of comparative efficiency. Such measures are: (a) a natural way of summarizing the information contained in the many univariate measures of performance that exist; and (b) likely to have more policy influence than any other single measurement instrument. They are a fundamental requirement to assure that health system money is spent wisely. The concerns discussed here therefore represent an urgent research agenda.

Notes

1. While we focus on hospital services as an expository device, it is important to keep in mind that more complex transformation processes exist in much of chronic care, preventive medicine and public health.
2. Some applications have sought to develop the mirror image 'production function' of health care organization performance, under which a single measure of an organization's output is modelled as a function of a range of organizational inputs. In general, this approach poses similar technical challenges, but is likely to be less useful from a value for money perspective.
3. It is worth noting that, using the conventional regression model, the coefficient on each explanatory variable in the cost function offers an estimate of the marginal price of producing the associated output, and therefore an estimate of the average implicit valuation of the output in the sample.
4. There was no consideration of the quality of outcomes in this model.

References

Aaron, H. (2008) Waste, we know you are out there, *New England Journal of Medicine*, 359(18): 1865–7.

Atkinson, A.B. (2005) *The Atkinson review: Final report. Measurement of government output and productivity for the national accounts*. Basingstoke: Palgrave Macmillan.

Bentley, T.G. et al. (2008) Waste in the U.S. health care system: a conceptual framework, *Milbank Quarterly*, 86(4): 629–59.

Briggs, A. and Gray, A. (2000) Using cost effectiveness information, *BMJ*, 320(7229): 246.

Busse, R., Schreyögg, J. and Smith, P. (2008) Variability in health care treatment costs amongst nine EU countries – results from the HealthBASKET project, *Health Economics*, 17(Suppl 1): S1–8.

CIHI (2010) *Canadian Hospital Reporting Project (CHRP)*. Ottawa: Canadian Institute For Health Information (http://www.cihi.ca/CIHI-ext-portal/internet/EN/Tabbed Content/health+system+performance/indicators/performance/cihi010657, accessed 16 July 2012).

Coelli, T., Rao, P. and Battese, G.E. (1998) *An introduction to efficiency and productivity analysis*. Boston, MA: Kluwer Academic Publishers.

Cylus, J.D. and Dickensheets, B.A. (2007) Hospital multifactor productivity: a presentation and analysis of two methodologies, *Health Care Financing Review*, 29(2): 49–64.

Davis, K., Schoen, C., Schoenbaum, S.C. (2007) *Mirror, Mirror on the Wall: An international update on the comparative performance of American Health Care*. New York: The Commonwealth Fund (http://www.commonwealthfund.org/Publications/Fund-Reports/2007/May/Mirror—Mirror-on-the-Wall—An-International-Update-on-the-Comparative-Performance-of-American-Healt.aspx, accessed 3 June 2012).

Dolan, P. (2008) Developing methods that really do value the 'Q' in the QALY, *Health Economics Policy and Law*, 3: 69–77.

Fetter, R. (1991) Diagnosis related groups: understanding hospital performance, *Interfaces*, 21(1): 6–26.

Fried, H.O., Lovell, C.A.K. and Shelton, S.S. (1993) *The measurement of productive efficiency: techniques and applications*. Oxford: Oxford University Press.

Goodman, C.A. and Mills, A.J. (1999) The evidence base on the cost-effectiveness of malaria control measures in Africa, *Health Policy and Planning*, 14(4): 301–12.

Häkkinen, U. and Joumard, I. (2007) *Cross-country analysis of efficiency in OECD health care sectors: options for research*. Paris: Organisation for Economic Co-operation and Development (Economics Department Working Papers).

Halsteinli, V., Kittelsen, S.A. and Magnussen, J. (2010) Productivity growth in outpatient child and adolescent mental health services: the impact of case-mix adjustment, *Social Science and Medicine*, 70(3): 439–46.

Hollingsworth, B. (2003) Non-parametric and parametric applications measuring efficiency in health care, *Health Care Management Science*, 6(4): 203–18.

Horton, S. et al. (1996) Breastfeeding promotion and priority setting in health, *Health Policy and Planning*, 11(2): 156–68.

Hussey, P.S. et al. (2009) A systematic review of health care efficiency measures, *Health Services Research*, 44(3): 784–805.

Jacobs, R., Smith, P. and Street, A. (2006) *Measuring efficiency in health care: analytic techniques and health policy*. Cambridge: Cambridge University Press.

Joumard, I. et al. (2008) *Health status determinants: lifestyle, environment, health care resources and efficiency*. Paris: Organisation for Economic Co-operation and Development (OECD Economics Department Working Paper, no. 627).

Kumbhakar, S.C. and Lovell, C.A.K. (2000) *Stochastic frontier analysis*. Cambridge: Cambridge University Press.

Linna, M., Häkkinen, U. and Magnussen, J. (2006) Comparing hospital cost efficiency between Norway and Finland, *Health Policy*, 77(3): 268–78.

Mason, A. et al. (2007) *International comparison of costs: an exploration of within- and between-country variations for ten healthcare services in nine EU member states*. Brussels: European Health Management Association (Deliverable 34, Phase III, Work Package 10 (WP10)).

McClellan, M. and Kessler, D (1999) A global analysis of technological change in health care: the case of heart attacks. The TECH Investigators, *Health Affairs (Millwood)*,18(3): 250–5.

McKinsey Global Institute (1996) *Health Care Productivity*. Los Angeles, CA: McKinsey Global Institute.

Mobley, L.R. and Magnussen, J. (1998) An international comparison of hospital efficiency: does institutional environment matter? *Applied Economics*, 30(8): 1089–100.

Mogyorosy, Z. and Smith, P.N. (2005) *The main methodological issues in costing health care services: A literature review*. York: Centre for Health Economics, University of York.

Moise, P., Jacobzone, S. and the ARD-IHD Experts Group (2003) *OECD study of cross-national differences in the treatment, costs and outcomes of ischaemic heart disease*. Paris: Organisation for Economic Co-operation and Development Publications (Health Working Papers).

Murray, C.J.L. and Evans, D.B. (eds) (2003) *Health Systems Performance Assessment: Debates, methods and empiricism*. Geneva: World Health Organization.

OECD (2003) *A Disease-based Comparison of Health Systems: What is best and at what cost?* Paris: Organisation for Economic Co-operation and Development Publishing.

OECD (2007) *Development of reliable health-specific purchasing power parities (PPPs)*. Paris: Organisation for Economic Co-operation and Development Publishing (http://www.oecd.org/document/36/0,3343,en_2649_33929_38503076_1_1_1_1,00.html, accessed 16 July 2012).

OECD (2010a) *Health care systems: Efficiency and policy settings*. Paris: Organisation for Economic Co-operation and Development Publishing (http://www.oecd-ilibrary.org/social-issues-migration-health/health-care-systems_9789264094901-en, accessed 25 September 2012).

OECD (2010b) *Value for money in health spending*. Paris: Organisation for Economic Co-operation and Development Publishing (OECD Health Policy Studies).

OECD (2012) *OECD Health Data 2012: Statistics and Indicators*. Paris: Organisation for Economic Co-operation and Development (http://www.oecd.org/document/30/0,3343,en_2649_34631_12968734_1_1_1_1,00.html, accessed 17 July 2012.)

Reinhardt, U.E., Hussey, P.S. and Anderson, G.F. (2002) Cross-national comparisons of health systems using OECD data, 1999, *Health Affairs*, 21(3): 169–81.

Retzlaff-Roberts, D., Chang, C.F. and Rubin, R.M. (2004) Technical efficiency in the use of health care resources: a comparison of OECD countries, *Health Policy*, 69(1): 55–72.

Schreyögg, J. et al. (2008) Cross-country comparisons of costs: the use of episode-specific transitive purchasing power parities with standardised cost categories, *Health Economics*, 17(Suppl 1): S95–103.

Smith, P.C. and Street, A. (2005) Measuring the efficiency of public services: the limits of analysis, *Journal of the Royal Statistical Society*, Series A (General) 168(2): 401–17.

Smith, P.C. (2009) *Measuring value for money in healthcare: concepts and tools*. London: Health Foundation (http://www.health.org.uk/publications/measuring-value-for-money-in-healthcare-concepts-and-tools, accessed 16 July 2012).

Steinmann, L. et al. (2004) Measuring and comparing the (in)efficiency of German and Swiss hospitals, *European Journal of Health Economics*, 5(3): 216–26.

Stone, M. (2002) How not to measure the efficiency of public services (and how one might), *Journal of the Royal Statistical Society*, Series A, 165(3): 405–34.

Street, A. et al. (2010) *Determinants of hospital costs and performance variation: Methods, models and variables for the EuroDRG project*. Berlin: Technische Universität Berlin (Working Papers in Health Policy and Management).

Technological Change in Health Care (TECH) Research Network (2001) Technological change around the world: Evidence from heart attack care, *Health Affairs (Millwood)*, 20(3): 25–42.

Thanassoulis, E. (2001) *Introduction to the theory and application of data envelopment analysis: a foundation text with integrated software*. Dordrecht: Kluwer Academic Publishers.

UK Centre for the Measurement of Government Activity (2008) *Public service productivity*. UK National Statistics Publication Hub (http://www.statistics.gov.uk/hub/government/central-and-local-government/public-service-productivity, accessed 16 July 2012).

Veillard, J. et al. (2005) A performance assessment framework for hospitals: the WHO Regional Office for Europe PATH project, *International Journal for Quality in Health Care*, 17(6): 487–96.

WHO (2000) *World Health Report 2000. Health systems: improving performance*. Geneva: World Health Organization.

WHO (2011) *Global Health Observatory Data Repository*. Geneva: World Health Organization (http://apps.who.int/ghodata, accessed 16 July 2012).

WHO Regional Office for Europe (2011) *European Health for all Database*. Copenhagen: World Health Organization Regional Office for Europe (http://data.euro.who.int/hfadb, accessed 16 July 2012).

Williams, A. (1985) Economics of coronary artery bypass grafting, *BMJ (Clinical Research Edition)*, 291(6491): 326–9.

chapter eleven

Commentary on International Health System Performance Information

Nick Fahy[1]

11.1 Introduction

In the context of the framework for HSPA set out in this publication, the aim of this chapter is to review the situation of data for international comparisons of health systems by the principal official international organizations working in this field – WHO, the EU and the OECD. Taking into account the dimensions of health system performance described in this book, it outlines areas of future development needed to help support international HSPA in the future.

There are, of course, other organizations that provide relevant data, such as the Commonwealth Fund, the Picker Institute and the Institute for Health Metrics and Evaluation (Commonwealth Fund, 2012; IHME, 2012; Picker Institute, 2012), as well as many others. A key advantage of publicly available international data from official sources though is that the involvement of countries in the definition and production of the data, and in their presentation and communication, also helps to ensure their subsequent acceptability and use by those public authorities; this is particularly important for sensitive comparisons such as for HSPA. This chapter will therefore focus on these principal official sources, while, of course, recognizing the valuable role of other sources in contributing to analysis of health systems performance more generally.

11.2 Background

Health systems are one of the core areas of national responsibility, and the role of all European and international organizations in this field is a supporting one. However, the potential for international comparisons to highlight issues and provide a basis for mutual learning has long been recognized, so there has been consistent interest in international data and comparisons, and a steady growth in action by international organizations to meet this need of their member countries.

Collecting and collating data on health has been part of WHO's global mandate since its establishment in 1948. For Europe, the WHO Regional Office for Europe hosts numerous health databases in the area of morbidity and mortality, communicable diseases, non-communicable diseases, environmental health, risk factors and health evidence. The best known among these databases is the Health For All database (WHO Regional Office for Europe, 2012a), which provides an overall dataset for health, with data for individual European countries going back to 1970, as well as specialized databases in other areas. The WHO Regional Office for Europe is currently establishing a single electronic access platform that will permit analyses of indicators across different databases.

Comparative data were at the heart of the origins of EU activity on health, with the Europe Against Cancer programmes. Health information and monitoring was part of the specific article for public health introduced in the EU treaties with the Maastricht Treaty in 1992 (Official Journal of the European Communities, 1992). The EU's statistical work is led by the EU statistical office, Eurostat (European Commission, 2012a), with additional work by the European Commission's directorates-general for Health and Consumers (European Commission, 2012c), and for Research and Innovation (European Commission, 2012d). The specific area of communicable disease is handled by the European Centre for Disease Prevention and Control (ECDC, 2012a), with its own legal provisions (Box 11.1).

The OECD's work on health data has similarly been growing over the past 25 years, initially starting with data collection on health expenditure and financing, being complemented with data collection on health care resources (human resources and physical/technical resources) and health care activities (OECD, 2012a). Since 2001, the OECD has launched a project on health care quality indicators to fill critical data gaps in this area, and its analytical work on different dimensions of the performance of health systems has expanded (OECD, 2012b).

All work on international comparative data faces similar challenges relating to: the differences in the organization of health systems between countries; the lack of shared definitions for even some of the most commonly used elements; problems of cross-population comparability of information (and difficulties in interpreting it); and the complexity of issues such as defining what constitutes 'good quality care' even within countries, let alone between them. Some of the efforts to overcome this and present comparisons of health systems at an international level have also revealed the complexities and risks of making international comparisons and, in particular, of attempting to reduce the complexity of health systems to single integrated indicators or ranks.

Despite these challenges, the progress that has been achieved is impressive, both in the scope of areas for which comparable international data on health are now available and in the degree to which comparability has been ensured. However, international data that would allow the kinds of comparisons of

Box 11.1 Communicable diseases: a model for data on health systems?

Communicable disease has been a priority area for European action on health information since the introduction of the Treaty article on public health in 1992. Unlike other areas of health data, which have been collected voluntarily, a specific legal provision was adopted by the EU in 1998 establishing a network for epidemiological surveillance of communicable disease and providing for rapid response to health threats (European Parliament and Council, 1998). On this basis, a set of disease-specific networks was established, putting in place agreed definitions and operational mechanisms for Europe-wide disease monitoring. This was followed by the creation of a specific agency – the ECDC – in 2005 in order to operate those specific surveillance networks and to identify, assess and communicate current and emerging threats to human health from infectious diseases more generally (European Parliament and Council, 2004). Its annual budget of over €57m and more than 250 staff (ECDC, 2010) is more than all the Commission's own resources for health data collection and communication combined, making this the clear focus of the EU's health data efforts.

Agreement was reached in 2008 on a framework regulation putting the collection of health statistics by the EU on a legal footing for the first time (European Parliament and Council, 2008). The first implementing regulation on causes of death was adopted in April 2011, and the Commission is preparing other implementing regulations covering other health data, which are expected to be adopted over the coming years. However, there is as yet no proposal for a similar agency to the ECDC to support this work in practice.

performance of health systems described in this publication have been one of the trickiest areas, being both technically complex and politically highly sensitive. Much therefore still remains to be done; this chapter will identify potential areas for development alongside the review of current progress.

11.3 Overall population health

The first challenge of international comparisons of health data has been to compare the overall health of populations – how long people live, when they become ill or die and of what.

Mortality and morbidity

Mortality statistics have been a core dataset for international health, with reasonable international comparability. Many countries track mortality data for their own domestic purposes, so the key challenge at international level has been focused on ensuring international comparability. Mortality and morbidity statistics are principally based on the ICD (WHO, 2012a). The establishment of the ICD as a common basis for comparable statistics has been a major achievement of WHO and earlier developers, and remains a key basis for comparable international data. For the EU, there is now a specific regulation (under the overall framework regulation described above) on causes of death statistics, on the basis of which a first collection of data took place in 2011.

In many countries, issues of timeliness, accuracy and level of population coverage of health information do still remain, even with this relatively well-established set of data. Although, in principle, data on mortality from the previous year should be available during the following year, in practice there are delays, meaning that the data available at any given time is typically from at least two years previously, and for some countries even further back (European Commission, 2012c).

There are, however, still countries in the European region that do not possess formal vital registration systems to systematically record and report causes of death and underlying diseases. Some countries have recently moved towards the establishment of such systems but still have low population coverage, particularly in rural areas. In other countries, vital events reporting is fragmented by being the responsibility of different governmental institutions, thus making the collection and reporting of information difficult and less reliable. Moreover, differences between countries (and indeed within countries) about how deaths are certified, recorded and allocated to the codes on which these statistics are based can be significant, and there are still some variations between countries in the overall systems being used (European Statistical Office, 2009). Steps are being taken to address these issues. For example, several countries are moving towards electronic systems for recording and collating deaths, which should also help to reduce the time and administration involved in providing mortality data. In addition, WHO, together with its partnership the Health Metrics Network, supports countries with a wide range of practical tools to assess and improve their health information systems and data (HMN, 2012). There are also collaborative initiatives towards improving the consistency and comparability of coding, such as the Iris project (now completed), which developed multi-language software for coding causes of death.

The current tenth version of the ICD is being revised, with the next iteration due by 2015 (WHO, 2012b). There are two key issues for continued comparability of data: continuity and clarity. To maintain comparability at an international level, it is vital to ensure that individual data series remain comparable over time. This does not prevent restructuring of the ICD, or indeed adding new codes, such as a code for *Helicobacter pylori* infection. For example, one major area of addition is in the field of rare diseases, where many new conditions will be properly integrated into the ICD for the first time, building on the work of Orphanet in particular (Orphanet, 2012a), and the logic of their integration may lead to some restructuring, such as adding a new chapter to the ICD on multi-systemic diseases. This need not create difficulties for international comparison, so long as there is a clear mapping of previous ICD codes onto the newer ones. Alongside this structural continuity, though, there remains the issue of clarity of interpretation. It is vital that definitions are clear enough that they can be understood and applied consistently in different countries if the resulting data are to be useful for comparison.

Development

In terms of future development, the key interest of policy is to know not just that somebody died, and of what, but *why*, which means being able to link this event to other factors. Given the substantial impact of inequalities on health, a key area for future development is to be able to link mortality data with socioeconomic data in order better to be able to compare progress towards addressing inequalities in health. There is already some analysis in this area, such as work by the European Commission linking life expectancy and educational level, which demonstrates a clear correlation with better-educated Europeans living longer (European Statistical Office, 2010). The OECD is also supporting the implementation of this methodology across the OECD countries. WHO has recently published an online atlas of health inequalities, based on existing data collections by Eurostat, which permits these analyses for 280 regions of countries in the EU. This tool allows and visually displays comparisons, including correlation analyses of health and non-health indicators (WHO Regional Office for Europe, 2012b). WHO is now working with countries outside the EU to participate in this effort.

However, a direct linkage of mortality data with socioeconomic status is not simply a question of passing additional data to the international level, as the mechanisms used for collecting mortality data at national level do not always include sufficient data about the person who died in order to be able to classify them by socioeconomic group. As countries move towards making the process of data collection electronic, enabling linkages between different types of data is one route through which this could be addressed.

Avoidable mortality

This brings us to the question of avoidable mortality. That people eventually die is inevitable; the key focus for policy and therefore for comparison is on deaths that could or should have been avoided. Within the context of HSPA, the focus is more specific still; rather than the potential for prevention through tackling health determinants (such as tobacco or alcohol), the key question is deaths that could or should have been prevented by health care system interventions, either through preventive or therapeutic efforts.

This has recently been assessed by a project on Avoidable Mortality In European Health Systems (AMIEHS, 2012), which evaluated the instances in which mortality can reasonably be considered 'avoidable' in the context of European health systems. Although this project made progress, the results suggest that identifying instances of 'avoidable' mortality in this way will require both more detailed analysis (e.g. linking to disease incidence and variations in quality of care within systems) and more detailed data (e.g. broken down by age, socioeconomic group and region, and linked to health care data), which suggests a need for further work if a set of indicators of amenable mortality is to be put in place.

If such indicators prove feasible, they could provide a basis for making existing mortality datasets more relevant for guiding policy. Since this calculation of avoidable mortality should be based on existing data on causes of death, it will have the advantage of effectively providing additional information for comparison with limited additional data collection by countries. Further investigation of this could be a priority area for HSPA.

Ill health and disability

The other key area which will be increasingly central to assessing the performance of health systems is the shift in patterns of ill health towards chronic conditions, which will make mortality data less useful as an overall indicator of population health. It will therefore become increasingly important to have data not only about deaths, but about ill health and disability as well.

At the aggregate level, when morbidity data are combined with mortality data, different measures of 'healthy life expectancy' can be calculated and reported. In estimating the global burden of disease, WHO uses the DALY (WHO, 2012c), which is a summary measure of population health, combining information on morbidity, disability and mortality, which is calculated using different sources of data, depending on condition, country and data availability. WHO also periodically calculates and reports an indicator of 'health-adjusted life expectancy', which measures the number of years a person can expect to live in full health, free from disease and disability. The EU has focused on 'healthy life-years', calculated through a combination of mortality data and self-reported limitations in activities, gathered as part of a Europe-wide survey on standards of income and living conditions (EU-SILC) (European Commission, 2012b). However, no matter which indicator is chosen, such aggregate composite measures of health involve some degree of choice about which data on health or disability status to use and how to value these different levels of health or disability status, and they are perhaps more useful in terms of their trends over time than in terms of their absolute levels.

More useful for policy would be comparable data about how the burden of disease is broken down among different conditions in different countries. WHO's Global Burden of Disease efforts are addressing precisely this issue but face huge data challenges at country level where modelling techniques are often used to describe disease patterns. The EU has started to explore the scope for pragmatic data collection based on simply using the best source available within different countries (even when these differ in their methodologies), but this has not been proceeding quickly due to a lack of resources at both national and European levels.

Tracer conditions

Given the size and complexity of putting in place comprehensive comparable data for HSPA, an interim option until such systems can be established would be to use tracer conditions, in order to give a cross-sectional picture of health systems. By focusing efforts more narrowly on key conditions, such as cardiovascular disease or diabetes, or rare diseases where comparable international data can shed light on wider processes, this could help to make detailed comparison both more feasible and possibly also more robust. This is probably best done through specific studies (including specific data collection) rather than through extending regular data collection. Such studies could, for example, be funded as part of health research, with specific requirements about data collection covering all appropriate countries.

11.4 Determinants, demographic and context

Health systems operate within different contexts, which affect how their performance should be assessed. In particular, HSPA needs to take account of the key determinants of health, especially those relating to preventable ill health. This reflects the Tallinn Charter (WHO Regional Office for Europe, 2012c), which states: "health systems are more than health care and include disease prevention, health promotion and efforts to influence other sectors to address health concerns in their policies" (paragraph 5).

The extent to which this is actually reflected in practice varies within countries. Nevertheless, including these broader elements in international comparisons of health system performance is important – it may indeed support action within countries to involve other sectors in promoting health where needed. In any event, the health system will be dealing with the effect of health determinants and, therefore, it is useful for HSPA to be considered broadly in this area.

Key determinants of health

WHO includes data on key health determinants in the Health For All database (WHO Regional Office for Europe, 2012a), such as the proportion of smokers, alcohol consumption and food availability, compiled from a variety of sources. The OECD similarly provides data on key determinants of health (OECD, 2011). For the EU, a more detailed list of indicators of determinants of health has been defined (which is included as part of the European Community Health Indicators) (European Commission, 2012e), covering issues such as body mass index, blood pressure, regular smokers, alcohol consumption, diet, physical activity and social support. However, although there has been much progress in the technical feasibility of collecting such data on a comparable basis across the EU (principally through specific surveys), in practice this list remains largely aspirational and providing regular and timely data for these indicators has been hampered by lack of resources.

The EU is also piloting a different approach of gathering data through examination involving a health professional (the *European Health Examination Survey*) (EHES, 2012) rather than through self-reported surveys. This has the potential to provide data that are more accurate and offer greater potential for analysis on a comparable basis, and thus to set the performance of different health systems in context more accurately.

Development

Historically, indicators on determinants of health have been focused on issues linked to individual behaviour and physical health – in particular, tobacco and alcohol use, diet and physical activity. However, two key additional determinants of health with a significant impact have become clearly identified in recent years, and determinants and indicators for these should be included in HSPA.

The first area for development concerning determinants is how these relate to health inequalities. The importance of the relationship between inequalities and social determinants of health has been recognized by WHO (WHO Regional Office for Europe, 2012d) and the EU (European Commission, 2009). The challenge for future development will be to integrate indicators that address the issue of inequalities, building on the expert work in this field. Part of this can be addressed through including an inequalities dimension in the indicators by also gathering socioeconomic data linked to existing health indicators. Some additional indicators addressing specific inequality issues may also be needed.

In its new European public health policy 'Health 2020' (WHO Regional Office for Europe, 2012e), the WHO Regional Office for Europe is addressing this issue. Based on a *European Review of Social Determinants of Health* and other commissioned studies, WHO together with its Member States is developing targets and indicators to measure progress in six major areas:

1. Governance for health and well-being;
2. Tackling the determinants of health and health inequalities;
3. Investing for healthy people (including well-being) and empowering communities;
4. Tackling systemic risk: the major burden of disease;
5. Creating healthy and supportive environments and assets for a healthy environment (including risk factors); and
6. Strengthening people-centred health systems.

These targets and indicators (around 12 in all) will be finalized by the next Regional Committee of Europe at its next session (RC62) in September 2012.

The second area for development is that of mental health and, closely associated with this, overall 'well-being'. Mental health has been increasingly recognized as constituting a major burden of ill health and as being substantially determined by factors outside health systems (Council of the European Union, 2011), including in many instances those linked to inequalities. Again, from a technical point of view, development in this area will depend on a combination of approaches, involving both the use of existing sources of data from other fields to provide indicators relevant to mental health (for example, linked to employment or justice) and the development of new indicators. In the area of 'well-being', the WHO Regional Office for Europe and numerous partners have embarked on an effort to quantify and set targets for well-being in the European Region. This will be reported on in 2013. However, the challenges in these fields are both technical and political, given sensitivities over both of these issues.

11.5 Health systems outcomes

The area of data about health outcomes is one of the most relevant, from a policy perspective, but also one of the most technically difficult to compare and the least developed.

Measuring outcomes

Before even considering comparability issues, there is a basic difficulty of defining what is to be considered a 'good' outcome in different cases and for different patients. Care providers have been understandably cautious about being compared on outcomes unless these can take into account the individual characteristics of the patient and their condition.

Ideally, data about the outcomes of health system interventions should be based on identifying individual patients and tracing them through the care process, in order to be able to see what happened and with what result, in the context of their particular condition and diagnosis – in other words, registry data. The leading field in which this has been achieved in a way that allows international comparisons to be made is cancer, and the impact of these data in bringing about widespread and fundamental policy changes across Europe has confirmed the power of such comparisons where they can be made (Coleman et al., 2008). Other areas can also provide similar comparable international data, such as for some rare diseases (Orphanet, 2012b). Comparable data are also required, for example, about communicable diseases within the EU (ECDC, 2012b). Such data remain the exception rather than the rule and continue to suffer from problems such as incompleteness of data and the lack of full capture of cases.

Health care quality indicators

An alternative approach has been to focus on a small number of indicators that could give an overall comparison of the quality of health systems. This has been the focus of the HCQI project taken forward by the OECD and co-financed by the EU (OECD, 2012c). These indicators address the process of providing care and a range of different outcomes (such as survival after cancer, heart attack or stroke). They have been the result of extensive international collaboration over at least ten years in order to develop indicators of quality that are both feasible and informative, and provide a good basis for comparison of quality between health systems.

Development

Principal burdens of disease

One obvious area for future development would be to amass better data for outcomes and quality indicators for the major burdens of disease – in particular, principal cause of death, key non-communicable diseases such as cardiovascular disease, and mental health (which, while both technically and politically tricky, represents a substantial burden of ill health).

The rise in chronic care also presents challenges for measuring outcomes that are not defined in terms of cure. There are different indicators of good care for some chronic conditions (for example, linked to deterioration or complications, some of which are already identified in the HCQI project), as well as the possibility of comparisons based on patients' own perceptions (see below). This area has been identified as a central challenge for health systems performance in the future (Council of European Union, 2010).

E-health – new types of data

The increasing implementation of ICT within health systems opens up an opportunity to gather data more efficiently and quickly, potentially including data that it has not been possible to collect at all on a large scale until now (at least not without prohibitive cost). Collecting data through registries, or similar means of tracking individuals through the health system, may provide the best data currently available, but this is inevitably complex to implement, generally requiring a dedicated data collection process alongside the actual process of care, as well as good linkages of different collection systems. However, information related to health care is increasingly stored and communicated electronically, and this creates the potential to gather data as part of the process of care itself.

This has substantial potential advantages. In principle, it could be both cheaper and quicker, and could also provide more sophisticated and better-linked data than much of the data currently available. However, there are also major challenges at a technical level, for example: how to extract data reliably from such sources and ensure that these data are sufficiently comparable; and how to ensure that the wide variety of systems already in place can be brought together for data purposes. There are also legal challenges: legitimate objectives of protecting people's personal data (and in particular their health data) have sometimes spilled over into obstructing the linking of data in a way that is still protected and manifestly in the public interest.

Nevertheless, this field holds the potential to fundamentally shift the way that data about health systems are collected, and this potential should be included in the objectives of ICT systems as they are introduced in health care and actions to support this, such as the next EU e-health action plan 2012–20 (European Commission, 2012f). There is scope for countries to work together in meeting both the technical and legal challenges outlined above, with work at the international level already underway within the European Commission and the OECD.

11.6 Patient experience

One important way of assessing health systems is to look at how well they perform from the perspective of the people they are intended to benefit. The traditional focus of health system data has been objective biological or administrative data, such as that described above. A different way of assessing performance is to ask patients themselves about their own perception of the performance of the health system through their experience of it, and to take this as an indicator of success.

This is, of course, a subjective perspective, although none the less real for that. Such data on patient experience can also help to provide insights into issues that are hard to measure in other ways, such as the responsiveness of the system, and the extent to which patients have been involved and engaged in their own care.

Comparability using such measures at the international level has its own issues, such as the extent to which variations reflect differences in experience or wider cultural differences. Nevertheless, this may be a useful area to explore for the future. It may be particularly relevant in providing indicators of success for chronic conditions, which will steadily become a more important area of health systems performance in the coming years. Recently, the OECD, in collaboration with the Commonwealth Fund, has tested a series of questions on patient experiences with ambulatory care on their use for international comparison.

11.7 Equity and variations

International comparisons of health system performance tend to focus on comparing the systems to each other at the country level. There are, however, important variations within systems that it is also important to reveal when assessing their overall performance.

Variations between people

The issue of inequalities has already been raised above with regard to determinants of health. An important part of addressing inequalities is to be able to compare the performance of health systems in meeting the needs of all their covered population, and thus to break down the performance of health systems according to other relevant attributes of patients, such as gender (which is already standardly the case wherever relevant).

The key issue here in Europe is the socioeconomic situation of users of health systems. There are already some data at EU level on unmet health care needs from the SILC survey, for example, aggregated by income and age. An ideal approach would be to link existing health data about users of health systems more generally to data about their socioeconomic status, in order to enable the benchmarks used for HSPA overall to be broken down by socioeconomic group. However, this is not straightforward as for many countries and data series it is not currently feasible to combine these two sources of data. Even where different data sources that could be combined from a technical point of view exist, this can be difficult legally due, in particular, to data protection rules (despite exceptions for statistics, health and research). Part of the ongoing work by international organizations concerning socioeconomic determinants of health should include looking at how to address these difficulties in the future.

In the short term, another approach is to use other sources to assess to what extent there is equal access to care. The OECD has used national health interview surveys (including those carried out as part of the first wave of the *European Health Interview Survey*) to assess income-related inequalities in the use of certain health services and to explore possible explanations, such as differences in the financing and organization of health systems (OECD, 2011). Future health interview surveys could be used to explore these issues further. Another approach could be to develop a specific longitudinal population cohort, broken down by socioeconomic group across different countries, and to track the performance of health systems in meeting their needs over time. If this could not be achieved across a full range of population and conditions, then again the concept of tracer conditions could be an interim solution, perhaps building on those areas described above where comparable registry data for Europe already exists.

Variations between regions

Another particularly European issue is that although international comparisons are historically made and compared between whole countries, in most European countries health systems are now primarily organized at regional level rather than at national level. Therefore, comparisons at national level without some regional breakdown are inherently limited in their utility, as they may – and do – conceal wide internal variation. This is clear from some of the data already described above, such as wide internal variations in health outcomes and costs, and has already been highlighted in some publications concerning regional variations, such as the EU's *Fifth Report on Economic, Social and Territorial Cohesion* (European Commission, 2010), itself drawing on Eurostat data, which already provides data at local (NUTS2) level.

This also underlines the utility of making such comparisons from a health perspective, as it provides a more specific evidence base for guiding investment within systems, and within the EU, at least, a potential additional argument for access to the EU structural funds to make those investments. Moreover, given that the underlying aim of international HSPA is to enable mutual learning, then it seems clear that such comparisons across the whole of the European region (53 countries, for the WHO) will need to develop a regional dimension.

In principle, there is no reason why this should be substantially more complex than for existing systems of nationally gathered data. After all, data are already collected across many countries (although this is not necessarily the case for everything – many countries either do not have disease registries or they do not cover the whole country). Rather than collecting different data, enabling regional comparisons can begin by simply sharing existing data at a sufficiently disaggregated level.

Some progress has already been made in developing and validating such regional-level comparisons, in particular through the ISARE project (ISARE, 2012) on regional health indicators, on which further work in this area could build. One key challenge will be to find better ways of presenting regional-level data and enabling meaningful comparisons, given that already comparing the large number of countries across the European region can make drawing conclusions difficult.

11.8 Financial protection

Related to the question of inequalities, one of the key objectives of EU health systems has been to ensure that health services are accessible to all, regardless of individuals' financial means.[2]

Some specific data are collected on the extent to which people find cost to act as a barrier to health care, and the cost of health care to them, in particular through the EU Household Budget and SILC surveys. This again is an area where the differences in the organization and administration of health systems between countries make comparisons difficult, as well as differences in expectations as to what constitutes normal access to health care.

One route towards a more detailed analysis would be to correlate information from social security and administrative sources (in particular, health insurers) and to identify the degree of financial exposure of individuals to health care costs from such data. This has proved difficult in the past, both technically in terms of combining the different data sources, and also in terms of the practical cooperation required between the different holders of data.

11.9 Inputs to health systems

One of the central elements of comparing performance is knowing what inputs are being made to the health system. Financial inputs have been one of the leading areas of international comparison and data collection. However, the key inputs affecting efficiency are staff and technology, and international data in these areas are less developed, although progress has been made.

System of Health Accounts

The core of international comparison of financial inputs to health systems is the System of Health Accounts (SHA), initially led by the OECD and now conducted in close collaboration with Eurostat and WHO (OECD, 2000). This is another area where countries do gather data for their own budgetary purposes; the challenge at international level has been focused on ensuring comparability. The enormous effort involved in achieving this illustrates the extent of variation between health systems, even in finding comparability for such superficially similar concepts as how much money is being spent and on what.

The SHA has also been one of the best examples of cooperation in health data comparison and has become an agreed tripartite system between the OECD, WHO and the EU (Eurostat), based on a single, shared data collection process. Since 2010, there has also been joint data collection between the OECD, the WHO Regional Office for Europe and Eurostat on non-monetary health care statistics (see next section).

Human resources for health and technology

Alongside money are the key inputs of human resources for health and technology; historically these have been less well compared at the international level. In the case of health personnel, this has principally been due to a lack of agreement about definitions of different types of staff, and also data sources that are focused on staff licensed to practice rather than those actually practising (the two numbers can be very different). Since 2010, a joint questionnaire between the OECD, WHO (Europe) and Eurostat has collected data on a range of health occupations, according to the concepts of: 'practising' (those providing care to patients); 'professionally active' (including both those who are practising and others who are working in health systems as managers, trainers, etc., although they may not provide direct care to patients); and all 'licensed to practice' (including those who may not actually be practising/ working in the system). Progress has already been achieved in data availability and comparability. The data collection is based, where possible, on the International Standard Classification of Occupations (ISCO-08). For the EU, at least, the definitions agreed for health professionals through the directive on mutual recognition of professional qualifications (European Parliament and Council, 2005) provide a common basis for comparison. Other work is being done in order to better understand issues related to health professionals (WHO Regional Office for Europe, 2012f), in particular regarding flows of health professionals from one country to another, which may also contribute to developing better data in this area. The collection of a minimum dataset on the international migration of health professionals may be included in future rounds of the joint questionnaire between the OECD, WHO and Eurostat.

The joint OECD/WHO/Eurostat questionnaire also includes a minimum dataset on diagnostic and therapeutic technologies (e.g. magnetic resonance imaging (MRI) and computed tomography (CT) scanners, radiotherapy equipment). However, although innovations in health-related technology and techniques have been central in driving both improvements and expenditure in modern times, calculating and comparing the contribution of these changes remains difficult. For example, reference estimates of the contribution of technology to overall changes in health system expenditure have taken the approach of calculating the effect of technology indirectly, as a residual after other effects have been accounted for, rather than measuring it directly (OECD, 2004). There are comparable data on major items of equipment, such as MRI units, plus some disease-specific analysis, but given the central contribution of technology to overall health system performance, this area remains a key challenge.

Development

Because these data tend to be collected through administrative structures, they are particularly influenced by the differences in organization between health systems. For example, detailed comparisons of expenditure for particular interventions have shown striking variations in health care treatment costs, but this requires detailed analysis of accounting issues, such as hospital overheads in different cases (Busse, Schreyögg & Smith, 2008). Planned development work for SHA includes estimating expenditure by disease. Given the variations that clearly exist, this is potentially a highly relevant area of performance comparison.

Another key area linked to performance of health systems will be the update of ICT, often described as "e-health". Given that a major objective for improving the productivity of health systems is better use of such technologies, developing better monitoring of their use in health systems would also seem to be a key priority for development. Proposals for improving comparability of data on e-health uptake through developing a 'model survey' have been outlined in the OECD–Commission project on the role of ICT in improving health sector efficiency (OECD, 2010a), and this could provide a basis for better comparability at international level.

One other growing indicator of health system performance concerns the phenomenon of people receiving care outside their own country, i.e. cross-border care. Although marginal in overall volume, this can be significant in specific regions or specialties. Eurostat already provides data on hospital discharges for non-residents, and the topic of cross-border care is also part of the planned future development of the SHA.

11.10 Efficiency

A shared priority for all health systems is efficiency; even if there are differences in resources allocated and priority areas, once resources are allocated to a goal they should be deployed as efficiently as possible.

However, making useful comparisons of efficiency is not straightforward. International comparisons can make macro comparisons about efficiency – in other words, compare the total amount of resources used and a global measure of health and health outcomes. But while this is good for newspaper headlines, it is not very helpful in guiding policy.

To be useful for policy purposes, comparisons of efficiency should be more focused on particular areas. For example, comparisons can be focused on: particular conditions or techniques, such as ischaemic heart disease (Moïse & Jacobzone, 2003); particular technologies (such as ICT, as discussed above); processes (such as health technology assessment (EunetHTA, 2012); improving coordination of care (Hofmarcher, Oxley & Rusticelli, 2007); or on the use of wider strategies, such as prevention (OECD, 2010b).

Such studies are complex and require significant resources, as well as depending on detailed data, which are not always available and are rarely straightforward to compare. However, they provide an insight into differences in efficiency of health system performance with sufficient precision to give a basis for practical responses and follow-up by policy-makers. This may be the best approach in this area, rather than focusing on developing further macro-level indicators of efficiency.

Diagnosis-related groups (DRGs)

As outlined above, efficiency is also a concern at the micro level, given the evidence of major variations both within and between health systems at the hospital level. Within many countries, DRGs are used as a mechanism to facilitate comparisons of costs and outputs between different providers. However, the DRGs used vary widely in their definition and implementation, and do not currently have a high degree of comparability at international level.

For the future, an EU-funded project is working to overcome this. The Euro-DRG project (Euro-DRG, 2012) is working towards providing a basis for hospital-level comparisons across European countries, focusing initially on twelve countries (Austria, the United Kingdom (England), Estonia, Finland, France, Germany, Ireland, the Netherlands, Poland, Portugal, Spain and Sweden). This potentially offers a way of achieving a sufficient level of detailed indicators to be a valuable basis for action, while still being broad enough that comparison at international level will be feasible.

11.11 Communicating and complementing international data

Even where comparable data that can enable HSPA exist, it is still essential to consider how best to interpret and communicate these data and what other information is needed to allow effective performance assessment.

Effective communication and reporting

Although this chapter has identified many areas in which more and better data are still required, much is already available. However, the full potential impact is not always achieved – sometimes available data are limited and/or generate comment and perceptions that are neither accurate nor helpful in improving health systems. How best to communicate assessments of health systems performance is not a trivial matter.

For example, although benchmarking and comparing performance in specific areas of detail with good comparable data can be useful, overall ranking of health systems in terms of some overall composite assessment of performance is rarely helpful, not least given the difficulties in drawing comparisons and differences in view of what 'good performance' means in any event. Yet, simply providing extensive volumes of data is also not helpful; data need to have some accompanying explanation to identify the key messages and issues they suggest in order to be effective. Accompanying examples and case studies are also powerful mechanisms in making abstract data more tangible. Formats combining these two elements, such as several WHO *World Health Reports* (WHO, 2012d) and the OECD *'Health at a glance'* series have proved particularly effective over time in communicating information effectively (OECD, 2011).

Two key challenges are how better to manage the complexity of inter-country comparisons (especially if a regional dimension is included), and how to make best use of more interactive information tools, such as those available in other areas (Gapminder, 2012).

Combining data with analysis

In any event, international data on HSPA have inherent limitations of variation and time lags in their production and can only be descriptive in nature. Such data are valuable, indeed vital, but not sufficient as an effective basis for policy. The effective translation of such and other information into policy remains a major challenge that goes beyond the scope of this chapter. Data need to be combined with analysis in order to provide a solid basis for action, with comparisons in data being used to identify areas that will be useful to study in more detail. These can then be analysed further through more detailed benchmarking of practices and detail on specific topics, as described in more detail in Chapter 4. Most importantly, countries need dedicated mechanisms for the translation of evidence into policy.

11.12 Priorities for future development

Partnership between international organizations

Historically, the different European and international organizations – principally WHO, the EU and the OECD – have gathered and developed data on health separately. These different systems had, and still have, somewhat different areas of mandate and concentration, reflecting the different mandates and responsibility of the different organizations. Each area of focus has its own unique value and, as they have each sought to respond to the challenges and needs of their member countries, these information systems have been working increasingly closely together to maximize synergies, avoid duplication and make best use of the limited funds available.

There are some examples where the information systems have already been brought together. In particular, as described above, the System of Health Accounts shows that an integrated tripartite system with a single data collection can reduce the administrative burden on member countries and make the best use of the resources of the international organizations themselves. Building on this success, the new joint questionnaire between the OECD, WHO (Europe) and Eurostat on non-monetary health care statistics has also helped to reduce the data collection burden on statistics regarding staff and technology, and is expected to be extended to cover health care activities in the coming years.

This also improves the credibility of the information provided; after all, when different international sources give somewhat different answers to what seem to policy-makers to be essentially the same question, the credibility of all those data sources is undermined.

The objective of working towards a single integrated information system for health in Europe was formally endorsed by the WHO European Region and the European Commission (WHO Regional Office for Europe, 2010) and work was begun by the two organizations in 2011. The OECD has membership which goes beyond the European region, but given the value already shown to all three organizations and their member countries by the tripartite agreement on the System of Health Accounts, there is clearly scope for all three organizations to work together towards this goal. This trilateral approach must be the most effective route to maximizing both the efficiency and the authority of international comparisons for health in general and HSPA in particular. Reflecting this, WHO has also invited the European Commission and OECD to partner with it in the development of a new European Health Information Strategy, which will be finalized by WHO Member States at the Regional Committee in 2013.

Development and improvement of data

From this review of the situation, although much has been achieved, there is much that still needs to be developed. Five areas in particular stand out: improving the coverage and quality of data; making existing data more relevant for policy; extending information coverage to other relevant issues; developing innovative methods to complement existing approaches; and improving the communication of data regarding health system performance.

Improving data and making them more relevant for policy

- Continuing development of internationally comparable data for avoidable mortality combining existing mortality data with analysis of avoidable mortality;
- Developing internationally comparable data for morbidity and disability;
- Extending data provision to international databases to include regional data in order to enable regional comparisons.

Identifying new indicators

- Developing specific indicators showing performance of health systems with regard to socioeconomic inequalities, building in particular on the work of the Commission on social determinants of health and the follow-up in Europe through the efforts of *Health 2020*.

Other areas that will also be important to address in the light of coming challenges include:

- Developing better specific indicators comparing the performance of health systems with regard to mental health, key non-communicable diseases and well-being;
- Implementing indicators for the application of ICT in health systems (e-health); and
- Developing indicators of health system performance in relation to chronic care.

Different methods to provide different insights

- Developing methods for using tracer conditions as an interim solution to provide a more detailed view of health system performance;
- Developing new methods for using data collected through e-health technologies, in particular data collected as part of the process of health care itself, to improve both efficiency and detail of data availability; and working together at the international level to meet the technical and legal challenges of doing so;
- Development of a Euro-DRG framework for benchmarking between providers; and
- In-depth cross-national studies comparing health systems efficiency in specific areas.

Better communication of health systems performance

- Piloting different reporting and communications formats and platforms for HSPA in order to develop empirical evidence about the most appropriate and effective mechanisms for communication and engagement with data, and to make best use of new technologies as they become available.

Notes

1 The author also wishes to thank Niek Klazinga and Gaetan Lafortune (OECD), Claudia Stein (WHO Regional Office for Europe), Stefan Schreck, Tuuli-Maria Mattila and Fabienne Lefebvre (European Commission) for their comments and suggestions on the chapter.
2 See Council conclusions on common values and principles in EU health systems adopted on 2 June 2006, OJ C 146, 22.6.2006, p.1.

References

AMIEHS (2012) *Avoidable Mortality in the European Union: Towards better indicators for the effectiveness of health systems*. Rotterdam: Avoidable Mortality in the European Union (http://amiehs.lshtm.ac.uk/, accessed 2 August 2012).

Busse, R., Schreyögg, J. and Smith, P.C. (2008) Variability in healthcare treatment costs amongst nine EU countries – results from the HealthBASKET project, *Health Economics*, 17(Suppl 1): S1–8.

Coleman, M.P. et al. (eds) (2008) *Responding to the challenge of cancer in Europe*. Ljubljana: Institute of Public Health of the Republic of Slovenia.

Commonwealth Fund (2012) Washington, DC: Commonwealth Fund (http://www.commonwealthfund.org/, accessed 17 July 2012).

Council of the European Union (2010) *Council conclusions: "Innovative approaches for chronic diseases in public health and healthcare systems"*. Brussels, 7 December 2010 (http://www.consilium.europa.eu/uedocs/cms_data/docs/pressdata/en/lsa/118282. pdf, accessed 2 August 2012).

Council of the European Union (2011) *Council conclusions on 'The European Pact for Mental Health and Well-being: results and future action'*, Luxembourg, 6 June 2011 (http://www.consilium.europa.eu/uedocs/cms_data/docs/pressdata/en/lsa/122389.pdf, accessed 2 August 2012).

ECDC (2010) *Annual Report of the Director*. Stockholm: European Centre for Disease Prevention and Control.

ECDC (2012a) Stockholm: European Centre for Disease Prevention and Control (http://ecdc.europa.eu/en/Pages/home.aspx, accessed 2 August 2012).

ECDC (2012b) *Surveillance*. Stockholm: European Centre for Disease Prevention and Control (http://ecdc.europa.eu/en/activities/surveillance/Pages/Activities_Surveillance.aspx, accessed 2 August 2012).

EHES (2012) *European Health Examination Survey*. Helsinki: National Institute for Health and Welfare (http://www.ehes.info/, accessed 2 August 2012).

EunetHTA (2012) Copenhagen: EunetHTA (http://www.eunethta.eu/, accessed 2 August 2012).

EuroDRG (2012) *EuroDRG Project: Diagnosis-related groups in Europe: Towards efficiency and quality*. Berlin: EuroDRG (http://www.eurodrg.eu/, accessed 2 August 2012).

European Commission (2009) Communication from the Commission to the European Parliament, the Council, the European Economic and Social Committee and the Committee of the Regions: *Solidarity in Health: reducing health inequalities in the EU*. (COM(2009)567 of 20.10.2009.) Brussels: European Commission.

European Commission (2010) *Fifth Report on Economic, Social and Territorial Cohesion*. Luxembourg: Publications Office of the European Union.

European Commission (2012a) Luxembourg: Eurostat, European Commission (http://epp.eurostat.ec.europa.eu/portal/page/portal/eurostat/home/, accessed 2 August 2012).

European Commission (2012b) *Healthy Life Years*. Public Health website. Brussels: European Commission (http://ec.europa.eu/health/indicators/healthy_life_years/index_en.htm, accessed 25 September 2012).

European Commission (2012c) *Indicators*. Public Health website. Brussels: European Commission (http://ec.europa.eu/health/indicators/policy/index_en.htm, accessed 2 August 2012).

European Commission (2012d) *Health Research*. Research and Innovation – Health website. Brussels: European Commission (http://ec.europa.eu/research/health/index_en.html, accessed 2 August 2012).

European Commission (2012e) *ECHI – list of indicators*. Public Health website. Brussels: European Commission (http://ec.europa.eu/research/health/index_en.html, accessed 2 August 2012).

European Commission (2012f) *eHealth Action Plan 2011–2020 public consultation*. Europe's Information Society website. Brussels: European Commission (http://ec.europa.eu/information_society/activities/health/ehealth_ap_consultation/index_en.htm, accessed 2 August 2012).

European Parliament and Council (1998) Decision No. 2119/98/EC of the European Parliament and of the Council of 24 September 1998 setting up a network for the epidemiological surveillance and control of communicable diseases in the Community. Luxembourg: Official Journal of the European Union.

European Parliament and Council (2004) Regulation (EC) No. 851/2004 of the European Parliament and of the Council of 21 April 2004 establishing a European centre for disease prevention and control. Luxembourg: Official Journal of the European Union.

European Parliament and Council (2005) Directive 2005/36/EC of the European Parliament and of the Council of 7 September 2005 on the recognition of professional qualifications. Luxembourg: Official Journal of the European Union.

European Parliament and Council (2008) Regulation (EC) No. 1338/2008 of the European Parliament and of the Council of 16 December 2008 on Community statistics on public health and health and safety at work. Luxembourg: Official Journal of the European Union.

European Statistical Office (Eurostat) (2009) *Health statistics – Atlas on mortality in the European Union.* Luxembourg: Office for Official Publications of the European Communities.

European Statistical Office (Eurostat) (2010) *Population and social conditions* (Eurostat, Statistics in Focus, 24/2012). (http://epp.eurostat.ec.europa.eu/cache/ITY_OFFPUB/KS-SF-10-024/EN/KS-SF-10-024-EN.PDF, accessed 2 August 2012).

Gapminder (2012) Stockholm: Gapminder (http://www.gapminder.org/, accessed 2 August 2012).

HMN (2012) *HMN Toolbox.* Geneva: Health Metrics Network (http://www.who.int/healthmetrics/tools/en/, accessed 2 August 2012).

Hofmarcher, M., Oxley, H. and Rusticelli, E. (2007) *Improved health system performance through better care coordination.* Paris: Organisation for Economic Co-operation and Development Publishing.

IHME (2012) Seattle, WA: Institute for Health Metrics and Evaluation (http://www.healthmetricsandevaluation.org/, accessed 17 July 2012).

ISARE (2012) Brussels: Indicateurs de santé des Régions Européennes Health Indicators in the European Regions (http://www.isare.org/projet.asp, accessed 2 August 2012).

Moïse, P. and Jacobzone, S. (2003) *OECD study of cross-national differences in the treatment, costs and outcomes of ischaemic heart disease.* Paris: Organisation for Economic Co-operation and Development Publishing.

OECD (2000) *A System of Health Accounts.* Paris: Organisation for Economic Co-operation and Development Publishing (http://www.oecd.org/health/healthpoliciesand data/1841456.pdf, accessed 25 September 2012).

OECD (2004) *Towards high-performing health systems.* Paris: Organisation for Economic Co-operation and Development Publishing.

OECD (2010a) *Improving health sector efficiency: the role of information and communication technologies.* Paris: Organisation for Economic Co-operation and Development Publishing.

OECD (2010b) *Obesity and the economics of prevention: fit not fat.* Paris: Organisation for Economic Co-operation and Development Publishing.

OECD (2011) *Health at Glance 2011: OECD Indicators.* Paris: Organisation for Economic Co-operation and Development Publishing (http://www.oecd.org/health/healthataglance, accessed 2 August 2012).

OECD (2012a) *OECD Health Data 2012.* Paris: Organisation for Economic Co-operation and Development Publishing (http://www.oecd.org/health/healthdata, accessed 2 August 2012).

OECD (2012b) *Health.* Paris: Organisation for Economic Co-operation and Development Publishing (http://www.oecd.org/health, accessed 2 August 2012).

OECD (2012c) *Health Care Quality Indicators.* Paris: Organisation for Economic Co-operation and Development Publishing (http://www.oecd.org/health/hcqi, accessed 2 August 2012).

Official Journal of the European Communities (1992) *Treaty on European Union.* Luxembourg: Official Journal of the European Communities (C 191, 29.07.1992).

Orphanet (2012a) *Orphanet: the portal for rare diseases and orphan drugs.* Paris: Orphanet (http://www.orpha.net/consor/cgi-bin/index.php, accessed 2 August 2012).

Orphanet (2012b) *Orphanet research and trials.* Paris: Orphanet (http://www.orpha.net/consor/cgi-bin/ResearchTrials_RegistriesMaterials.php?lng=EN, accessed 2 August 2012).

Picker Institute Europe (2012) Oxford: Picker Institute Europe (http://www.pickereurope.org/, accessed 17 July 2012).

WHO (2012a) *International Classification of Diseases (ICD).* Geneva: World Health Organization (http://www.who.int/classifications/icd/en/, accessed 2 August 2012).

WHO (2012b) *The International Classification of Diseases 11th Revision is due by 2015.* Geneva: World Health Organization (http://www.who.int/classifications/icd/revision/en/index.html, accessed 2 August 2012).

WHO (2012c) *Health statistics and health information systems: Global Burden of Disease* (http://www.who.int/healthinfo/global_burden_disease/en/, accessed 2 August 2012).

WHO (2012d) *The World Health Report.* Geneva: World Health Organization (http://www.who.int/whr/en/, accessed 2 August 2012).

WHO Regional Office for Europe (2010) EUR/RC60/12 Add. 1. Regional Committee for Europe, Moscow, Russian Federation, 13–16 September 2010 (http://www.euro.who.int/en/who-we-are/governance/regional-committee-for-europe/past-sessions/sixtieth-session/documentation/working-documents/eurrc6012-add.-1, accessed 2 August 2012).

WHO Regional Office for Europe (2012a) European Health for All database (HFA-DB) Copenhagen: World Health Organization Regional Office for Europe (http://www.euro.who.int/en/what-we-do/data-and-evidence/databases/european-health-for-all-database-hfa-db2, accessed 17 July 2012).

WHO Regional Office for Europe (2012b) *Equity in Health: Inequalities in health system performance and their social determinants in Europe.* Copenhagen: World Health Organization Regional Office for Europe (http://data.euro.who.int/equity, accessed 2 August 2012).

WHO Regional Office for Europe (2012c) *The Tallinn Charter: Health Systems for Health and Wealth.* Copenhagen: World Health Organization Regional Office for Europe (http://www.euro.who.int/en/what-we-do/conferences/who-european-ministerial-conference-on-health-systems/documentation/conference-documents/the-tallinn-charter-health-systems-for-health-and-wealth, accessed 2 August 2012).

WHO Regional Office for Europe (2012d) *Social determinants.* Copenhagen: World Health Organization Regional Office for Europe (http://www.euro.who.int/en/what-we-do/health-topics/health-determinants/socioeconomic-determinants, accessed 2 August 2012).

WHO Regional Office for Europe (2012e) *Health 2020.* Copenhagen: World Health Organization Regional Office for Europe (http://www.euro.who.int/en/what-we-do/event/first-meeting-of-the-european-health-policy-forum/health-2020, accessed 2 August 2012).

WHO Regional Office for Europe (2012) *PROMeTHEUS – Health PROfessional Mobility in THe European Union Study.* Copenhagen: World Health Organization Regional Office for Europe (http://www.euro.who.int/en/who-we-are/partners/observatory/activities/research-studies-and-projects/prometheus, accessed 26 September 2012).

chapter twelve

Conclusions

Irene Papanicolas and Peter C. Smith

12.1 Introduction

In 1997, Rudolf Klein wrote: "the cross-national exchange of ideas and experience in health care reform has, in recent years, reached epidemic proportions" (Klein, 1997). Fifteen years later the amount of information available on cross-country comparisons of health systems has grown even further – both in terms of the comparisons published by international organizations (such as WHO, 2000; Smith, 2002; Commonwealth Fund, 2006; Mattke et al., 2006; HCP, 2009; Mladovsky et al., 2009; Joumard, André & Nicq, 2010; OECD, 2010a, 2010b; Paris, Devaux & Wei, 2010; WHO, 2011) and in terms of the comparative studies published in the health policy and health services research literature (such as Reinhardt, Hussey & Anderson, 2002; Starfield, Shi & Mackino, 2005; Busse, Schreyögg & Smith, 2008; Kotzian, 2008; Busse et al., 2011; Schreyögg, Stargadt & Tiemann, 2011).

Early international health system comparisons (Goldmann, 1946; Mountin & Perrot, 1947; Roemer, 1960; Abel-Smith, 1963; Andersen, 1963; Abel-Smith, 1967) were motivated by an interest in cross-country learning and the application of these lessons to national policy (Nolte, Wait & McKee, 2006; Nolte et al., 2008). Yet, despite the proliferation of international comparison, and its continued promise for national improvement, there is concern that the useful exchange of knowledge and mutual learning is much less prevalent than might be expected (Klein, 1997; Marmor, Freeman & Okma, 2005; Nolte et al., 2008). Too often, international comparisons have been made in areas where there is convenient availability of routinely collected information, rather than in areas of policy importance. Moreover, comparisons can be misleading when not accompanied by an understanding, or explanation, of key differences in national settings, leading to the potential for important misinterpretations. Finally, just as comparisons can be used for information and learning to support constructive debate on national policies, so can they be misused, either knowingly or unknowingly.

In this chapter we aim to summarize the key lessons that have emerged from this volume on the state of the art in international comparisons across different performance domains. As more information becomes available to policy-makers, managers, patients and citizens, more guidance is necessary to understand what knowledge can be extracted from this information and how it can be used for improvement. By bringing together what we do and do not know about information available in each domain, we can better understand what can be gained from international benchmarks.

The chapter begins by emphasizing the role of a conceptual framework in international comparisons to clarify what is, and is not, being measured, and to enumerate possible endogenous and exogenous influences on attainment. We then examine the key lessons that have emerged from recent international comparisons, in conjunction with experience from other sectors, with a view to informing future progress. For each of the performance domains reviewed in this volume, we consider: the key challenges for comparison; what progress has been made towards performing better comparisons; and possibilities for further development. We conclude by bringing together lessons from all these areas to consider how to identify potential areas for improvement from international comparisons.

12.2 The role of conceptual frameworks in international comparisons

The objectives and focus of international comparisons of health system performance have varied. Some initiatives have attempted to evaluate the whole system, while others are restricted to a particular domain; some seek to evaluate the success of a particular reform in different settings, while others compare overall performance of key policy goals. Whatever the purpose of the comparison, given the diverse nature of national health systems, a conceptual framework is needed to provide clarity for the analytical, technical and operational thinking required to draw meaningful comparisons.

Chapter 2 reviewed the different types of frameworks that exist, noting that they can be for different purposes (Table 12.1). Depending on the framework adopted for the international comparison, different aspects of health systems will be compared. Some key areas that require attention from any operational framework are:

- identification of the boundaries of the health system;
- identification and clear conceptualization of final and intermediate health system goals; and
- identification of the key factors (within or outside the boundaries of the health system) that will influence the attainment of these goals.

In constructing the conceptual framework, it is essential to define the boundaries of what is being measured. A clear definition of boundaries will facilitate the specification of objectives, determine which indicators to include in the system, and how to interpret these for accountability and management purposes. Once boundaries have been set, the key objectives of the health

Table 12.1 Types of frameworks

Type of framework	What it is	International example(s)	When to use
Descriptive framework	Provides a basic description of the health system and the components it is made up of, yet does not explain why any particular health system would perform better than another.	Joumard, André & Nicq (2010); Thomson et al. (2011); Paris, Devaux & Wei (2010); Wendt, Frisina & Rothgang (2009).	To understand/compare the different structural and organizational features that make up a particular health system as well as the differences in national settings.
Analytic framework	Goes beyond describing what exists in a health system to also analyse the functional components of a system.	WHO (2000); Arah et al. (2003); Roberts (2008)	To understand/compare differential performance on final and intermediate goals and which factors may influence these.
Deterministic framework	Tries to determine what factors influence the performance of the health system, in order to identify which reforms, interventions or policies are most successful.	IHP (2008); WHO (2008)	To understand/compare differential performance of particular reform, interventions or policies on selected indicators of performance.

Adapted from: Hsiao & Sidat, 2008.

system should be identified and clearly defined. The framework should also reflect aspects of health system design, such as: the payment system; market structure; accountability and governance arrangements; IT infrastructure; and regulation. These factors may be useful in understanding underlying production processes that may contribute to good or bad performance, and may also be helpful in identifying the most suitable indicators for assessment and comparison. For example, if a DRG payment system is used, it may make sense to ensure that certain performance measures are consistent with the DRG codes so that provider performance can be linked directly with expenditure, in order to make judgements about efficiency (Smith et al., 2009). In international comparisons, in particular, it is likely that differences in national setting, as well as system organization and structure, will play an important part in variations (Box 12.1), and so recognition of these factors becomes even more important (Marshall et al., 2003).

When outlining the objectives of the health system, policy-makers should consider areas of high priority that are difficult to conceptualize and measure.

Box 12.1 Health system design – an important variable in international comparisons of health system performance

Most health systems share broadly similar goals (such as health improvement and responsiveness) and face similar challenges (such as ageing populations and rising costs), thus there is scope for mutual learning across countries. However, no two health systems are the same; health systems and health policy differ in every country with regards to the design of the health care system, the structure and organization of the functions that make up the health system (such as financing arrangements, input generation or service delivery), as well as the differences in national setting and patient populations. Thus, in order to be able to learn *what* findings can be translated across countries, and *how* to interpret variations in performance, it is necessary to understand how these features differ across countries.

There is little comparative work on health system design and setting, and part of the difficulty in carrying out such work is the pace of change due to new reforms. The most notable work in this area is carried out by the European Observatory on Health Systems and Policies through their Health Systems in Transition (HiT) series, which is periodically updated and carried out for many countries worldwide. Less work exists that systematically assesses performance with regards to health system design. Various classifications of healthy system design have been identified in the literature, which focus on identifying a group of similar institutional features, often relevant to financing structure, service delivery or welfare state design (Esping-Andersen, 1987; Bambra, 2005, 2007; Wendt, Frisina & Rothgang, 2009; Joumard, André & Nicq, 2010).

International comparisons lack consistent cross-country data on health care institutions as well as empirical characterizations of health systems. Some recent efforts have been made to address these areas, such as the work recently published by the OECD (Joumard, André & Nicq, 2010) and the Commonwealth Fund (Thomson et al., 2011). The former examines the links between policy settings and health care system efficiency, using the classification of countries; while the latter provides comparable overviews of cross-country data of 14 health systems.

Highlighting the importance of such areas in a framework can provide the necessary impetus to develop better measurement, which in turn can lead to increased awareness and improvement of the domain. Examples of such areas are responsiveness and efficiency. The concept of responsiveness, introduced in *WHR2000*, is now included in most frameworks. This, in turn, has driven enhanced data collection and analysis in order to make information in this area more readily available. The area of efficiency remains less developed, as there is still a lack of consensus concerning its conceptualization, and a lack of metrics to capture the concept adequately. Yet, recognition of the importance of system efficiency has led to increased research, which in time may provide more suitable solutions to this problem of measurement (Chapter 10). Benchmarking in all sectors frequently focuses on efficiency and cost reductions. Many of the most discussed international comparisons of health systems have attempted to compare 'value for money' across national health systems (WHO, 2000; Feachem, Sekhri & White, 2002). Given the current financial situation, this interest is likely to become more pronounced as countries seek to identify ways in which they can do more for less (or perhaps less for less) (OECD, 2010b). This makes the search for conceptual clarity and better indicators of efficiency particularly urgent.

In seeking to understand the link between performance on key objectives and system processes and characteristics, it is also important to take into consideration the dynamic nature of a health system. All health systems are dynamic entities; performance in one period will influence performance in other periods. Most outcomes of the system are a result not only of efforts put in the time period being measured but also from factors that operate with a time lag, such as behaviour over the lifecycle or previous contact with the health system. Likewise, physical resources, such as hospitals and medication available in a current period, are a result of investments made in previous years and will in part contribute to future attainment. Any framework should therefore, in principle, seek to capture the dynamic processes that make up the health system. Work in this area has hitherto been very limited.

One final consideration in the development of a conceptual framework for comparative purposes is the increasing need to harmonize national data with international practice and standardized definitions of indicators being internationally compared. International organizations can play a key role in leading this process and in providing guidance and tools that can assist in standardizing definitions and harmonizing data collection techniques.

12.3 Lessons learned from existing international comparisons

International comparisons in health and other sectors

There is great potential to learn from the successes and failures of past benchmarking exercises, both in health and other sectors. In Chapter 4, Neely makes the distinction between performance benchmarking (establishing performance standards) and practice benchmarking (establishing the reasons why organizations achieve the level of performance they do). Both types of benchmarking occur in international comparisons, yet the latter has been most prevalent in health (Berwick, 1996; Walshe, 2003). However, experience from other sectors suggests that it is practice benchmarking that leads to more policy learning and improvement.

Clearly, performance benchmarking and practice benchmarking are inter-related. Establishing performance benchmarks is often a prerequisite for understanding the underlying practices, but there are particular challenges to integrating performance and practice benchmarking, especially in the govern-mental sector. The primary challenge is that – for reasons of accountability and transparency – benchmarking in the public sector often becomes competitive. It frequently appears that benchmarking data are being used by government bodies to highlight how well they are performing relative to their peers, or by international or national bodies to promote a policy idea, rather than as a means of looking for ways to improve. This behaviour is also observed in international comparisons of health systems. The result is that responses to benchmarking become defensive – in the form of justifying policy choices or seeking to discredit the benchmarking analysis – rather than a constructive process of searching for new ideas and ways of working.

The successes and failures of *WHR2000* provide important lessons on how to conduct performance and practice benchmarking of health systems. While conducted as a practice benchmarking exercise, in the spirit of identifying which functions of health systems contribute to improved performance, the rankings presented by the report also created defensive responses towards the exercise itself. The Scientific Peer Review Group (SPRG) noted that summary rankings are more likely to capture the attention of key decision-makers and to promote action. The report's emphasis on system performance has indeed had a far-reaching impact amongst policy-makers and academics, and has had a catalytic effect on research into improving data collection and methodology for comparisons. However, the debate it generated was not always constructive, as countries sought to justify their own ranking. In contrast, it is noteworthy that the subsequent OECD performance framework (Hurst & Jee-Hughes, 2001) refrained from summarizing through a ranking exercise, and has instead provided a range of disaggregated comparative statistics for its Member States.

Some commentators have questioned the legitimacy of international organizations such as WHO undertaking HSPA. However, many nations have since expressed interest in collaborating with WHO to assess the performance of their own health systems, and to use this evidence to improve performance. Since 2000, the role of WHO and other international organizations in HSPA has been more clearly defined as global exporters of international standards. WHO has assisted many countries with developing frameworks for HSPA, often based upon the framework used in *WHR2000* (WHO Regional Office for Europe, 2012). As there was general consensus upon this framework, and the intrinsic and instrumental goals it defines, the principal debate in HSPA has been able to move from questions of 'what to measure' to 'how to measure it'.

As noted above, a persistent criticism of most international comparisons is that they provide only a static 'snapshot' of the health system, failing to capture the dynamic nature of health system performance discussed above, especially with respect to public health actions. Some developments have been addressed towards this issue, for example, in the field of tracer conditions and effective coverage (Box 12.2). However, we feel this aspect of HSPA remains underdeveloped both conceptually and practically.

International comparisons in performance domains

The data collection techniques and methodological tools used for performance measurement have developed considerably over the past decade. New and enhanced datasets have been developed, and are updated regularly. For example, the last decade has seen considerable development in the measurement of patient-reported outcomes, patient satisfaction measures and patient

Box 12.2 Effective coverage

Shengelia et al. (2005) define effective coverage as "the fraction of maximum possible health gain an individual with a health care need can expect to receive from the health system". Effective coverage has three main theoretical underpinnings: access; utilization; and effectiveness (WHO, 2001; Shengelia et al., 2005). Access refers to the availability, accessibility, affordability and acceptability of health services. Utilization serves as a sort of proxy for demand for health services, given access. Effectiveness is a function of several variables such as: efficacy of health care; the extent to which health interventions are available; inputs (quality and quantity of resources); quality assurance mechanisms; patient compliance and health behaviour; and external factors (i.e. socioeconomic and environmental factors). As an indicator, effective coverage can identify the effectiveness of current health system activities and the areas where more investment should be made in the future. It is a potentially important indicator in HSPA, as it is directly linked to the health system and can serve as an important contemporary measure of future performance.

The WHO (2001) consultation on effective coverage identified five different aspects of coverage that can be measured, to determine where problems lie in achieving effective coverage, and thus target policy accordingly. Each of these areas should be measured for various socioeconomic groups, recognizing that coverage tends to be lower for those with lower socioeconomic status (WHO, 2001):

Availability coverage:

- The proportion of people for whom sufficient resources and technologies have been made available;
- The ratio of resources to the total population in need;
- The proportion of facilities that offer specific resources, drugs, technologies, etc.

Accessibility coverage:

- The proportion of people for whom health services are accessible in terms of their distance or travel time.

Acceptability coverage:

- The proportion of people for whom interventions are acceptable (cultural acceptability, beliefs, religion, gender, etc);
- The proportion of people for whom health services are affordable.

Contact coverage:

- The proportion of the population who have contacted a health service provider.

Effective coverage:

- The proportion of people who have received effective interventions. The interventions for which effective coverage is measured should be chosen according to the following criteria:
  o Ability to produce a significant health gain in a short time;
  o The size of the health problem at regional, country and global levels;
  o Evidence of the effectiveness of a health intervention, and its credibility;
  o Correspondence to the national health priorities and policies, and objective needs;
  o Balance between different modalities of health care, preventive to curative, and between different types of illness: communicable, non-communicable, life-cycle related health conditions etc;
  o Cost–benefit ratio of obtaining information at the country level;
  o Ability to link the global processes with country priorities for the benefit of the latter.

The intention is that the measurement of effective coverage allows capacity-building opportunities that will enable the health system to improve future performance through informed decision-making and management. This indicator allows for a more comprehensive and dynamic assessment of the health system that can be more informative for comparisons than static indicators, which do not provide a clear understanding of what is driving good or bad performance.

Source: ECHO, 2001

experience measures. Indicators such as avoidable mortality, which seek to measure the contribution of health care to health, are also being better developed and more frequently used. Some indicators are now being selected through rigorous selection mechanisms that aim to identify how appropriate they are, rather than how readily available they are. In addition, risk adjustment techniques have become more advanced, and allow us to better control for exogenous factors that may lead to changes in performance. However, a challenge that remains for international comparisons is how to provide data in a way that it is better able to support policy decisions, i.e. are there better ways to collect, analyse or present data to inform national policy-makers on where potential improvements can be made?

This section summarizes the state of the art in the measurement of the key health system dimensions reviewed in this volume. It also highlights: the key methodological issues that have arisen when selecting indicators and analysing data; the progress that has been made; and the priorities for future work.

Population health

Population measures of health are useful for examining overall population health and the global burden of disease; however, they are influenced by many factors which lie outside of the health system, such as socioeconomic status or environment, and thus may not provide a clear picture of health system performance alone. Efforts have been made to combine these broad measures of population health with information on population morbidity, e.g. health- and disability-adjusted life expectancy. These types of indicators have been met with criticism on the grounds of methodological limitations, as well as the inherent value judgements they make, which may not capture the heterogeneity in perceptions of quality of life, or be representative across countries or people (Rosén, 2001; Anand et al., 2003). More recently, there has been considerable development of indicators that are better able to capture the contribution of the health system to population health through indicators such as avoidable mortality or tracers (Chapter 5).

Avoidable mortality (or causes of death that should be avoided in the presence of timely and effective health care) represents an alternative measure of population health that can be better attributed to the health system, broader public health policies and also changes in lifestyles (Nolte & McKee, 2004). As Figure 12.1 indicates, the relative performance of countries changes considerably when comparing amenable mortality (without ischaemic heart disease) to a more generic indicator of population health such as DALE. Indeed, in Figure 12.1, no country retained the same rank for both indicators, and 12 of the 19 countries evaluated dropped more than two ranks. This figure nicely illustrates the importance of boundaries in making assessments about health system performance.

While there has been considerable development in the range of population health measures, which allows better distinction between the contribution of health care and extraneous factors, progress is still required in order to make international comparisons more meaningful. Issues to be resolved include the availability and coding of data, particularly on cause of death where there is a lack of comparability across countries and over time. Coding is also influenced by changes between versions of the ICD and national coding rules, often reflecting whether automated coding is used or not. New developments in technology, such as EHR and multi-language software, will allow for better and more consistent coding across countries. Policy-makers looking to understand changes in the health status of their population should also make greater use of tracer conditions, by which the everyday experiences of those in need of care can be understood and addressed. The potential gains from relatively straightforward international standardization are considerable.

Yet, not all of the problems facing population health indicators may have a ready solution and so what is important is to understand these factors and to take them into account in interpreting data, particularly in the context of comparing health systems. Some of the most important issues to consider in the interpretation of data relate to the difficulty of attribution, not only as regards other factors that can influence health status, but also in distinguishing changes in the ability of the health system to prevent death once disease has occurred from changing the incidence of that disease, thus complicating attribution. Moreover, observed changes in mortality from particular causes can reflect changes in any one, or a combination of, innovation, coverage or quality. These can be difficult to distinguish. Finally, in the analysis of national policy, it is important to consider the varying, and often diffuse, lag periods

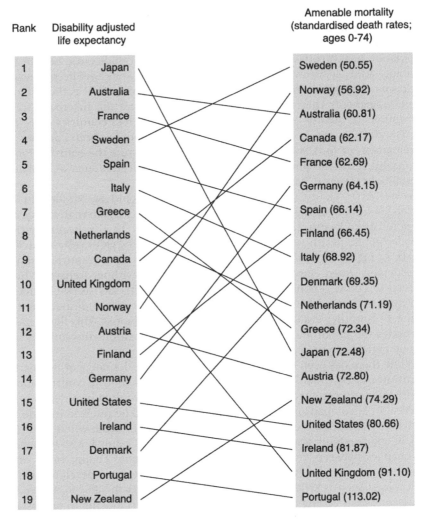

Figure 12.1 Country rankings for DALE and amenable mortality
Source: Nolte & McKee, 2003.

between the introduction of a policy or treatment innovation and a change in outcome.

Health services outcomes

Many international comparisons of health system performance are interested in the value added by different health services or health service outcomes. Table 12.2 summarizes the broad areas of services under consideration, and the comparability considerations to which they give rise. Internationally, one of the key sources of comparable data in this area is made available by the OECD,

Table 12.2 Main indicators for health service outcomes

Main indicators	Policy uses	Limitations
Hospital outcome indicators: e.g. HSMRs, case-fatality rates for AMI and stroke, patient safety indicators and hospital readmission rates	Hospitals are considered by many policy-makers to be the epicentre of the health care system – these indicators consider the contribution hospitals have to health outcomes over time.	HSMRs do not account for preventable deaths and the observation that a majority of deaths are unavoidable. Differences across hospital systems and records make comparability across hospitals and countries difficult. Lack of data collection at the individual level and lack of supporting information for which to case-adjust indicators pose issues for reliability and comparability of indicators. Readmission indicators pose problems of comparability due to different definitions of time frames and type of readmission investigated as well limitations in case-mix. More information is needed to determine the actual relationship between readmissions and the quality of care.
Patient-reported outcome measures (PROMs): e.g. SF36, EQ-5D	PROMS are useful as they are not only able to capture and regularly assess aspects of health that are of most concern to patients but are argued to be essential for the assessment of patient need and communication between patient and provider in routine care.	Individualized instruments are very time-consuming and often involve complex interviews. Uptake largely hindered by comparability issues, especially in content validity and the relative importance of different criteria. Questionnaires are considered costly and time-consuming. May be regarded as 'soft information' by some stakeholders.
Indicators for long-term care: e.g. process indicators, client experiences, nursing-related outcomes (bed sores, patient falls), outcomes of targeted illnesses (diabetes, dementia, etc.).	Measuring the quality of long-term care services is of high importance given the global ageing population trend and the present morbidity and disability patterns associated with chronic diseases.	Complexity of chronic care and the different levels and settings of service provision hampers the identification of possible quality indicators, and creates difficulties in standardized data collection and reporting conventions. It is hard to pinpoint medical outcome measures to the performance of long-term care institutions; as a result, nursing-related indicators are usually the only ones used. Outcomes of targeted illnesses (such as avoidable admissions for diabetic patients) may be as much an indicator for other areas, such as GP or specialist care.

(Continued)

Table 12.2 Main indicators for health service outcomes (*Continued*)

Main indicators	Policy uses	Limitations
Indicators for primary care: e.g. avoidable events, preventable admissions, process indicators	The significance of primary care lies in its effectiveness in preventing illness and death, and in its association with a more equitable distribution of health in populations.	The wide variation in payment and contractual organization for primary care services across countries inevitably translates into differences in the scope of data collection possible. Despite progress in the international collection of data, the most robust source for deriving indicators in primary care remains hospital administrative data; this does not provide a complete assessment of a primary care system's quality of care. Collection of data on avoidable admissions and adherence to processes relating to specific clinical areas (e.g. diabetes, asthma, COPD) is sufficiently relevant to policy and scientifically sound for potential use in international data collection but still of limited availability across countries.
Indicators for mental health: e.g. unplanned schizophrenia and bipolar disorder readmission rates	Mental health problems are common, affecting all sections of society and every age group.	Variation of organization across countries makes the assessment of the quality of mental health care services for evidence-based policy difficult. The availability of national indicator data suitable for international comparison is extremely limited due to: the complex nature of mental health disorders; differences in diagnostic and therapeutic practices; institutional government barriers; as well as differences in the coding and reporting of mental health care within and between countries.
Indicators for preventive care: e.g. screening rates	Screening is of great interest to policy-makers because of the significant bearing it may have on survival prospect.	There are many methodological issues relevant to the data collection for and comparability of cancer screening indicators in combination with other cancer outcome information, such as five-year survival rates and cancer mortality rates, including: data sourcing (e.g. surveys vs registries); heterogeneity in cancer survival and screening reporting periods; age standardization; the extent to which country data are nationally representative; and perhaps most importantly, a lack of cancer staging data.

AMI: acute myocardial infarction; COPD: chronic obstructive pulmonary disease; HSMRs: hospital standardized mortality rates; PROM: patient-reported outcome measure.

Adapted from: Chapter 6.

through their Health Care Quality Indicators project, initiated in 2001 with the long-term objective of developing a set of indicators that could be used to investigate the quality of health care across countries using comparable data (Mattke et al., 2006). In the conceptual framework defining the project, quality is defined as "the degree to which health services for individuals and populations increase the likelihood of desired health outcomes and are consistent with current professional knowledge" (Kelley & Hurst, 2006). The indicators available consist mainly of process and outcome measures for the most important disease, risk and client groups at the population level, and their preventative, curing or caring interventions. There are limited data available, both nationally and especially internationally, to evaluate morbidity outcomes, and this is seen as the key issue needing attention in the years to come, especially given the increasing incidence of mental illness, chronic conditions and multiple comorbidities across the world.

Further development in measuring health outcomes is conditional on the enhancement and expansion of current data sources. There have been some initiatives to explore the potential for better utilization of existing data for policy improvement through linkages, both at the national and international levels, such as the PERFECT, EuroHOPE and ECHO projects (Box 12.3). This will usually require: the availability of good patient-level data; further use of UPIs to link various data sources; the use of secondary diagnoses codes, present-at-admission codes and standardization of procedure codes, to increase the potential for case-mix adjustments for outcome measures; and the further development and testing of new measures such as resident assessment instrument (RAI), PROMS and other measures that can use EHR and patient surveys as their main data source. Contingent on privacy and data protection regulation, and supported by the necessary R&D to test reliability and validity, health outcome measures, capturing health services outcomes, will become an increasingly important part of HSPA. Chapter 11 considers these in more detail.

Equity

Equity in health care is a goal embraced by most industrialized countries, and is recognized as an overarching objective that spans the health dimension in most conceptual frameworks. Yet, any attempt to measure and compare equity across health systems requires careful definition of the precise equity concept under scrutiny. The literature on equity in health is often focused either on equity in health status (*substantive equity*) or on equity in treatment within the health care system (*procedural equity*) (Aday, Begley & Lairson, 2004). The measurement requirements and challenges, as well as the potential policy implications, are very different in these two areas (Table 12.3). Large improvements in international comparisons of equity, both substantive and procedural, can be made through improvements in availability and quality of population health and health service outcome data. Most notably, efforts to link various databases, such as those described in Box 12.3, will provide policy-makers with more information as to the source and extent of inequities both within and outside the health system. Future developments on the collection of morbidity data, as

Box 12.3 PERFECT, EuroHOPE and ECHO projects

The following research projects have explored methods to create databases for comparative performance within and across countries. Using registry data for selected conditions, and linking data across different points in the treatment pathway, these projects are able better to understand why variations in health services outcomes occur and how to direct policy towards improvement.

PERFECT

The aim of the PERFECT project is to develop performance indicators that can be used for the assessment and evaluation of health policy. These data can be used to create regional hospital-level benchmarks that allow policy-makers to evaluate the entire episode of patient care (Figure 12.2) for selected conditions, and thus understand and learn from best practices. The episode of care refers to the entire treatment from the beginning of the disease to the end of treatment over any organizational boundaries. Part of the difficulty, but also the strength, of this approach involves collecting and linking the data from different registries that capture the events and outcomes occurring at each point in the treatment episode. This includes: population-level data from all producers of specialized health care; data on care of the elderly; prescribed medicines; cost data; and death statistics.

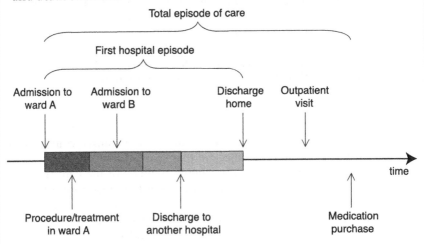

Figure 12.2 An example of events within an episode of care

Source: Peltola et al., 2011.

The project was undertaken in Finland, using Finnish registries for selected conditions with sufficient significance in terms of costs and disease burden and where specialized medical care plays a key role (stroke, hip fracture, low-birth-weight infants, breast cancer, schizophrenia, AMI, and hip and knee replacements). The evaluation and monitoring of conditions using this approach provides useful information for benchmarking and performance assessment and evaluation. For example, the evidence from the hip analysis indicates that the details of the surgical treatment of hip fractures are not nearly as critical in terms of effectiveness as the multidisciplinary rehabilitation phase. Indeed, the results of this study were used to update the care guidelines for hip fracture treatment in Finland.

Sources: Häkkinen et al., 2011; Peltola et al., 2011; Sund et al., 2011.

EuroHOPE

The EuroHOPE project is the successor to the PERFECT project, beginning in 2010 and funded by the EU FP7 programme. It aims to extend the methodology used in the PERFECT project to other European countries (Finland, Sweden, Scotland, Italy, Netherlands, Norway and Hungary) in order to evaluate the performance of European health care systems in terms of outcomes, quality, use of resources and costs. One of the key aims of the project is to develop methods for international comparisons, using the PERFECT methodology that allows for routine evaluations using registry data. This will allow clear improvements to be identified across and within countries, and facilitate cross-learning.

Source: EuroHOPE, 2012.

ECHO

The ECHO project derives from the Spanish Atlas VPM Project. This project was a nationwide health services research (HSR) programme concerning the analysis of unwarranted regional variations in medical practice and health care outcomes in Spain. The idea was to use the study of these variations to provide national policy-makers and managers with information that could be used for health service improvement.

In order to facilitate this process, the project collected patient-level hospital data from the various regional authorities and made them available to policy-makers, managers and other stakeholders through a central database on the Atlas website where they could conduct research on key issues themselves. The project team also conducted research on issues such as unwarranted variations in general surgery, orthopaedics, paediatric hospitalizations, cardiovascular procedures, mental health hospital care, oncologic surgery, avoidable hospitalizations, C-section rates, and patient safety or mortality in cardiovascular procedures.

In 2010, European FP7 Funding was obtained to repeat the project on a European scale, to bring together national hospital databases of several European countries, in the form of the ECHO project. Participating countries include: Spain, Portugal, Slovenia, England, Denmark and Austria.

Source: ECHO, 2001.

Table 12.3 Main indicators for equity

Main indicators	Policy uses	Limitations
Substantive equity		
Equity in health outcomes: i.e. distribution of health amongst different groups. Constructed from indicators of health status and socioeconomic variables.	The main goal of the health systems would be to decrease the gap between health outcomes that are systematically related to socioeconomic status and, hence, focusing on reducing socioeconomic inequalities in health outcomes is the usual performance measure in the health systems. There is also substantial evidence on inequalities in health across many population groups (region, ethnicity, gender, language).	Measures are limited by the availability of outcome indicators available, as well as their linkage to socioeconomic variables. Numerous surveys include outcome and socioeconomic information but the reliability of subjective measures of health status raises important methodological challenges that relate to the potential reporting bias that could appear. Longitudinal data are lacking, especially for a comparative analysis making it difficult to understand changes over time. Objective measures, such as physicians' assessments or hospital stays, are best for comparative purposes. However, the availability of objective measures of health, such as biomarkers, is limited. Biomarkers may still be subject to bias and are not included in longitudinal data. Standardization of biomarker data collection across countries is also an issue.
Equity in access or utilization: i.e. distribution of access or utilization of health care for equal amounts of need amongst different groups. Constructed from indicators of access, utilization, need, unmet need and socioeconomic variables.	The main focus of equity of access or utilization is to measure whether individuals with the same level of need are receiving the same level of health care.	Often the terms access and utilization are used interchangeably, implying that an individual's use of health services is proof that he/she can access these services. However, utilization is not equivalent to access. Utilization and need are often captured by survey information, which can suffer from reporting bias as well as comparability issues across countries. Few data are collected longitudinally, and there are large gaps on data to inform on environmental factors.

Equity in financing: i.e. distribution of financing of health care amongst different groups. Constructed from indicators of expenditure and income.	The main focus on equity of financing is to determine whether the health system is progressive (namely, how much larger payments are as a share of income for the poor than for the better-off).	The tabulation of average incomes and health care payments by income groups has been used in the literature. However, this methodology is not able to establish how much more progressive one system is than another.
Equity in responsiveness, i.e. distribution of responsiveness amongst different groups. Constructed from information on responsiveness and socioeconomic indicators.	Responsiveness of the health care system has been defined as the extent to which health services are aligned with user preferences in domains such as patient autonomy, choice and quality of amenities. Equity in this area considers the distribution of this health system goal across groups in the population.	There is still a lack of clarity on what is meant by responsiveness, resulting in numerous different, conflicting measures within and across countries.

Adapted from: Chapter 7.

well as the wider availability of longitudinal information across all areas, will yield a better understanding of the nature of inequities, whether they persist over time and how they are influenced by policy changes both within and outside the health system (Chapter 7).

Financial protection

While procedural equity takes into account the extent to which financial barriers to access exist within a health system, the area of financial protection in health is often studied as a distinct policy concern. It is concerned with the extent to which households are protected from the risk of becoming impoverished as a result of expenditure on health care. This area has received considerable policy attention and development of thinking in the past decade; *WHR2000* identified it as one of the main objectives of any health system (WHO, 2000) and in 2010 it was the topic of the *World Health Report*, which emphasized the need for all health systems to move towards universal coverage (WHO, 2010). Evidence suggests that, while many high-income countries have sought to address this issue through the introduction and strengthening of universal health insurance, variations in measures of financial protection between countries and over time persist (WHO Regional Office for Europe, 2009). Moreover, the issue is far more acute in many lower-income countries, where there is massive variation in the extent to which households (especially the poor) enjoy some degree of financial protection.

The main indicators used to measure financial protection in health are based on people's out-of-pocket expenditures on health care and their relation to some income threshold (Chapter 8). The simplest of these is the percentage of out-of-pocket payments for care in any given country. While this gives some indication of the lack of coverage of health care by the system, it does not provide any information about who is making these payments, whether they are for necessary care, and what impact they have on household income. Thus, two other indicators have been developed that are able to relate a household's out-of-pocket spending to a threshold defined in terms of living standards in the absence of the spending: the first defines spending as catastrophic if it exceeds a certain percentage of the living standards measure; the second defines spending as impoverishing if it makes the difference between a household being above or below the poverty line (Wagstaff, 2009).

While such indicators are better able to capture the extent to which payments in health care influence household income, they too are limited in what they measure. There is a notable gap in the measurement of the long-term effects that may arise, especially if households have borrowed money to pay for health care, or have lost earnings due to ill health. Furthermore, a lack of financial protection may inhibit some people from seeking appropriate health care when they are sick. Yet conventional measures of financial protection will not suggest any catastrophic implications for people denied access in this way. A priority for future work is to integrate indicators of financial impoverishment due to illness with indicators of poor health caused by financial barriers to access to health services.

Finally, to best assess the above indicators of financial protection, it is important that policy-makers have a good understanding of the organization of the health system being assessed, especially with regards to its financing arrangements (Box 12.4), as well as any relevant reforms. This is crucial to understanding why financial protection is unsatisfactory, and designing mechanisms for improving the situation.

Box 12.4   Financing arrangements in health systems

The WHR2000 categorized the financing function of health systems into the following: collection of funds; pooling of resources; and purchasing of services. While this categorization was generally met with approval, it was felt that metrics should be created in order to generate objective evidence in this area that would allow policy-makers to determine the effectiveness of different financing mechanisms in achieving the overarching health system goals (Anand et al., 2003). Through a series of consultations and technical work WHO, together with feedback from the SPRG, proposed a set of potential indicators to measure how well the system collects, pools and allocates funds to service provision (Table 12.4).

Table 12.4 Measurement of financing function

Revenue Collection

- Formal sector share of GDP;
- Natural resource revenues as a share of total public sector income;
- Public sector expenditures as a share of GDP;
- External health sector aid as a share of total public health expenditure;
- The share of public health expenditures in total public expenditure;
- Total health expenditure (per capital level and share of GDP);
- The share of total health expenditures that are pre-paid (as against those which are paid out-of-pocket at time of service).

Pooling

- Mean and concentration index of share of co-payments to total health expenditure in each pool;
- Mean and concentration index of membership in each pool;
- Mean and concentration index of per capita spending in each pool.

Purchasing

- Number of purchasers;
- Means and distribution of total expenditure across purchasers;
- Mean and distribution of the number of providers who are contracted or hired by each purchaser;
- Share of total funds allocated by inputs (e.g. salaries and traditional budgets), outputs (e.g. fee for service), and outcomes (e.g. capitation).

Adapted from: Anand et al., 2003.

While these indicators provide a starting point, the SPRG recommended further research and development of indicators and suggested the incorporation of further measures in the following areas of financing:

- A minimum threshold of funding for the health sector, if there is one;
- The costs of revenue collection;
- The size of the uncovered population (people who do not belong to any pool or who are eligible for free public service);
- The progressivity of the financing system;
- The differences in benefit packages between pools;
- Information on risk distribution amongst pools;
- Information on overlapping pools;
- Incentives generated by payment mechanisms that influence the costs, quality, amount and type of health service provided;
- Information on the transparency and accountability of the financing function;
- The source of funds, including external aid;
- Incentives for research vs. policy guidance;

Links to other goals, such as provision, coverage and responsiveness.

Patient experience

There remains a lack of conceptual clarity as to what the concept of patient experience encompasses and this domain is therefore underdeveloped. It can embrace concepts as diverse as timeliness and convenience of access to health care; treatment with consideration of respect and dignity; and attention to individual preferences and values. Moreover, there is interest not only in the absolute level of responsiveness in a system, but also in how it is distributed amongst different groups in the population.

WHR2000 highlighted the importance of this domain through the introduction of the concept of 'responsiveness' (Murray & Frenk, 2000). Responsiveness captures aspects of patient satisfaction and acceptability on the one hand and patient experience on the other, highlighting the need for distinct areas for measurement. Measurement initiatives have included the subsequent *World Health Surveys* and the work of (amongst others) the OECD, Commonwealth Fund, the European Union and the Picker Institute. These have provided useful information on cross-country comparison, but their diversity of approaches highlights the need for international harmonization before robust comparisons can be made.

Given the subjective nature of patient experience and patient satisfaction, the main sources of information for this are patient or general population surveys. It is important that the sampling frame is consistent across countries (for example, an inpatient survey might pick up different subsets of the population if countries have different policies on disease treatment). There is also a need to address possible response biases for respondents from different countries, for example, if expectations vary systematically between countries. Tools such as anchoring vignettes show promise in correcting for these variations.

Finally, it may not always be clear how to interpret cross-country benchmarks of patient satisfaction or patient experience. High patient satisfaction in one country might signify something quite different from high satisfaction in another (Box 12.5), depending on national norms and expectations. Comparisons of performance across countries, and the associated policy inferences, should therefore be undertaken with great care.

Efficiency

While efficiency and productivity are major areas of interest in both national and international comparisons, clarity on conceptualization and measurement in these dimensions is less developed than most other areas of performance assessment (Chapter 10). The core idea of efficiency is easy to understand in principle – maximizing output relative to input – yet it often becomes more

Box 12.5   Interpreting performance information across settings

What do high patient satisfaction rankings tell us about overall health system performance?

In early 2012, two studies were released examining how patient satisfaction was related to other outcomes in a hospital setting. In February 2012, a team of researchers investigating English data found that hospitals with better patient ratings were hospitals with lower death and readmission rates (Greaves et al., 2012). A month later, a team of researchers investigating United States data found that higher patient satisfaction was associated with higher use of health care and increased mortality (Fenton et al., 2012).

These conflicting findings pose problems for the interpretation of patient experience information across countries – is high patient experience indicative of good or bad performance? However, it is quite possible that the variation observed between the two studies is related to the very different health system structures – suggesting that performance information should always be considered relative to national setting, and not independent of context. Indeed, Fenton et al. (2012) suggest that a possible explanation for the negative association between patient satisfaction and mortality in their study is that the health care marketplace in the United States puts considerable emphasis on patient satisfaction scores and online reviews. Thus, physicians are eager to please their patients and may be acceding to more patient requests for tests, treatments and medication than they would otherwise.

In order to make international benchmarks more meaningful for national improvement, it might therefore be more meaningful to compare countries with similar health system structures and to provide some initial indication of what different levels of performance are likely to be associated with.

difficult to define when applied to a concrete situation. The production process underlying health systems is intrinsically complex and poorly understood, making it difficult to develop measures that reliably capture efficiency. International comparison is especially challenging, given the variations in what is considered to fall within the boundaries of a 'health system'. Combined with key gaps in data availability, the scope for misleading and contested comparisons is evident (Black, 2012).

In its broadest form, health system efficiency seeks to assess attainment on all the individual domains of performance discussed above in relation to the resources consumed. Given the challenges in each of the domains, it is hardly surprising to find that initiatives such as *WHR2000* give rise to such controversy. In particular, a significant element of many health system outcomes is attributable not to health system interventions but to external factors (social capital, income levels, environment, or the work of other agencies) and also the result of the combination of health system actions over a number of years, which cannot be attributed to the inputs in a single period.

Satisfactory measurement of whole system efficiency therefore relies on resolution of many issues in individual performance domains. For this reason, it may be the case that – for the foreseeable future – a more feasible and useful strategy might be to examine efficiency by scrutinizing the operation of specific parts of the health system. For example, indicators such as the average 'length of inpatient stay' have been collected in many settings over a long period. Of course, the use of such metrics requires considerable analytic care to ensure that like is being compared with like – some countries might treat a larger proportion of patients outside the hospital setting. Approaches such as the Health Basket patient 'vignettes' might offer some scope for standardization, particularly if they can be extended to situations outside the hospital setting.

While efficiency measurement at the health system level is extremely useful for international comparisons, the methods necessary for robust measurement still need refinement before they can be used to inform policy. More work needs to be done to refine the methodologies used for measurement, as well as to provide good quality and comparable data on the outputs, inputs and environmental factors necessary for risk adjustment. In the meantime, it is important for policy-makers to find a balance between whole system measures and more fragmented efficiency measures, especially given complex and variable production processes within and across countries. Efficiency measurement at different levels of analysis can be very informative for international comparisons, particularly through a focus on disease costing or programme budgeting, which allows comparisons to focus on a similar process across health systems (Box 12.6).

12.4 Using international comparisons for improvement

If undertaken carefully, health system performance comparison offers a powerful resource for identifying weaknesses and suggesting relevant reforms. The progress that has been achieved is impressive, both in the scope of areas

Box 12.6 Using diagnostic-related groups (DRGs) for efficiency
comparisons

DRGs were initially designed as a classification tool, proposed by Robert
Fetter and colleagues in 1980, as a way of comparing and controlling
hospital costs (Fetter et al., 1980). The basic idea is that by dividing
patients into diagnostic groups, which are weighted according to factors
influencing the cost of treatment, relative case groups can be constructed
to reflect the difference in the resource utilization of hospitals. These
variations can be indicative of differential efficiency across providers and
thus direct policy-makers to areas where they can improve performance,
but also areas of best practice where potential efficiency gains can be
identified.

In 1983, DRGs were used to form the basis of Medicare and Medicaid's
Prospective Payment System (PPS), where they were used as a means to
reimburse hospitals by activity. Under this type of reimbursement system
hospitals are paid for the activities they perform, thus encouraging
them to respond to patient preferences and demands and operate more
efficiently. In order to do this, DRGs in each country need to accurately
reflect the resources and costs of treating a group of similar patients.

Since 1983, many countries have adopted DRG type payment systems,
including Australia, Austria, France, Germany and the UK. Given their
international application, researchers have gone back to the initial idea
of using DRGs as comparative tools that can be used to better understand
and measure the production process at the hospital level, through
comparisons across DRGs and reimbursement rates. The European funded
EuroDRG project (2007–11) explored the potential for cross-country
comparison and learning, using DRGs as a tool for comparison.

The key findings of the project can be found in the edited volume
Diagnosis-Related Groups in Europe (Busse et al., 2011).

Given the heterogeneity of classifications and coding across countries,
it is difficult to use them as a tool for efficiency comparisons. However
they show potential for international reporting and benchmarking in the
future as long as an international classification can be developed that
provides a level of aggregation for groups that is both feasible and policy-
relevant in a wide range of countries.

Source: EuroDRG, 2012.

for which comparable international data on health are now available and in
the degree to which comparability has been improved. However, the science
of international comparison is still at a developmental stage. Policy-makers
therefore need to be made aware of both the strengths and limitations of health
system comparison. This section considers the key requirements necessary to
create comparable indicators that address the needs of policy-makers. These
are likely to be: appropriate methods of summarizing complex information; a

narrative that highlights the key issues and uncertainties; a diagnosis of why the reported variations are arising; and the implications for policy action.

Appropriate methods of summarizing complex information

In order to benchmark health systems, whether for a particular dimension of performance or for overall performance, policy-makers must rely on a few meaningful indicators. The role of a conceptual framework is to help organize thinking to identify priorities for new developments, and to ensure that collection and analysis efforts are not misdirected or duplicated. The eventual requirement for meaningful international comparison is to develop an optimal portfolio of performance metrics, in the light of health systems' differential organizational structures and accountability arrangements, as well as the variable levels of resources and analytic capacity available within countries. Even when analytic resources are limited, policy-makers should be aware of the major contribution that comparison can offer in improving quality and avoiding waste. The intention is to provide policy-makers with a holistic view of population needs, the services provided and outcomes achieved, and to offer guidance on the reasons for any variation. Thus, indicators should be chosen with regard to their ability to measure what has been identified as important, rather than merely reflecting what is readily available. This will serve to make the measurement exercise robust and will also help to highlight areas where further development is necessary.

This volume attempts to identify the state of the art in measurement in key domains of health system performance in order to assist policy-makers in selecting and interpreting indicators for international comparison. Each chapter has reviewed the main indicators that are available for international comparisons, existing challenges and the way forward. The issues identified are summarized in Table 12.5 below.

There are various ongoing initiatives and developments that have the potential to add further value to international comparisons, as reviewed in detail in Chapter 11. One very large area of development is that of ICT, often described within the EU context in particular as "e-health", which has the potential to greatly improve data collected at the system level. Moreover, as increasing numbers of people seek health care outside their own country, especially within Europe, there is a growing need for better comparability at the international level (Legido-Quigley et al., 2011). However, the very fine levels of detail needed to make such comparisons useful add still further to the methodological and practical challenges discussed above.

Narratives that identify key issues and uncertainties

As highlighted in Table 12.5, one of the key challenges faced in international comparisons is controlling for the heterogeneity in national settings and identifying the underlying processes and characteristics that give rise to better performance. Despite their diversity, there are still practices that one system can

Table 12.5 Key resources and challenges

Dimension	Challenges for international comparison	Way forward
Population health	Many measures fail to distinguish the contribution of the health system. Many countries' mortality data are lacking in timeliness and accuracy. Problems of comparability among countries and over time, reflecting changes in and differences between international and national coding rules. Large gaps in availability of evidence on the effectiveness of treatments reducing mortality.	The development of EHR and the development of multi-language software to assist with coding to deal with the problems in timeliness and accuracy of mortality data. The development of internationally comparable clinical databases that provide risk-adjusted information on individual outcomes of treatment that can help disentangle attribution. Greater use of tracer conditions which enable a better understanding of everyday experience of those in need of care.
Health service outcomes	Lack of well-defined boundaries of 'health systems' and 'health services'. Gaps in understanding of the relationships between measurements on the micro-, meso- and macro-levels of the health system. Limited set of dimensions captured by outcome measures with a marked lack of measures on disabilities or discomfort. Intermediate process measures show potential for complementing outcome indicators but when used on their own may not be as meaningful to stakeholders. Lack of available, good-quality and comparative data at the patient level. International comparison is complicated by different organizational settings and reporting conventions across systems.	Creating more registry data, which identify individual patients and trace them through the care process. Focus on a small number of indicators, which could give an overall comparison of the quality of health systems, such as the HCQI project taken forward by the OECD and co-financed by the EU. Find ways to measure outcomes that are not defined in terms of cure, which are important for the measurement of chronic disease and long-term care. Find ways to assess health systems based on how well they perform from the perspective of the people they are intended to benefit.

(Continued)

Table 12.5 Key resources and challenges *(Continued)*

Dimension	Challenges for international comparison	Way forward
Equity	Lack of existing datasets that provide a longitudinal perspective.	Better collection of indicators on determinants of health.
	Limited evidence has been recorded on how sensitive inequalities are to the inclusion of environmental effects.	Invest in well-designed evaluative studies of major interventions to reduce health inequalities and equity to access in health care, taking advantage of natural experiments (changes in employment opportunities, housing provision or cigarette pricing).
	Limited understanding of the factors explaining the health production process and sources of inequalities, including the role of mental conditions along with cognitive biases in measuring self-reported health.	
	Wide use of self-reported measures of health status given their availability in harmonized datasets, which allow international comparisons, but have important limitations that are aggravated for the lack of measures of calibration available in some datasets but not in others.	Put processes in place to ensure the availability and comparability of data, as well as harmonization of definition and collection instruments.
	Inadequate identification of what stands behind measures of socioeconomic position, namely, different income sources and measures of wealth and social environmental controls which differ across the life-cycle.	Invest in data linkages to allow desegregation by socioeconomic status and better monitoring of health inequalities across countries.
Fairness in financing	The construction of indicators depends crucially on adequately defining and measuring households' true capacity to pay for health care, which is not straightforward.	Invest in data collection of household income and spending patterns.
	Indicators only account for the short-term impacts of financial hardship and ignore the influence of coping strategies (such as selling assets or borrowing money to pay for care), with their longer-term consequences for household welfare.	Research to develop metrics better suited to capture the intertemporal financial consequences of illness arising from coping strategies.
	Indicators do not take into consideration the consequences of lost income due to illness for the measured degree of financial protection.	Search for practical alternatives to account for the effect of financial barriers to health care access in financial protection analyses.
	Indicators do not give information about (and are likely to be affected by) the extent of financial barriers to access to health care.	

Dimension	Challenges for international comparison	Way forward
Responsiveness	Lack of conceptual clarity as to what constitutes responsiveness.	Agree on a working international definition of responsiveness on which to base measures.
	Lack of clarity creates confusion as to what is measured and how.	
	Surveys on satisfaction are very sensitive to question wording, sampling and demographic factors.	Incorporate tools that allow for some correction of the bias produced by differences in experience or wider cultural differences.
Efficiency	The production process underlying health systems is intrinsically complex and poorly understood. Most measures make simplifying assumptions that may sometimes result in misleading data.	Improve data collection on key inputs, which affect efficiency, such as staff and technology, where international data is underdeveloped.
	Outputs are generally multidimensional and therefore preference weights are needed if they are aggregated into a single measure of attainment. The choice of such weights is intrinsically political and contentious.	Research to find suitable metrics that measure organizational factors and administrative structures, which influence inputs and outputs.
	A fundamental challenge in developing an efficiency measure is ensuring that the output being captured is directly and fully dependent on the inputs that are included in the measurement.	Improve clarification on the type of efficiency being measured by different indicators.
	Environmental factors, policy constraints, population characteristics and other factors may be largely responsible for determining health outcomes, yet it is difficult to incorporate all possible determinants appropriately into an efficiency assessment.	Improve the conceptualization of the production process in order to better harmonize data collection efforts.
	From an accounting perspective, the assignment of inputs and associated costs to specific health system activities is fundamentally problematic, often relying on arbitrary accounting rules or other questionable assignments.	Improve collection of high-quality comparable data on outputs, inputs and environmental factors necessary for risk adjustments.
	Although researchers have developed indicators that seek to measure full production processes, these measures are often not the most informative for policy-makers looking to identify and address inefficiencies.	Invest in research to refine methodologies for whole-system efficiency measurement.
	Many outputs are the results of years of health system endeavour, and cannot be attributed to inputs in a single period.	Find a balance between whole-system measures and more fragmented efficiency measures.
		More consideration of how indicators take static and dynamic elements of inputs and outputs into account.

EHR: electronic health records; HCQI: health care quality indicators.

Adapted from: Chapter 11.

learn from another. The key to such learning is to identify those areas where meaningful comparisons can be made and those where more caution is appropriate. The weight placed on comparisons can be influenced through the narrative that is used to discuss issues and uncertainties. If comparisons are to be treated as a process of learning, the first step to encouraging meaningful benchmarking is to adopt useful presentation mechanisms that highlight and explain uncertainties and variations.

The presentation of comparisons has hitherto not always been especially helpful for policy-makers. Neither the bald presentation of league tables nor a detailed list of caveats is well suited to securing appropriate policy responses. Two types of risk arise from poor presentation of comparisons: uncritical acceptance of results and potentially costly and inappropriate reforms of the health system; or rejection of the comparisons as inadequate, and a consequent lost opportunity for reform. In either case, the key issue is the need to focus on the policy-maker's action, and to ensure that it is well-informed, acknowledges the inevitable uncertainty, and is proportionate. There are many different methods to summarize and present data in order to best showcase the key issues behind them. Box 12.7 demonstrates how different modes of presentation can be used to highlight different issues for a range of audiences.

In any presentation, an important consideration is that many of the indicators used for international comparison contain implicit value judgements that should be subjected to careful scrutiny. These value judgements are often unavoidable and occur as a result of having to prioritize which data to collect, how to analyse them and deciding what to present. For example, these judgements may inform the indicators and weights that make up a summary measure of system-level performance or the ethical perspective adopted when evaluating equity in health systems. Policy-makers, at the very least, need to be aware that certain value judgements have been made, at all levels of analysis, and to take these into account when interpreting the information they are given, by considering what assumptions have been made to construct the indicator they are studying. Awareness about these judgements will help to guide policy-makers to the areas where they should dig deeper in order to understand what a relative ranking means, and where there is potential for improvement.

Understanding variations

There are a number of reasons why variations in reported performance might arise, and it is important that any comparison seeks to understand the sources of variation. The policy actions arising from different causes might be quite different, ranging from the collection of new data, improved data audit and commissioning new analysis, to reassessing priorities or health system reforms designed to address genuine weaknesses in performance. Box 12.8 summarizes some of the more important reasons for variation.

If genuine performance variations are identified, policy-makers will often wish to know which characteristics of the health systems under scrutiny are giving rise to the good and bad performance, and whether specific reforms in other countries have been effective. As noted above, comparative data on

Box 12.7 Different perspectives on performance

- **Means or distributions**
  Means give information on the average performance of each country but distributions allow comparisons to be made on the variations in performance across countries.

- **Single indicators or composite measures**
  Composite indicators give information on multiple dimensions of performance but may be complex to interpret, less informative on which domain's performance is good or bad, and can raise methodological issues from the manner in which they are constructed.

- **Generic or condition/diagnosis/procedure-specific**
  Generic measures tend to be more easily available and are less at risk of small number problems, but the latter may be more informative for policy-makers.

- **Measures along care pathways**
  These types of measures can be very useful to identify which areas of the pathway countries perform differently in, but are not easily measurable using available data.

- **Never events or sentinel events**
  These are measures of events that should never occur or rare events, but require clear definitions across countries and reliable monitoring systems.

- **Measures in relation to a standard or in comparison to other countries**
  Benchmarks can be presented in different ways depending on what is of interest. Comparisons can be made within a set of similar countries or all countries. They can be in relation to each other's performance at one period or over multiple time periods; absolute performance; or performance relative to a particular target.

- **Longitudinal or cross-sectional data**
  Comparing trend data across countries may be more useful for identifying areas of potential improvement but often this is not readily available and may have more comparability issues.

Adapted from: Raleigh & Foot, 2010.

---

health system characteristics are currently very weak, and it is furthermore especially difficult to confirm that there is causality from system characteristics to performance. This is a core area for further development that we discuss further in the following section.

Health system reforms are usually very difficult to evaluate convincingly, because they are rarely implemented as randomized experiments. Furthermore, the authors of the reforms are sometimes reluctant to expose their innovations

Box 12.8 Possible sources of variations in cross-country performance indicators

---

Comparability issues

1. The data used for comparison are lacking or incorrect. For example:

- No recent data are available for some countries, so older data are used instead.
- No data are available on an area being measured, so proxies are used instead.

2. The definition of the indicator is not standardized across countries. For example:

- Waiting times are compared across countries, but the start of the period of waiting is measured differently across countries (e.g. in one country it begins when the patient first makes contact with the system; in another it begins when the patient is first referred to a specialist, etc.).
- Hospital length of stay is compared across countries, but due to different system design features the hospitals have different thresholds for admission/discharge.
- Patient experience is measured by comparing surveys conducted on different country populations (patients vs general population).

3. The coding of the indicator is not standardized across countries or measurement instruments, leading to cross-country bias. For example:

- Mortality for a certain condition is compared when countries apply differential coding patterns for that condition.
- Self-assessed health is compared across countries using household surveys, which use different scales to measure how healthy the respondent is (e.g. very good, good, bad, very bad vs excellent, very good, good, bad, very bad).
- In cost data, payments are not adjusted for differences in purchasing power parity.
- In surveys, linguistic differences in translated questions influence respondents' answers.

Measurement issues

4. The indicator does not measure what it purports to measure. For example:

- Data quality is poor, or derived from an unrepresentative sample.
- The indicator is not adjusted for external factors known to influence it, such as demographic factors or socioeconomic deprivation.
- There is a time-lag in data collection.
- Uncertainty arises from a small number of observations, leading to high random error in estimates.

Performance issues

5. The indicator suggests good or bad performance in a certain area.

The international benchmark for the indicator indicates it is at the lower end of the spectrum because performance in this area is lower than the rest of the peer group.

to proper evaluation, given the risk that the results may be disappointing. Therefore, analysts often rely on non-experimental comparisons between jurisdictions that implement the reforms and those that do not, indicating an important role for comparable data across health systems (Rice and Jones, 2011).

Notwithstanding the need for continual monitoring and updating of methods, it is important to note that data collection is an expensive endeavour. Resources can be wasted if proper thought is not given to whether and how data collection should be expanded or limited to best measure in line with intentions (Naylor, Iron & Handa, 2002). Information innovations should be subject to the same cost-effectiveness criteria as other health technologies, and implemented fully only after proper testing and assurance that they will offer good value for money. Moreover, there are often large amounts of data available from existing sources that might be better exploited for health analysis, perhaps through data linkage; this may, in some circumstances, provide opportunities for quicker and more cost-effective solutions to performance assessment than investing in completely new data collection or enhancement initiatives.

Drawing implications for policy actions

International comparisons of health systems and policy learning are related activities. There are examples of instances where international comparisons have led to health system reform; for example, the *WHR2000* exercise is reported to have fed into health care reform initiatives in China, Mexico, the Islamic Republic of Iran and elsewhere (Murray & Frenk, 2010). Yet it often appears that more time and effort is made in drawing comparisons than in understanding the reasons behind these variations or searching for methods to improve system performance across settings. While international comparisons are an important mechanism for holding national policy-makers and politicians to account, they also offer the potential to promote mutual learning.

Given the large diversity in health systems, the transfer of successful processes from one nation to another will often be challenging, requiring careful consideration of alignment of the innovation with the whole system. An example of this is the recent adoption of DRGs in many European countries as a basis for provider payment mechanisms. In some cases, even the case groupings themselves have been directly imported from overseas. Yet their underlying operation differs considerably depending on the national setting, history and organization of the health system (Busse et al., 2011). The successful integration of overseas policies into a local system often involves a degree of transformation to ensure compatibility with existing structures.

The Health Systems in Transition (HiT) series of health system profiles carried out systematically by the European Observatory on Health Systems and Policies provides a solid basis of qualitative data from which policy-makers and researchers can derive information on national health systems that can complement quantitative analysis. Such sources of comparative descriptive information can yield extremely useful insights when seeking to understand the meaning behind quantitative differences in performance.

Although it is likely that much learning will come from the scrutiny of reforms in similar systems, experience in other sectors suggests that there is scope for learning from quite different experiences (Chapter 4). The benchmarking of the English NHS and Kaiser Permanente in the last decade also shows the potential for such interactions and mutual learning between very different systems (Ham, 2010). Newer initiatives of this sort exist for cross-country learning in specific areas of the health system, such as health technology assessment (HTA). In 2008, the National Institute of Clinical Excellence (NICE), a pioneer in the application of clinical and cost–effectiveness information to medicine, set up NICE International as a not-for-profit offshoot of the main organization to assist policy-makers in other countries in adopting and using clinical guidelines, HTA methods and evidence.[1] Another area where there seems to be considerable interest and potential for cross-country learning of this sort is in the development of e-health initiatives and how these can inform better care pathways.

The successful integration of overseas policies into a local system often involves a degree of adaptation to ensure compatibility with existing structures. Even if potentially valuable health system practices and characteristics of other systems can be identified, there remains the question of whether, and how successfully, features can be translated into another health system. Such translation is not straightforward; can be costly and disruptive; and can yield disappointing results if not undertaken with care. Practices – and their impact – are often context-dependent. They are shaped by national characteristics, system design, history and adaptation. It is therefore most important that reforms should be designed with the context in mind, and that promising new practices are, where appropriate, aligned with the existing health system feature and properly evaluated to ensure that they are yielding the expected benefits.

12.5 Future priorities and way forward

Given the increasing demand for and availability of information comparing the performance of health systems, it is important that policy-makers consider what makes comparisons most useful for health system improvement. While there can be no definitive guide, the experience set out in this book suggests that the following guidelines are important for the creation and interpretation of international comparisons.

- International health system performance comparisons have the potential to provide a rich source of evidence as well as to influence policy. However, comparisons that are not conducted with properly validated measures and unbiased policy interpretation may prompt adverse policy impacts, so caution is required in the selection of indicators, the methodologies used and the interpretations made. Policy-makers should ensure that:
  - o Definitions of performance indicators are clear and consistent, and fit into a clear conceptual framework that is suitable for the comparison being made.
  - o The metrics used in international comparison enjoy widespread acceptance and are defined in unambiguous terms that are consistent with most countries' data collection systems.
  - o Variations in the demographic, social, cultural and economic circumstances of nations are adjusted for, where possible. This will allow for more meaningful comparison and assessment of the drivers of variations across systems.
  - o The advantages and disadvantages of using 'single number' measures of whole health system performance are carefully considered. While offering a more rounded view of performance, these types of measures have limited scope for policy action, and may distract policy-makers from seeking out and remedying the parts of their system that require attention.
- While efforts should continue to improve and broaden data collection efforts, policy-makers should also make themselves familiar with the limitations of existing indicators in order to be able to interpret them appropriately.
- Lessons from benchmarking activities in other sectors suggest that, when applied to health systems, benchmarking will be most effective if it: focuses on practice as well as performance; is grounded in the broader change process; is well structured and planned in order to engage stakeholders; and carefully considers how performance is linked to resource allocation.
- International comparisons are useful in identifying areas of potential improvement for policy-makers. The improvements themselves will take more work at the national level for policy-makers to understand characteristics and processes that contribute to relative levels of performance. These efforts can include analysis of existing data, collections of new indicators that do not exist, and visits to other countries to better understand other practices that may be beneficial.

International comparison is, without question, an important potential driver of health system improvement. At its best it can offer a unique tool for policy-makers interested in understanding whether their health system is performing as well as it could, and in identifying promising reforms for securing improvements. Furthermore, such comparison serves a crucial governance role, in allowing citizens to hold their governments, professions and other accountable parties properly to account for their performance as guardians of the health system. However, although the science of comparison is advancing rapidly, there is still great potential for misinterpretation and abuse of comparative information. Therefore, as this book has sought to show, there remains a large and important agenda for action to improve the practice of comparisons. Nevertheless, the potential gains – in the form of improved health and accountability – are enormous.

Note

1 See http://www.inpharm.com/news/170898/work-nice-international.

References

Abel-Smith, B. (1963) *Paying for health services: a study of the costs and sources of finance in six countries.* Geneva: World Health Organization (Public Health Papers, no. 17).

Abel-Smith, B. (1967) *An international study of health expenditure and its relevance for health planning.* Geneva: World Health Organization (Public Health Papers, no. 32).

Aday, L.A. et al. (2004) *Evaluating the Healthcare System: Effectiveness, efficiency, and equity,* 3rd edn. Chicago: Health Administration Press.

Anand, S. et al. (2003) Report of the Scientific Peer Review Group on health systems performance assessment, in C.J.L. Murray and D.B. Evans (eds) *Health Systems Performance Assessment: Debates, methods and empiricism.* Geneva: World Health Organization.

Anderson, O.W. (1963) Medical care: its social and organizational aspects. Health-service systems in the United States and other countries – critical comparisons, *New England Journal of Medicine*, 269: 896–900.

Arah, O.A. et al. (2003) Conceptual frameworks for health systems performance: a quest for effectiveness, quality, and improvement, *International Journal for Quality in Health Care*, 15: 377–98.

Bambra, C. (2005) Cash versus services: 'worlds of welfare' and the decommodification of cash benefits and health care services, *Journal of Social Policy*, 34(2):195–213.

Bambra, C. (2007) Going beyond the three worlds of welfare capitalism: regime theory and public health research, *Journal of Epidemiology and Community Health*, 61: 1098–102.

Berwick, D.M. (1996) A primer on leading the improvement of systems, *BMJ*, 312(7031): 619–22.

Black, N. (2012) Declining health care productivity: the making of a myth, *The Lancet*, 379(9821): 1167–9.

Burau, V. and Blank, R. (2006) Comparing health policy: an assessment of typologies of health systems, *Journal of Comparative Policy Analysis*, 8(1): 63–76.

Busse, R., Schreyögg, J. and Smith, P.C. (2008) Variability in healthcare treatment costs amongst nine EU countries – results from the HealthBASKET project, *Health Economics*, 17(Suppl 1): S1–8.

Busse, R. et al. (2011) *Diagnosis-related groups in Europe: Moving towards transparency, efficiency and quality in hospitals.* Maidenhead: McGraw-Hill Education (WHO European Observatory on Health Systems and Policies Series).

Commonwealth Fund (2006) *Framework for a high performance health system for the United States.* New York: The Commonwealth Fund.

Delnoij, D. et al. (2000) Does general practitioner gatekeeping curb health care expenditure? *Journal of Health Services Research and Policy*, 5(1): 22–6.

ECHO (2001) *What is the ECHO Project?* Zaragoza: European Collaboration for Healthcare Optimization (http://www.echo–health.eu/, accessed 26 September 2012).

Esping-Andersen, G. (1987) *The Three Worlds of Welfare Capitalism.* Princeton, NJ: Princeton University Press.

EuroDRG (2012) *EuroDRG Project: Diagnosis-related groups in Europe: Towards efficiency and quality.* Berlin: EuroDRG (http://www.eurodrg.eu/, accessed 26 September 2012).

EuroHOPE (2012) *What is the EuroHOPE project?* Helsinki: EuroHOPE (http://www.eurohope.info/, accessed 26 September 2012).

Feachem, R.G., Sekhri, N.K. and White, K.L. (2002) Getting more for their dollar: a comparison of the NHS with California's Kaiser Permanente, *BMJ*, 324(7330): 135–41.

Fenton, J.J. et al. (2012) The cost of satisfaction: a national study of patient satisfaction, health care utilization, expenditures, and mortality. *Archives of Internal Medicine*, 172(5): 405–11.

Fetter, R.B. et al. (1980) Case mix definition by diagnosis-related groups, *Medical Care*, 18(Suppl 2): 1–53.

Goldmann, F. (1946) Foreign programs of medical care and their lessons, *New England Journal of Medicine*, 234: 155–60.

Greaves, F. et al. (2012) Associations between Web-based patient ratings and objective measures of hospital quality, *Archives of Internal Medicine*, 172(5): 435–6.

Häkkinen, U. et al. (2011) Analysing current trends in care of acute myocardial infarction using PERFECT data, *Annals of Medicine*, 43(Suppl): S14–21.

Ham, C. (2010) *Working together for health: Achievements and challenges in the Kaiser NHS Beacon Sites Programme.* Birmingham: Health Services Management Centre.

HCP (2009) *Euro Consumer Heart Index report.* Brussels: Health Consumer Powerhouse.

Hsiao, W.H. and Sidat, B. (2008) *Health systems: Concepts and deterministic models of performance.* Background paper prepared for the Workshop on Research Agendas on Global Health Systems, Harvard University, December 3–5, 2008.

Hurst, J. and Jee-Hughes, M. (2001) *Performance measurement and performance management in OECD health systems.* Paris: Organisation for Economic Co-operation and Development Publishing (OECD Labour Market and Social Policy Occasional Paper, no. 47).

IHP (2008) *Monitoring performance and evaluating progress in the scale-up for better health: A proposed common framework.* Document prepared by the monitoring and evaluating working group of the International Health Partnership and Related Initiatives (IHP+), led by the WHO and the World Bank.

Joumard, I., André, C. and Nicq, C. (2010) *Health care systems: efficiency and institutions.* Paris: Organisation for Economic Co-operation and Development (OECD Economics Department Working Paper, no. 769).

Kelley, E. and Hurst, J. (2006) *Health Care Quality Indicators project: Conceptual framework paper.* Paris: Organisation for Economic Co-operation and Development Publishing (OECD Health Working Paper, no. 23).

Klein, R. (1997) Learning from others: shall the last be the first? *Journal of Health Politics, Policy and Law,* 22(5): 1267–78.

Kotzian, P. (2008) Control and performance of health care systems. A comparative analysis of 19 OECD countries, *International Journal of Health Planning and Management,* 23(3): 235–57.

Kroneman, M.W., Maarse, H. and van der Zee, J. (2006) Direct access in primary care and patient satisfaction: a European Study, *Health Policy*, 76(1): 72–9.

Legido-Quigley, H. et al. (2011) Cross-border healthcare in the European Union: clarifying patients' rights, *BMJ*, 342: d296.

Marmor, T.R., Freeman, R. and Okma, K. (2005) Comparative perspectives and policy learning in the world of health care, *Journal of Comparative Policy Analysis*, 7(4): 331–48.

Marshall, M.N. et al. (2003) Can health care quality indicators be transferred between countries? *Quality and Safety in Health Care*, 12(1): 8–12.

Mattke, S. et al. (2006) *Health Care Quality Indicators project: Initial indicators report.* Paris: Organisation for Economic Co-operation and Development Publishing (OECD Health Working Paper, no. 22).

Mladovsky, P. et al. (2009) *Health in the European Union: trends and analysis.* Copenhagen: WHO Regional Office for Europe (European Observatory on Health Systems and Policies).

Mountin, J.W. and Perrott, G.S. (1947) Health insurance programs and plans of western Europe: summary of observations, *Public Health Reports*, 62(11): 369–99.

Murray, C.J.L. and Frenk, J. (2000) A framework for assessing the performance of health systems, *Bulletin of the World Health Organization*, 78(6): 717–30.

Murray, C.J.L. and Frenk, J. (2010) Ranking 37th – measuring the performance of the U.S. health care system, *New England Journal of Medicine*, 362(2): 98–9.

Naylor, C.D., Iron, K. and Handa, K. (2002) Measuring health system performance: problems and opportunities in the era of assessment and accountability, in P.C. Smith (eds) *'Measuring up': Improving health system performance in OECD countries.* Paris: Organisation for Economic Co-operation and Development.

Neuhauser, D. (2004) Assessing health quality: the case for tracers, *Journal of Health Services Research and Policy*, 9(4): 246–7.

Nolte, E. and McKee, M. (2003) Measuring the health of nations: analysis of mortality amenable to health care, *BMJ*, 327(7424): 1129.

Nolte, E. and McKee, M. (2004) *Does healthcare save lives? Avoidable mortality revisited.* London: Nuffield Trust (http://www.nuffieldtrust.org.uk/sites/files/nuffield/publication/does-healthcare-save-lives-mar04.pdf, accessed 25 September 2012).

Nolte, E., Wait, S. and McKee, M. (2006) *Investing in health: Benchmarking health systems.* London: The Nuffield Trust.

Nolte, E. et al. (2008) Learning from other countries: an on-call facility for health care policy, *Journal of Health Services Research and Policy*, 13(Suppl): 58–64.

OECD (2010a) *Improving value in health care: measuring quality.* Paris: Organisation for Economic Co-operation and Development (http://www.oecd.org/health/hcqi, accessed on 23 April 2012).

OECD (2010b) *Value for money in health spending.* Paris: Organisation for Economic Co-operation and Development (OECD Health Policy Series).

Paris, V., Devaux, M. and Wei, L. (2010) *Health systems institutional characteristics: a survey of 29 OECD countries.* Paris: Organisation for Economic Co-operation and Development (Publishing CD Health Working Papers, no. 50) (http://dx.doi.org/10.1787/5kmfxfq9qbnr-en, accessed 8 June 2012).

Peltola, M. et al. (2011) A methodological approach for register-based evaluation of cost and outcomes in health care, *Annals of Medicine*, 43(Suppl) S4–13.

Raleigh, V.S. and Foot, C. (2010) *Getting the measure of quality: Opportunities and challenges.* London: The King's Fund.

Reinhardt, U.E., Hussey, P.S. and Anderson, G.F. (2002) Cross-national comparisons of health systems using OECD data, 1999, *Health Affairs (Millwood)*, 21(3): 169–81.

Rice, N. and Jones, A.M. Economic analysis of health policies, in S. Glied and P.C. Smith (eds) (2011) *The Oxford Handbook of Health Economics.* Oxford: Oxford University Press.

Roberts, M.J. et al. (2008) *Getting health reform right: A guide to improving performance and equity.* Oxford: Oxford University Press.

Roemer, M.I. (1960) Health departments and medical care – a world scanning, *American Journal of Public Health*, 50: 154–60.

Rosén, M. (2001) Can the WHO Health Report improve the performance of health systems? *Scandinavian Journal of Public Health*, 29(1): 76–80.

Schreyögg, J., Stargardt, T. and Tiemann, O. (2011) Costs and quality of hospitals in different health care systems: a multi-level approach with propensity score matching, *Health Economics*, 20(1): 85–100.

Shengelia, B. et al. (2005) Access, utilization, quality, and effective coverage: an integrated conceptual framework and measurement strategy, *Social Science and Medicine*, 61(1): 97–109.

Smith, P.C. (2002) Developing composite indicators for assessing health system efficiency, in P.C. Smith (ed.) *'Measuring up': Improving health system performance in OECD countries*. Paris: Organisation for Economic Co-operation and Development.

Smith, P.C. et al. (2009) *Performance measurement for health system improvement: Experiences, challenges and prospects*. Cambridge: Cambridge University Press.

Starfield, B., Shi, L. and Mackino, J. (2005) Contribution of primary care to health systems and health, *The Milbank Quarterly*, 83(3): 457–502.

Sund, R. et al. (2011) Monitoring the performance of hip fracture treatment in Finland, *Annals of Medicine*, 43(Suppl): S39–46.

Thomson, S. et al. (eds) (2011) *International Profiles of Health Care Systems*. New York: The Commonwealth Fund.

Wagstaff, A. (2009) Financial protection, in P.C. Smith et al. (eds) *Performance measurement for health system improvement: Experiences, challenges and prospects*. Cambridge: Cambridge University Press.

Walshe, K. (2003) International comparisons of quality of health care: what do they tell us? *Quality and Safety in Health Care*, 12(1): 4–5.

Wendt, C., Frisina, L. and Rothgang, H. (2009) Healthcare system types: a conceptual framework for comparison, *Social Policy and Administration*, 43(1): 70–90.

WHO (2000) *The World Health Report 2000 – Health systems: improving performance*. Geneva: World Health Organization.

WHO (2001) *Draft report of technical consultation on effective coverage in health systems*. 27–29 August 2001, Rio De Janeiro, Brazil (http://www.who.int/health-systems-performance/technical_consultations/effcov_report.pdf, accessed 8 June 2012).

WHO (2008) *A framework to monitor and evaluate implementation*. Geneva: World Health Organization Document Production Services (http://www.who.int/dietphysicalactivity/M&E-ENG-09.pdf, accessed 8 June 2012).

WHO (2010a) *The World Health Report 2010. Health systems financing: the path to universal coverage*. Geneva: World Health Organization.

WHO (2011) *World Health Statistics 2011*. Geneva: World Health Organization.

WHO Regional Office for Europe (2009) *The European Health Report 2009: Health and health systems*. Copenhagen: World Health Organization Regional Office for Europe.

WHO Regional Office for Europe (2012) *Case studies on health system performance assessment: A long-standing development in Europe*. Copenhagen: World Health Organization Regional Office for Europe.

Index

abbreviations xxiii–xxv
access
  defining 203
  equity 202–7
  financial barriers 237–42
  health systems 202–7
  inequity indices 206–7
  measuring 204–7
  needs 203–4, 205
  rates 206
  regression methods 206
  terminology 40
  unmet needs 203–4, 205
acute myocardial infarction (AMI), case-
    fatality rates 161–4, 165
administrative databases, health services
    outcomes 177
age/disease-specific indicators, population
    health 132–7
Ageing-Related Diseases (ARD) study, health
    systems efficiency 291–4
allocative efficiency, health systems
    efficiency 284–6
ambition, benchmarking 123
amenable mortality, population health
    145–9, 343, 344
AMI *see* acute myocardial infarction
AMIEHS *see* Avoidable Mortality in European
    Health Systems

analytic methods, health systems efficiency
    297–303
analytic techniques, health systems
    efficiency 305–6
analytical international frameworks 46–8,
    337
appendectomy, health systems efficiency 293
architecture, health systems 41–5, 48, 50
ARD *see* Ageing-Related Diseases study
assessment of initiatives, international
    comparisons of health systems 97–102
attribution, international comparisons of
    health systems 104–5
avoidable mortality, population health
    145–9, 317–18, 342–4
Avoidable Mortality in European Health
    Systems (AMIEHS), key domain of
    performance, HSPA 16, 17

Behavioral Healthcare Framework,
    international frameworks 51–4
benchmarking 113–26
  ambition blocking 123
  benchmarking cycle 124
  benefits 117–21
  Commonwealth Fund Framework for a
    High Performance System 2006: 85
  criticisms 123
  defining 113–15

Dutch National Institute for Public Health
and the Environment (RIVM) 5
European Community Health Indicators
(ECHI) Project 5
good practices 121–2
implications 124–5
innovation blocking 123
international comparisons 5, 367
lessons to date 12, 13
National Health Service (NHS) 5–7
National Scorecard 5
Open Method of Coordination (OMC)
(2000) 55
performance (results) benchmarking
115–16, 117
policy influence 5
positive impact 123–4
practice (process) benchmarking 115–16,
117
process (practice) benchmarking 115–16,
117
professionalism 123
purpose 116–20
requirements 102
results (performance) benchmarking
115–16, 117
scope 113–15
shortcomings 122–3
system responsibility 123
United States health system 5
United States Veterans Health
Administration 5
value from 121–2
bipolar disorder 170–3
birth and death statistics, health services
outcomes 176
boundaries
equity 184–5
health systems 14–15, 33–5, 50
implications 33–5
breast cancer
population health 137, 138
screening 173, 174, 291–3
burdens of disease, health systems outcomes
322

cancer services
England 3–4
international comparisons 3–4
policy influence 3–4
capacity to pay, financial protection 227–9,
232, 234, 236
catastrophic spending on health care,
financial protection 227–30, 231–5,
237–42, 246–7
Commonwealth Fund Framework for a High
Performance System 2006:
benchmarking 85
existing health system performance
assessment initiatives 85
international frameworks 66–7

Commonwealth Fund International Health
Policy Survey (IHPS)
comparative methodology 272–3
financial protection 244–5
interpretation of data differences 272–3
methodological considerations 272–3
patient experience 272–6
satisfaction 272–6
communicable diseases, international health
system performance information 314–15
concentration curve/index, health outcomes
194–6
conceptual frameworks, international
comparisons of health systems 336–9
conceptual models, health systems efficiency
303–5
Control Knobs Framework 2003:,
international frameworks 61–3
coping strategies, financial protection 232
correlation measures, health outcomes 193
cross-border health care, international
comparisons 4
current developments, performance
measurement 1–2
current measures of future performance,
international comparisons of health
systems 105–6

DALYs see disability-adjusted life years
data collection
communicating international data 328–9
complementing international data 328–9
international health system performance
information 313–15, 330–1
World Health Organization (WHO) 79
data improvement, international health
system performance information 330–1
data issues, health systems efficiency 306–7
data issues, financial protection 242–6
availability 245
Commonwealth Fund International Health
Policy Survey (IHPS) 244–5
comparability 245–6
European Union Statistics on Income and
Living Conditions (EU-SILC) 243–4
Household Budget Survey (HBS) 243–4
International Household Survey Network
(IHSN) 245
Living Standards Measurement Study
(LSMS) 243
minimum requirements 242–3
quality 245
sources of data 243
World Health Survey (WHS) 244
data limitations, health outcomes 201
data problems
administrative databases 177
birth and death statistics 176
electronic health records (EHRs) 177
health services outcomes 176–8
health systems performance 176–8

methodological problems 177–8
national registries 176
population surveys 177
data quality, international comparisons 367
decomposition analysis, health outcomes
  196–7
descriptive international frameworks 46–8,
  337
descriptive methods, health systems
  efficiency 302–3
design, health systems 337–9
determinants of health
  developments 320–1
  international health system performance
    information 319–21
deterministic and predictive international
  frameworks 46–8, 337
diagnosis-related groups (DRGs)
  efficiency 288–9, 328, 357
  health systems efficiency 288–9
  international health system performance
    information 328
direct spending on health care, financial
  protection 226–7, 228
disability, population health 139–41,
  318–19
disability-adjusted life years (DALYs),
  population health 139–41
discretionary vs essential spending, financial
  protection 232
distributional effects, financial protection
  235
DRGs *see* diagnosis-related groups
Dutch National Institute for Public
  Health and the Environment (RIVM),
  international benchmarks 5
dynamic effects, international comparisons
  of health systems 105–6

e-health
  health systems outcomes 322
  health systems performance assessment
    (HSPA) 25
ECHI *see* European Community Health
  Indicators Project
ECHIM *see* European Community Health
  Indicators Monitoring project
ECHO project, health services outcomes 347,
  348–51
effective coverage, health systems
  performance assessment (HSPA) 340,
  341–2
efficiency
  see also health systems efficiency
  diagnosis-related groups (DRGs) 288–9,
    328, 357
  international comparisons 361
  international comparisons in performance
    domains 355–6, 357
  international comparisons of health
    systems 106–7

international health system performance
  information 327–8
key domain of performance, HSPA 22–4
terminology 39
EGIPSS *see* Integrated Performance Model for
  the Health Care System (1998)
electronic health records (EHRs), health
  services outcomes 177
England, cancer services 3–4
equality, vs equity 183–4
equity 183–222
  access, health systems 202–7
  boundaries 184–5
  defining 183–4
  vs equality 183–4
  ethical paradigms 184, 185
  financing 208–10
  health outcomes 186–201
  health system goals 210
  health systems 201–10
  international comparisons 360
  international health system performance
    information 323–5
  key domain of performance, HSPA 17–20
  key issues, international comparisons
    211–13
  lessons to date 347–52
  paradigms 184, 185
  policy recommendations 213–16
  procedural equity 215
  substantive equity 214–15
  terminology 40
  World Health Survey (WHS) 213
equity-efficiency trade-off, health outcomes
  197–8
essential vs discretionary spending, financial
  protection 232
ethical paradigms, equity 184, 185
EU-SILC *see* European Union Statistics on
  Income and Living Conditions
Euro Health Consumer Index
  existing health system performance
    assessment initiatives 89–91
  Health Consumer Powerhouse (HCP)
    89–91
Eurobarometer surveys, satisfaction 256–7,
  258–9
EuroHOPE project, health services outcomes
  347, 348–51
European Community Health Indicators
  (ECHI) Project 83–4
  international benchmarks 5
  national performance assessment 49
European Community Health Indicators
  Monitoring (ECHIM) project 83–4
European Observatory on Health Systems
  and Policies
  Health Systems in Transition (HiT) reports
    76, 366
  international comparisons of health
    systems 76

European Union, existing health system
performance assessment initiatives
83–5, 86–8
European Union Statistics on Income and
Living Conditions (EU-SILC), financial
protection 243–4
*Everybody's Business: Strengthening health
systems to improve health outcomes*, World
Health Organization (WHO) 8
existing frameworks
see also international frameworks
Behavioral Healthcare Framework 51–4
Commonwealth Fund Framework for a
High Performance System 2006: 66–7
Control Knobs Framework 2003: 61–3
Framework for Assessing Behavioral
Healthcare 1998: 51–4
Health Care Quality Indicators (HCQI)
Framework 2006: 63–5
Integrated Performance Model for the
Health Care System (EGIPSS) (1998) 54–5
international frameworks 51–72
International Health Partnership and
Related Initiatives (IHP+) Framework
2008: 70–2
OECD Framework 2001: 58–61
OECD Health Care Quality Indicators
(HCQI) Framework 2006: 63–5
Open Method of Coordination (OMC)
(2000) 55–6
'systems thinking' frameworks 69–70
WHO (2000) Framework 56–8
WHO Building Blocks 2007: 67–9
existing health system performance
assessment initiatives 76–92
Commonwealth Fund Framework for a
High Performance System 2006: 85
Euro Health Consumer Index 89–91
European Union 83–5, 86–8
Health Consumer Powerhouse (HCP)
89–91
National Institute for Health and Welfare
92
Nordic Collaboration 91–2
Nordic hospital comparison study group
(NHCSG) 92
Nordic Medico-Statistical Committee
(NOMESKO) 92
Northern Dimension Partnership in Public
Health and Social Wellbeing (NDPHS) 92
Organization for Economic Cooperation
and Development (OECD) 78–82
World Health Organization (WHO) 76–8
expectations, responsiveness 263–5
experience, patient *see* patient experience

financial protection 223–54
access barriers 237–42
capacity to pay 227–9, 232, 234, 236
catastrophic spending on health care
227–30, 231–5, 237–42, 246–7

Commonwealth Fund International Health
Policy Survey (IHPS) 244–5
coping strategies 232
data issues 242–6
direct spending on health care 226–7, 228
distributional effects 235
essential vs discretionary spending 232
European Union Statistics on Income and
Living Conditions (EU-SILC) 243–4
financial barriers to access 237–42
financial barriers to unmet needs 237–42
health systems performance 223–6, 246–7
Household Budget Survey (HBS) 243–4
impoverishing spending on health care
230–5, 237–42, 246–7
indicators 235–51
international comparisons in performance
domains 352–4
International Health Policy Survey (IHPS)
244–5
international health system performance
information 325
International Household Survey Network
(IHSN) 245
key domain of performance, HSPA 20, 21
Living Standards Measurement Study
(LSMS) 243
longer-term financial consequences of
health spending 233, 237
loss of earnings 233–4
measuring 226–35
methodological challenges 235–46
need for 223–4
out-of-pocket spending on health care
226–7, 228
policy concern 224–5
policy uses/abuses 246–7
pooling 224, 225
positive impact 225
poverty line 230–5
poverty trap 225
pre-payment 224, 225
research priorities 235–46
securing 224
sources of data 243
subsistence spending 236
unmet needs 234–5, 237–42
World Health Survey (WHS) 244
financing
equity 208–10
fairness 360
Gini coefficient 209
health systems 41–5, 208–10
international comparisons 360
international frameworks 41–5
Kakwani progressivity index 209–10
Lorenz curve 209
methodological techniques 208–10
Framework for Assessing Behavioral
Healthcare 1998:, international
frameworks 51–4

frameworks, international *see* international
    frameworks
future priorities, international comparisons
    366–8

gap measures, health outcomes 192–3
general practitioners, patient experience
    267–72
Gini coefficient
    financing 209
    health outcomes 193–6
    Kakwani progressivity index 209
goals
    health systems 35–41, 50, 76–8, 127, 210
    international frameworks 35–41

HALE *see* health-adjusted life expectancy
HCP *see* Health Consumer Powerhouse
HCQI *see* Health Care Quality Indicators
    Framework 2006:
health, terminology 38
health-adjusted life expectancy (HALE),
    population health 139–40
health care contribution
    inventory approach 142–3
    population health 141–4
    production function 142–4
health care payments *see* financial protection
health care quality indicators, health systems
    outcomes 321
Health Care Quality Indicators (HCQI)
    Framework 2006: 78–82, 168
    international frameworks 63–5
    key domain of performance, HSPA 18
Health Consumer Powerhouse (HCP)
    Euro Health Consumer Index 89–91
    existing health system performance
        assessment initiatives 89–91
health outcomes
    concentration curve/index 194–6
    correlation measures 193
    data limitations 201
    decomposition analysis 196–7
    equity 186–201
    equity-efficiency trade-off 197–8
    gap measures 192–3
    Gini coefficient 193–6
    health status 186–91
    inequalities 186–201
    key variables 186–92
    long-term care services 166–7
    long-term inequalities in health 198–201
    Lorenz curve 193–6
    measurement techniques 192–3
    measuring 185–201
    mobility index (MI) 198–201
    objective measures 187–91
    preventive care 173
    regression measures 193
    screening 173, 174
    self-assessed health (SAH) 187–9

social determinants 186, 187
socioeconomic variables 191–2
subjective measures 187–91
survey data 189–90
variables 186–92
variation 191–2
vignettes 190–1
health policy information (WHO Europe) 79
health services outcomes 157–81
    acute myocardial infarction (AMI), case-
        fatality rates 161–4, 165
    administrative databases 177
    birth and death statistics 176
    comparisons 157–81
    data problems 176–8
    ECHO project 347, 348–51
    electronic health records (EHRs) 177
    EuroHOPE project 347, 348–51
    *Everybody's Business: Strengthening health
        systems to improve health outcomes* 8, 76–8
    health systems performance 158–60
    health systems performance assessment
        (HSPA) 344–7
    indicators 344–7
    international comparisons 359
    key domain of performance, HSPA 16–17
    lessons to date 344–7, 348–9
    methodological problems 177–8
    multidimensional 159–60
    national registries 176
    patient-reported outcome measures
        (PROMS) 173–6
    patient safety indicators 164–6
    PERFECT project 347, 348–51
    population surveys 177
    readmission rates 166
    stroke, case-fatality rates 161–4, 165
health status, health outcomes 186–91
health systems
    see also health systems performance; health
        systems performance assessment (HSPA)
    access 202–7
    architecture 41–5, 48, 50
    boundaries 14–15, 33–5, 50
    defining 128–9
    design 337–9
    equity 201–10
    financing 41–5, 208–10
    goals 35–41, 50, 76–8, 127, 210
    inequities 201–10
    Kakwani progressivity index 209–10
    key terms 37–40
    leadership/governance 41–5
    needs 203–4, 205
    objectives 35–41
    patient experience 255–79
    patient satisfaction 255–79
    performance measurement 45–8
    purpose 35–41
    resource generation 41–5
    responsiveness 255–79

risk factors 41–5
satisfaction 255–79
scope 128–9
service provision 41–5
unmet needs 203–4, 205
World Health Survey (WHS) 213
health systems efficiency 281–312
see also international comparisons of
health systems
Ageing-Related Diseases (ARD) study 291–4
allocative efficiency 284–6
analytic methods 297–303
analytic techniques 305–6
appendectomy 293
common data 287–9
comparative measures 281–312
conceptual models 303–5
data issues 306–7
debates 303–7
descriptive methods 302–3
diagnosis-related groups (DRGs) 288–9
difficulties with methodologies 309
examples, efficiency indicators 289–97
explanatory variables 297, 298–9
gaps 303–7
HealthBASKET project 293–4
indicators 287–97
international comparisons of health
systems 106–7
issues 303–7
macro-level data 288
mammography 291–3
measuring 287–97
methodological problems 309
models/modeling 307–9
multiple data items 289
outcomes, transforming inputs into 282–4
vs performance measurement 286–7
production process, hospital care 282–4,
289–97
vs productivity measurement 286–7
productivity measurement 305–6
quality-adjusted life years (QALYs) 284–5,
290
risk adjustment 288
statistical methods 301
technical efficiency 284–6
variables, explanatory 297, 298–9
World Health Report 2000 (WHR2000) 297
Health Systems in Transition (HiT) reports
European Observatory on Health Systems
and Policies 76, 366
international comparisons 366
health systems outcomes
burdens of disease 322
developments 322
e-health 322
health care quality indicators 321
international health system performance
information 321–2
measuring outcomes 321

health systems performance
see also international comparisons of
health systems
data problems 176–8
financial protection 223–6, 246–7
health services outcomes 158–60
hospital services contribution 160–6
mental health care contribution 170–3
patient-reported outcome measures
(PROMS) 173–6
policy uses/abuses 246–7
preventive care 173
primary healthcare contribution 167–70
health systems performance assessment
(HSPA)
see also international comparisons of
health systems; international health
system performance information
distribution of health outcomes 9
e-health 25
effective coverage 340, 341–2
health services outcomes 344–7
international frameworks 31–74
international organizations' roles 7–9
key domains of performance 12–24
lessons to date 10–12, 13, 340–56
methodological debates 10–11
objectives 7–9
policy influence 10–11
population health 342–4
potential 2
World Health Report 2000 (WHR2000)
32–48, 76–8
HealthBASKET project
health systems efficiency 293–4
international comparisons of health
systems 86, 93–5, 107
hip fracture, international comparisons 5–7
hip replacement, international comparisons
5–7
HiT reports *see* Health Systems in Transition
reports
hospital services
acute myocardial infarction (AMI), case-
fatality rates 161–4, 165
avoidable hospital admission rates 169
contribution to health systems
performance 160–6
hospital-standardized mortality rates
(HSMRs) 160–1
patient safety indicators 164–6
readmission rates 166
stroke, case-fatality rates 161–4
hospital-standardized mortality rates
(HSMRs) 160–1
Household Budget Survey (HBS), financial
protection 243–4
HSMRs *see* hospital-standardized mortality
rates
HSPA *see* health systems performance
assessment

human resources, international health
system performance information 326

IHD *see* ischaemic heart disease
IHP+ *see* International Health Partnership
and Related Initiatives Framework 2008:
IHPS *see* International Health Policy Survey
IHSN *see* International Household Survey
Network
impoverishing spending on health care,
financial protection 230–5, 237–42,
246–7
inequity indices, access 206–7
information, performance *see* international
health system performance information
information technology
see also e-health
international comparisons 4–5
innovation, benchmarking 123
inpatient care
patient experience 266–7
survey data 266–7
inputs to health systems
developments 327
human resources 326
international health system performance
information 325–7
System of Health Accounts (SHA) 325–6
Integrated Performance Model for the
Health Care System (EGIPSS) (1998),
international frameworks 54–5
international comparisons
benchmarking 5, 367
cancer services 3–4
cross-border health care 4
data quality 367
efficiency 361
equity 360
financing 360
frameworks 7–9, 31–74
future priorities 366–8
in health sector, lessons to date 339–40
health services outcomes 359
Health Systems in Transition (HiT) reports
366
hip fracture 5–7
hip replacement 5–7
for improvement 356–66
increased interest 4
information technology 4–5
international benchmarks 5
interpreting performance information 355
knee replacement 5–7
limitations 367
narratives 358–61
performance indicators, variation 362–5
performance measurement 362–5
policy actions 365–6
policy influence 2–7, 367
population health 359
purpose 2–7

responsiveness 361
satisfaction 355
summarizing complex information 358–61
variation 362–5
international comparisons in performance
domains
ECHO project 347, 348–51
effective coverage 340, 341–2
efficiency 355–6, 357
EuroHOPE project 347, 348–51
financial protection 352–4
health services outcomes 344–7
lessons to date 340–56
patient experience 354–5
PERFECT project 347, 348–51
population health 342–4
international comparisons of health systems
75–112
assessment of initiatives 97–102
attribution 104–5
conceptual frameworks 336–9
current measures of future performance
105–6
dynamic effects 105–6
early 335
efficiency 106–7
European Observatory on Health Systems
and Policies 76
existing health system performance
assessment initiatives 76–92
Health Systems in Transition (HiT) reports
76
HealthBASKET project 86, 93–5, 107
key issues 101–8, 211–13
lessons to date 339–56
limitations 108
metrics 103–4
Organization for Economic Cooperation
and Development (OECD) 101–2
productivity measurement 106–7
whole system vs fragmentary comparison
102–3
World Health Report 2000 (WHR2000)
97–101
World Health Survey (WHS) 95–7
international frameworks 7–9, 31–74
see also existing frameworks
analytical international frameworks 46–8,
337
Behavioral Healthcare Framework 51–4
classifying 45–8
Commonwealth Fund Framework for a
High Performance System 2006: 66–7
Control Knobs Framework 2003: 61–3
criteria 32–48
descriptive international frameworks 46–8,
337
deterministic and predictive international
frameworks 46–8, 337
developing 32–48
existing frameworks 51–72

financing 41–5
Framework for Assessing Behavioral
　Healthcare 1998: 51–4
goals 35–41
Health Care Quality Indicators (HCQI)
　Framework 2006: 63–5
Integrated Performance Model for the
　Health Care System (EGIPSS) (1998) 54–5
International Health Partnership and
　Related Initiatives (IHP+) Framework
　2008: 70–2
international organizations' roles 7–9
monitoring and evaluation (M&E) 46–8
Murray and Frenk (2000): WHO Framework
　56–8
national performance assessment 48–9
objectives 9, 35–41
OECD Framework 2001: 58–61
OECD Health Care Quality Indicators
　(HCQI) Framework 2006: 63–5
Open Method of Coordination (OMC)
　(2000) 55–6
resource generation 41–5
risk factors 41–5
service provision 41–5
'systems thinking' frameworks 69–70
types 336–9
WHO (2000) Framework 56–8
WHO Building Blocks 2007: 67–9
World Health Report 2000 (WHR2000) 32
International Health Partnership and Related
　Initiatives (IHP+) Framework 2008:,
　international frameworks 70–2
International Health Policy Survey (IHPS)
　comparative methodology 272–3
　financial protection 244–5
　interpretation of data differences 272–3
　methodological considerations 272–3
　patient experience 272–6
　satisfaction 272–6
international health system performance
　information 313–34
　see also existing health system performance
　assessment initiatives; health
　systems performance; health systems
　performance assessment (HSPA)
communicable diseases 314–15
communicating international data 328–9
complementing international data 328–9
data collection 313–15, 330–1
data improvement 330–1
determinants of health 319–21
diagnosis-related groups (DRGs) 328
efficiency 327–8
equity 323–5
financial protection 325
health systems outcomes 321–2
human resources 326
inputs to health systems 325–7
partnerships 329–30
patient experience 323

population health 315–19
priorities for development 329–31
System of Health Accounts (SHA) 325–6
variation 323–5
International Household Survey Network
　(IHSN), financial protection 245
international organizations' roles, health
　systems performance assessment (HSPA)
　7–9
inventory approach, health care contribution
　142–3
ischaemic heart disease (IHD)
　major factors 129–31
　population health 129–31, 133–6

Kaiser Permanente
　mutual learning 5–7
　National Health Service (NHS) 5–7
　United States health system 5–7
Kakwani progressivity index
　financing 209–10
　Gini coefficient 209
　health systems 209–10
　Lorenz curve 209
key domains of performance, HSPA 12–24
　Avoidable Mortality in European Health
　　Systems (AMIEHS) 16, 17
　boundaries 14–15
　efficiency 22–4
　equity 17–20
　financial protection 20, 21
　Health Care Quality Indicators (HCQI)
　　Framework 2006: 18
　health services outcomes 16–17
　population health 15–16
key issues, international comparisons
　equity 211–13
　health systems 101–8, 211–13
　narratives 358–61
key terms
　access 40
　efficiency 39
　equity 40
　health 38
　health systems 37–40
　quality 38
　responsiveness 39
key variables, health outcomes 186–92
knee replacement, international comparisons
　5–7

leadership/governance, health systems
　41–5
lessons to date
　benchmarking 12, 13
　equity 347–52
　health services outcomes 344–7, 348–9
　health systems performance assessment
　　(HSPA) 10–12, 13, 340–56
　international comparisons in health sector
　　339–40

international comparisons in performance domains 340–56
international comparisons of health systems 339–56
population health 342–4
World Health Report 2000 (*WHR2000*) 340
Living Standards Measurement Study (LSMS), financial protection 243
long-term care services, health outcomes 166–7
long-term inequalities in health
health outcomes 198–201
mobility index (MI) 198–201
longer-term financial consequences of health spending, financial protection 233, 237
Lorenz curve
financing 209
health outcomes 193–6
Kakwani progressivity index 209
loss of earnings, financial protection 233–4
LSMS *see* Living Standards Measurement Study

macro-level data, health systems efficiency 288
mammography 173, 174
health systems efficiency 291–3
mental health care
bipolar disorder 170–3
health systems performance 170–3
schizophrenia 170–3
methodological challenges, financial protection 235–46
methodological debates, health systems performance assessment (HSPA) 10–11
methodological problems
health services outcomes 177–8
health systems efficiency 309
metrics, international comparisons of health systems 103–4
mobility index (MI)
health outcomes 198–201
long-term inequalities in health 198–201
models/modeling
health systems efficiency 307–9
Integrated Performance Model for the Health Care System (EGIPSS) (1998) 54–5
monitoring and evaluation (M&E) international frameworks 46–8
morbidity
measuring 137–9
population health 132–9, 315–18
mortality
acute myocardial infarction (AMI), case-fatality rates 161–4, 165
amenable mortality 145–9, 343, 344
avoidable mortality 145–9, 317–18, 342–4
Avoidable Mortality in European Health Systems (AMIEHS) 16, 17
developments 317

population health 132–7, 145–9, 315–18, 342–4
stroke, case-fatality rates 161–4
Murray and Frenk (2000): WHO Framework, international frameworks 56–8
mutual learning
Kaiser Permanente 5–7
National Health Service (NHS) 5–7
United States health system 5–7

narratives, key issues, international comparisons 358–61
National Health Service (NHS)
international benchmarks 5–7
Kaiser Permanente 5–7
mutual learning 5–7
National Institute for Health and Welfare, existing health system performance assessment initiatives 92
national performance assessment
European Community Health Indicators (ECHI) Project 49
international frameworks 48–9
national registries, health services outcomes 176
National Scorecard
international benchmarks 5
United States health system 5
NDPHS *see* Northern Dimension Partnership in Public Health and Social Wellbeing
needs
see also unmet needs
access 203–4, 205
defining 204
health systems 203–4
NHCSG *see* Nordic hospital comparison study group
NOMESKO *see* Nordic Medico-Statistical Committee
Nordic Collaboration, existing health system performance assessment initiatives 91–2
Nordic hospital comparison study group (NHCSG), existing health system performance assessment initiatives 92
Nordic Medico-Statistical Committee (NOMESKO), existing health system performance assessment initiatives 92
Northern Dimension Partnership in Public Health and Social Wellbeing (NDPHS), existing health system performance assessment initiatives 92

objective measures, health outcomes 187–91
objectives
health systems 35–41
health systems performance assessment (HSPA) 7–9
international frameworks 9, 35–41
OECD *see* Organization for Economic Cooperation and Development

Open Method of Coordination (OMC) (2000)
benchmarking 55
international frameworks 55–6
Organisation for Economic Co-operation and
Development (OECD)
existing health system performance
assessment initiatives 78–82
international comparisons of health
systems 101–2
OECD Framework 2001: 58–61, 78–82
OECD Health Care Quality Indicators
(HCQI) Framework 2006: 18, 63–5,
78–82, 168
out-of-pocket spending on health care,
financial protection 226–7, 228
outcomes
see also health outcomes; health services
outcomes
health systems outcomes 321–2
measurement, population health 127–8
transforming inputs into 282–4

partnerships, international health system
performance information 329–30
patient experience
Commonwealth Fund International Health
Policy Survey (IHPS) 272–6
general practitioners 267–72
health systems 255–79
inpatient care 266–7
international comparisons in performance
domains 354–5
International Health Policy Survey (IHPS)
272–6
international health system performance
information 323
survey data 266–7
patient-reported outcome measures (PROMS)
health services outcomes 173–6
health systems performance 173–6
Short Form 36 (SF36) 175
patient safety indicators
health services outcomes 164–6
hospital services 164–6
patient satisfaction, health systems 255–79
payment, health care see financial protection
PERFECT project, health services outcomes
347, 348–51
performance assessment tools, World Health
Organization (WHO) 79
performance information see international
health system performance information
performance measurement
see also health systems performance
current developments 1–2
health systems 45–8
vs health systems efficiency 286–7
international comparisons 362–5
perspectives 362–5
performance (results) benchmarking 115–16,
117

policy actions, international comparisons
365–6
policy influence
cancer services 3–4
health systems performance assessment
(HSPA) 10–11
international benchmarks 5
international comparisons 2–7, 367
policy recommendations
equity 213–16
procedural equity 215
substantive equity 214–15
policy uses/abuses, financial protection
246–7
pooling, financial protection 224, 225
population health 127–56
age/disease-specific indicators 132–7
amenable mortality 145–9, 343, 344
avoidable mortality 145–9, 317–18, 342–4
breast cancer 137, 138
determinants 129–32
disability 139–41, 318–19
disability-adjusted life years (DALYs)
139–41
generic indicators 132
health-adjusted life expectancy (HALE)
139–40
health care contribution 141–4
health systems performance assessment
(HSPA) 342–4
ill health 318–19
international comparisons 359
international health system performance
information 315–19
inventory approach 142–3
ischaemic heart disease (IHD) 129–31,
133–6
key domain of performance, HSPA 15–16
lessons to date 342–4
measuring 132–41
morbidity 132–9, 315–18
mortality 132–7, 145–9, 315–18, 342–4
outcomes measurement 127–8
production function 142–4
risk factors 132–7
sudden infant death syndrome (SIDS) 131
summary measures 139–41
tracer concept 150–1, 318–19
population surveys, health services outcomes
177
poverty line, financial protection 230–5
poverty trap, financial protection 225
practice (process) benchmarking 115–16,
117
pre-payment, financial protection 224,
225
preventive care
health outcomes 173
screening 173, 174
primary healthcare contribution, health
systems performance 167–70

priorities for development, international health system performance information 329–31
priorities, future, international comparisons 366–8
procedural equity, policy recommendations 215
process (practice) benchmarking 115–16, 117
production function, health care contribution 142–4
production process, hospital care, health systems efficiency 282–4, 289–97
productivity measurement
vs health systems efficiency 286–7
health systems efficiency 305–6
international comparisons of health systems 106–7
professionalism, benchmarking 123
PROMS see patient-reported outcome measures

QALYs see quality-adjusted life years
quality
data quality, international comparisons 367
terminology 38
quality-adjusted life years (QALYs), health systems efficiency 284–5, 290

Rapid Assessment Protocol for Insulin Access (RAPIA), tracer concept 151
readmission rates
health services outcomes 166
hospital services 166
regression measures, health outcomes 193
regression methods, access 206
research priorities, financial protection 235–46
resource generation
health systems 41–5
international frameworks 41–5
responsiveness
conceptual issues 255–6
expectations 263–5
health care expenditure 265
health systems 255–79
international comparisons 361
to legitimate expectations 257–65
measurement issues 255–6
survey data 257–65
terminology 39, 255–6
World Health Report 2000 (WHR2000) 257–65
World Health Survey (WHS) 257–65
results (performance) benchmarking 115–16, 117
risk adjustment, health systems efficiency 288
risk factors
health systems 41–5
international frameworks 41–5
population health 132–7

RIVM see Dutch National Institute for Public Health and the Environment

SAH see self-assessed health
satisfaction
Commonwealth Fund International Health Policy Survey (IHPS) 272–6
conceptual issues 255–6
Eurobarometer surveys 256–7, 258–9
health systems 255–79
international comparisons 355
International Health Policy Survey (IHPS) 272–6
measurement issues 255–6
survey data 256–7, 258–9
terminology 255–6
schizophrenia 170–3
screening
breast cancer 173, 174, 291–3
health outcomes 173, 174
preventive care 173, 174
self-assessed health (SAH), health outcomes 187–9
service provision
health systems 41–5
international frameworks 41–5
SF36 see Short Form 36
SHA see System of Health Accounts
Short Form 36 (SF36), patient-reported outcome measures (PROMS) 175
SIDS see sudden infant death syndrome
social determinants, health outcomes 186, 187
socioeconomic variables, health outcomes 191–2
sources of data, financial protection 243
statistical methods, health systems efficiency 301
stroke, case-fatality rates 161–4
subjective measures, health outcomes 187–91
subsistence spending, financial protection 236
substantive equity, policy recommendations 214–15
sudden infant death syndrome (SIDS), population health 131
summarizing complex information, international comparisons 358–61
survey data
see also Commonwealth Fund International Health Policy Survey (IHPS); International Health Policy Survey (IHPS); World Health Report 2000 (WHR2000); World Health Survey (WHS)
Eurobarometer surveys 256–7, 258–9
health outcomes 189–90
inpatient care 266–7
patient experience 266–7
responsiveness 257–65

satisfaction 256–7, 258–9
unmet needs 205
World Health Organization (WHO) 79
System of Health Accounts (SHA),
    international health system performance
    information 325–6
system responsibility, benchmarking 123
'systems thinking' frameworks, international
    frameworks 69–70

technical efficiency, health systems efficiency
    284–6
tracer concept
    population health 150–1, 318–19
    Rapid Assessment Protocol for Insulin
    Access (RAPIA) 151

United States health system
    international benchmarks 5
    Kaiser Permanente 5–7
    mutual learning 5–7
    National Scorecard 5
United States Veterans Health
    Administration, international
    benchmarks 5
unmet needs
    access 203–4, 205
    financial protection 234–5, 237–42
    health systems 203–4, 205
    survey data 205

variables
    explanatory variables, health systems
    efficiency 297, 298–9
    health outcomes 186–92
variation
    cross-country performance indicators
    362–5
    health outcomes 191–2
    international comparisons 362–5
    international health system performance
    information 323–5
    between people 323–4

between regions 324–5
understanding 362–5
vignettes, health outcomes 190–1

whole system vs fragmentary comparison,
    international comparisons of health
    systems 102–3
WHR2000 see World Health Report 2000
WHS see World Health Survey
World Health Organization (WHO)
    data collection 79
    *Everybody's Business: Strengthening health
    systems to improve health outcomes* 8, 76–8
    existing health system performance
    assessment initiatives 76–8
    health policy information (WHO Europe)
    79
    international organizations' roles 8
    Murray and Frenk (2000): WHO Framework
    56–8, 76–8
    performance assessment tools 79
    survey data 79
    WHO (2000) Framework 56–8, 76–8
    WHO Building Blocks Framework 2007:
    67–9, 76–8
    WHO statistical databases 79
World Health Report 2000 (WHR2000) 8
    criticisms 97–101
    debates 10–11
    defining 'health systems' 129
    health systems efficiency 297
    health systems goals 127
    health systems performance assessment
    (HSPA) 32–48, 76–8
    lessons to date 340
    responsiveness 257–65
World Health Survey (WHS)
    equity 213
    financial protection 244
    health systems 213
    international comparisons of health
    systems 95–7
    responsiveness 257–65